The Future of
Antibiotherapy and
Antibiotic Research

Based on the Proceedings of the Second Rhône-Poulenc
Round Table Conference entitled "Antibiotics of the Future",
held in Paris from 13-15 February, 1980.

The Future of Antibiotherapy and Antibiotic Research

Edited by

L. NINET
P. E. BOST
D. H. BOUANCHAUD
J. FLORENT

Centre Nicolas Grillet
Rhône – Poulenc
Vitry-sur-Seine, France

1981

ACADEMIC PRESS

A Subsidiary of Harcourt Brace Jovanovich, Publishers

London   New York   Toronto   Sydney   San Francisco

ACADEMIC PRESS INC. (LONDON) LTD.
24/28 Oval Road,
London NW1

United States Edition published by
ACADEMIC PRESS INC.
111 Fifth Avenue
New York, New York 10003

British Library Cataloguing in Publication Data
The Future of Antibiotherapy and Antibiotic Research.
1. Antibiotics — Congresses
I. Ninet, L
615'.329   RM265.2   80-41959

ISBN 0-12-519780-2

Printed in Great Britain by
Mackays of Chatham Ltd

Contributors

Acar, Jacques   Professeur de Microbiologie, Université Paris VI, Service de Microbiologie. Hôpital St. Joseph, 7, rue Pierre Larousse, 75014 Paris, France.

Bastin, Raymond   Professeur, Université Paris VII, Chef de Clinique des Maladies Infectieuses, Hôpital Claude Bernard, 10, avenue de la Porte d'Aubervilliers, 75019 Paris, France.

Bergan, Tom   Assoc. Professor, Department of Microbiology, Institute of Pharmacy, University of Oslo, P.O. Box 1108 Blindern, Oslo 3, Norway.

Braude, Raphael c/o Commonwealth Agricultural Bureaux, Pig News and Information, Lane End House, Shinfield, Reading RG2 9BB, Great Britain.

Braun, Volkmar   Professor of Microbiology, Microbiology Department, University of Tübingen, 28 Auf der Morgenstelle, D 7400 Tübingen, Federal Republic of Germany.

Chabanon, Gérard   Chef de Travaux à la Faculté de Médecine, Laboratoire Central de Bactériologie-Virologie, C.H.U. Toulouse Rangueil, Chemin du Vallon, 31054 Toulouse, France.

Chabbert, Yves   Professeur, Directeur du Département de Bactériologie, Institut Pasteur, 25, rue du Docteur Roux, 75015 Paris, France.

Davies, Julian   Professor of Biochemistry, Department of Biochemistry, College of Agricultural and Life Sciences, University of Wisconsin, 420, Henry Mall, Madison, Wisconsin 53706, U.S.A.

Demain, Arnold L.   Professor of Industrial Microbiology, Department of Nutrition and Food Science, Massachussetts Institute of Technology, Cambridge, Massachussetts 02139, U.S.A.

Duval, Jean   Professeur, Université Paris XII, Chef du Laboratoire de Bactériologie et de Virologie, Unité de Médecine, Hôpital Henri Mondor, 51, avenue du Maréchal de Lattre de Tassigny, 94010 Créteil, France.

Frottier, Jacques   Professeur, Université Paris VII, Clinique des Maladies Infectieuses B, Hôpital Claude Bernard, 10, avenue de la Porte d'Aubervilliers, 75019 Paris, France.

Gilvarg, Charles   Professor, Department of Biochemical Sciences, Princeton University, Princeton, New Jersey 08544, U.S.A.

Hopwood, David A.   Professor, Head of Department of Genetics, John Innes Institute, Colney Lane, Norwich NR4 7UH, Great Britain.

Humbert, Guy   Professeur, Ecole de Médecine. Université de Haute Normandie, Département des Maladies Infectieuses, Hôpital Charles Nicolle, 76038 Rouen, France.

Kunin, Calvin M. Professor, Chairman, Department of Medicine, The Ohio State University Hospital, N-1013, 410 West 10th Avenue, Colombus, Ohio 43210, U.S.A.

Labia, Roger Maître de Recherches au C.N.R.S., Centre d'Etudes et de Recherches de Chimie Organique Appliquée, 2 à 8, rue Henry Dunant, 94320 Thiais, France.

Lagrange, Philippe Professeur, Unité d'Immunophysiologie Cellulaire, Institut Pasteur, 25, rue du Docteur Roux, 75015 Paris, France.

Lechevalier, Hubert A. Professor, Waksman Institute of Microbiology, Rutgers University, P.O. Box 759, Piscataway, New Jersey 08854, U.S.A.

Le Goffic, François Professeur, Directeur du Centre d'Etudes et de Recherches de Chimie Organique Appliquée, C.N.R.S., 2 à 8, rue Henry Dunant, 94320 Thiais, France.

Milhaud, Guy Professeur, Service de Pharmacie et de Toxicologie, Ecole Nationale Vétérinaire d'Alfort, 7, avenue du Général de Gaulle, 94704 Maisons-Alfort, France.

Omura, Satoshi Professor, Director, Microbial Chemistry, The Kitasato Institute, 5-9-1 Shirokane, Minato-ku, Tokyo 108, Japan.

Richmond, Mark Henry Professor of Bacteriology, Department of Bacteriology, Medical School, University Walk, Bristol BS8 1TD, Great Britain.

Rinehart, Kenneth L. Professor of Chemistry, Rogers Adams Laboratory, School of Chemical Sciences, University of Illinois, Urbana, Illinois 61801, U.S.A.

Ruckebusch, Yves Professeur, Laboratoire de Physiologie et de Pharmaco-dynamie, Ecole Nationale Vétérinaire de Toulouse, 23, Chemin des Capelles, 31076 Toulouse, France.

Sabath, Léon D. Professor, Head of Section of Infectious Diseases, University of Minnesota, School of Medicine, Minneapolis, Minnesota 55455, U.S.A.

Sande, Merle A. Professor of Medicine, San Francisco General Hospital and University of California, San Francisco Medical School, San Francisco, California, U.S.A.

Sebald, Madeleine Professeur, Unité des Anaérobies, Département de Bactériologie, Institut Pasteur, 28, rue du Docteur Roux, 75015 Paris, France.

Tomasz, Alexander Professor, Department of Microbiology, The Rockefeller University, 1230 York Avenue, New York, N.Y. 10021, U.S.A.

Trouet, André Professeur, Faculté de Médecine, Université Catholique de Louvain, Institut International de Pathologie Cellulaire et Moléculaire, 7539, avenue Hippocrate, Bruxelles B 1200, Belgique.

Vazquez, David Professor, Center of Molecular Biology. Faculty of Sciences, Autonomous University of Madrid, Canto Blanco, Madrid 34, Spain.

Williams, John David Professor, Department of Medical Microbiology, The London Hospital Medical College, University of London, Turner Street, London E1 2AD, Great Britain.

Participants

Bénazet, Francis   Professeur Agrégé, Directeur du Département de Bactériologie et de Parasitologie, Rhône-Poulenc, Centre Nicolas Grillet, Vitry-sur-Seine, France.

Blondel, Jean-Claude   Direction des Recherches, Rhône-Poulenc Santé, Paris, France.

Bobichon, Louis   Directeur des Recherches Biochimiques, Rhône-Poulenc S.A , Paris, France.

Bost, Pierre Etienne   Département de Biochimie, Rhône-Poulenc, Centre Nicolas Grillet, Vitry-sur-Seine, France.

Bouanchaud, Daniel   Service de Bactériologie, Rhône-Poulenc, Centre Nicolas Grillet, Vitry-sur-Seine, France.

Bourat, Guy   Direction des Recherches et du Développement, Rhône-Poulenc S.A., Paris, France.

Bourdon, Raymond   Professeur, Conseiller Pharmaceutique, Président de l'Institut de Biopharmacie, Rhône-Poulenc Santé, Paris, France.

Boutelier, Raymonde   Directeur Produits, Laboratoire Roger Bellon, Neuilly-sur-Seine, France.

Collier, John   Pharmaceutical Research and Development, May and Baker Ltd., Dagenham, Essex, Great Britain.

Courvalin, Patrice   Unité de Bactériologie Médicale, Institut Pasteur, Paris, France.

Debarre, François   Direction des Recherches, Rhône-Poulenc Santé, Paris, France.

Djebbar, Françoise   Développement Médical, Rhône-Poulenc Santé, Paris, France.

Eiglier, Marianne   Direction des Recherches, Rhône-Poulenc Santé, Paris, France.

Ferrando, Raymond   Professeur, Directeur du Département de Nutrition et d'Alimentation, Ecole Nationale Vétérinaire d'Alfort, Maisons-Alfort, France.

Fillastre, Jean-Paul   Professeur, Service de Néphrologie, Faculté de Médecine, Université de Haute Normandie, Rouen, France.

Firth, Mary   Medical and Scientific Tape Transcription, 49 Woodstock Avenue, London NW11 9RG, Great Britain.

Florent, Jean   Département de Biochimie, Rhône-Poulenc, Centre Nicolas Grillet, Vitry-sur-Seine, France.

Fouché, Jean Directeur des Recherches Techniques, Rhône-Poulenc, Vitry-sur-Seine, France.

Géro, Stephan Directeur de Recherches au C.N.R.S., Institut de Chimie des Substances Naturelles, Gif-sur-Yvette, France.

Halliday, Robert Director of Research, Norwich-Eaton Pharmaceuticals, Norwich, New York 18 815, U.S.A.

Heijenoort, Jean van Maître de Recherches au C.N.R.S., Institut de Biochimie, Orsay, France.

Jeambourquin, Raoul Directeur du Centre Nicolas Grillet, Rhône-Poulenc, Vitry-sur-Seine, France.

Jeanmart, Claude Directeur des Recherches de l'Alimentation Equilibrée, Commentry, France.

Jollès, Georges Directeur des Recherches, Rhône-Poulenc Santé, Paris, France.

Julou, Louis Directeur des Recherches Biologiques Pharmaceutiques, Rhône-Poulenc, Centre Nicolas Grillet, Vitry-sur-Seine, France.

Kernbaum, Serge Département des Maladies Infectieuses et Tropicales, Hôpital Saint-Louis, Paris, France.

Lallemand, Jean-Yves Maître de Recherches au C.N.R.S., Laboratoire de Chimie, Ecole Normale Supérieure, Paris, France.

Lechevalier, Mary Waksman Institute of Microbiology, Rutgers University, Piscataway, New Jersey, U.S.A.

Leroy, Jean-Pierre Service de Parasitologie, Rhône-Poulenc, Centre Nicolas Grillet, Vitry-sur-Seine, France.

Le Roy, Pierre Département de Chimie, Rhône-Poulenc, Centre Nicolas Grillet, Vitry-sur-Seine, France.

Lombardi, Bernard Département de Biochimie, Rhône-Poulenc, Centre Nicolas Grillet, Vitry-sur-Seine, France.

Lukacs, Gabor Maître de Recherches au C.N.R.S., Institut de Chimie des Substances Naturelles, Gif-sur-Yvette, France.

Lunel, Jean Département de Biochimie, Rhône-Poulenc, Centre Nicolas Grillet, Vitry-sur-Seine, France.

Mancy, Denise Département de Biochimie, Rhône-Poulenc, Centre Nicolas Grillet, Vitry-sur-Seine, France.

Mariat, François Professeur, Unité de Mycologie, Institut Pasteur, Paris, France.

Messer, Marcel Directeur des Recherches Chimiques et Biochimiques Pharmaceutiques, Rhône-Poulenc, Centre Nicolas Grillet, Vitry-sur-Seine, France.

Modai, Jacques Professeur, Clinique des Maladies Infectieuses, Hôpital Claude Bernard, Paris, France.

Moutonnier, Claude Département de Chimie, Rhône-Poulenc, Centre Nicolas Grillet, Vitry-sur-Seine, France.

Ninet, Léon Directeur du Département de Biochimie, Rhône-Poulenc, Centre Nicolas Grillet, Vitry-sur-Seine, France.

Pascal, Claude Direction des Recherches Analytiques, Rhône-Poulenc, Centre Nicolas Grillet, Vitry-sur-Seine, France.

Pascard, Claudine Directeur de Recherches au C.N.R.S., Institut de Chimie des Substances Naturelles, Gif-sur-Yvette, France.

Pasquier, Pierre   Directeur des Recherches Thérapeutiques, Rhône-Poulenc Santé, Paris, France.

Potier, Pierre   Directeur de Recherches au C.N.R.S., Co-Directeur de l'Institut de Chimie des Substances Naturelles, Gif-sur-Yvette, France.

Roussel, Christian   Direction des Recherches, Santé Animale, Rhône-Poulenc Santé, Paris, France.

Royer, Pierre   Département Vétérinaire, SPECIA, Paris, France.

Salem, Allan   Pharmaceutical Research and Development, May and Baker Ltd., Dagenham, Essex, Great Britain.

Theilleux, Jacques   Département de Biochimie, Rhône-Poulenc, Centre Nicolas Grillet, Vitry-sur-Seine, France.

Tissier, Anne-Marie   Département Anti-Infectieux, SPECIA, Paris, France.

Videau, Daniel   Département d'Analyse Biologique, Institut de Biopharmacie, Rhône-Poulenc Santé, Paris, France.

Vildé, Jean-Louis   Professeur, Clinique des Maladies Infectieuses B, Hôpital Claude Bernard, Paris, France.

Waldvogel, Francis   Professeur de Microbiologie Clinique, Hôpital Cantonal, Genève, Suisse.

Woehrle, Roger   Directeur Adjoint des Recherches Thérapeutiques, Rhône-Poulenc Santé, Lyon, France.

Wooldridge, K.R.H.   Pharmaceutical Research Manager, May and Baker Ltd., Dagenham, Essex, Great Britain.

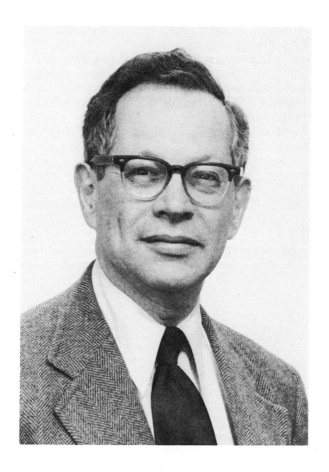

In memory of David Perlman
1920–1980

Edward Kremers Professor of Pharmaceutical Biochemistry
University of Wisconsin Madison – Wisconsin

His greviously mourned death deprived all the
participants in the Rhône-Poulenc Round Table
Conference of his exceptional knowledge and
his attentive friendship.

Preface

This volume contains the Proceedings of the Second Rhône-Poulenc Round Table, held in Paris in February 1980. The aim of this meeting was to evaluate the needs for new antimicrobial agents in human and animal medicine and to analyse those parts of our present knowledge which could be used to improve the performance of existing drugs and guide the search for new ones, especially natural antibiotics. In this respect, several renowned scientists, coming from all parts of the world and from different disciplines, met for three days to present their work and exchange their knowledge and ideas.

The reader will not find in this book the infallible means of discovering the "miracle antibiotic" or of drawing its structure, nor a complete picture of all the possible methods of tackling the problem. Perhaps through theories expressed here, some well established and others just emerging, he will realise the paucity of our general knowledge and appreciate the huge gaps to be filled in order ultimately to win the battle against infectious diseases. Perhaps he will also become acquainted with the intensive efforts that have already been made and are still being made by universities and industry in this direction.

It is our real pleasure to thank warmly all the contributors and participants who agreed to attend the meeting and to work actively together, in a friendly atmosphere of free discussion. We are particularly indebted to Drs. J. Acar, Y. Chabbert, J. Davies, A. Demain, F. Le Goffic and M. Richmond for their generous advice and kind help, before and during the conference. It would take too long to name all our colleagues of the Rhône-Poulenc Group of Companies who assisted us so efficiently in the organisation of the meeting. We wish to extend our hearty thanks to all of them, and especially to Miss M. Eiglier and Mrs. N. Gérard and to Mr. J.C. Blondel. Finally, this conference would not have been held without the initiative, the confidence, and the constant moral and financial support of the Research Manager of the Health Division of the Rhône-Poulenc Group, Dr. G. Jollès, to whom we express our deep gratitude.

The transcription of several presentations and of all the discussions, has been efficiently carried out by Dr. Mary Firth, and the translation of all the French communications by Dr. Allan Salem, with the cooperation of Miss S. Copping, Mrs. J. Schock, Mrs. M. Tantet, Mrs. M. Dorizon, Mrs. R. Hollevoet and Miss L. Yaghdjian. Mr. J.-P. Labbé and Mr. M. Lomont have taken special care over the general presentation of the figures. The help of all these people, together with the expert and kind assistance of the staff of Academic Press Inc. (London) are gratefully acknowledged.

May, 1981   L.N., P.E.B., D.H.B. and J.F.

Opening Remarks

Dr. G. JOLLES

It is a great privilege for me today to open the second Rhône-Poulenc Round Table Conference on the Antibiotics of the Future.

The present time is certainly very rich in scientific events of all kinds, from major congresses including several thousand participants such as the Chemotherapy Conference last Autumn in Boston, to very exclusive meetings to which only specialists with the highest credentials are admitted.

Our objective today is neither to compete with these two types of meeting nor to find a half-way point between these two extremes. In fact, our primary goal is to do something else, something more pragmatic: the objective of our Round Table Conference is to try to create, on a broad and particularly topical issue of Pharmaceutical Research, a contact between top fundamental scientists and researchers of the Industry who want to initiate important therapeutic advances for tomorrow.

Two years ago for our first Round Table, the topic we chose was the Pharmacology of Immunoregulation. Immunology is currently undergoing rapid evolution and if major fundamental progress has so far been achieved, the transfer of all that new knowledge to the level of practical medicine and drug design has certainly not yet been achieved; this was therefore a question, the clarification of which could prove particularly useful.

However, the topic we chose for today's meeting, antibiotic therapy, may seem somewhat surprising because it includes a great number of positive achievements. What progress has been made since Fleming's and Waksman's discoveries, and how many compounds have been discovered, from cephalosporins to macrolides, from aminoglycosides to synergistins! Pharmacopoeias are full of antibiotics; excellent products have been discovered and have given rise to numerous "me too" drugs. Next to the antibiotics, there are also the synthetic antimicrobials ranging from sulphonamides to nalidixic and pipemidic acids.

Now, what can we still expect from antibiotics? Don't we have everything we need against infective diseases until the end of this century? Those who frequently meet with clinicians know quite well that everything is not yet solved in this field and it is true also that in medicine and in chemotherapy, as everywhere else, there is a steady and stepwise evolution.

If one looks into the future, it is certain that microbial infections will remain an enemy of every day life, it is certain that we shall need antibiotics and antimicrobials to fight them, but is it just as certain that it will *always* be the same antibiotics, that it will *only* be the same antibiotics?

I would compare the Conference on Immunoregulation we organised two years ago with the thoughts a young person may have while contemplating passionately his future which seems most promising. But today's conference on antibiotics makes me think rather of a middle-aged woman who has beautiful years full of success behind her and who is wondering whether yesterday's success will be just as rewarding tomorrow.

In a way, such considerations are very close to today's meeting programme: we intend to make a broad survey of the present situation, then look into the future and prepare adequate action.

In the first part entitled "Analysis of the present situation: needs, constraints and objectives for the future", we would like, first of all, those whose activities are closer to clinical practice to make a general review of the present status of antibiotic therapy; this should eventually lead them to identify the strong and weak points of antibiotics currently available and to determine the future needs. We have also included Animal Health because we want this review to be exhaustive.

In the second and third parts, suggestions should essentially be directed towards a research programme adapted to these needs for the future. In the second part, "Methods of selection and assessment of drugs", the new research pathways opened up by scientific progress should be reviewed, with particular emphasis on the knowledge of those mechanisms of action which may give rise to substantial innovations. The last contributions will deal with new methods of extraction of antibiotics, their screening and early identification, and also genetics and bioconversions.

In order to cement the various lectures within the framework of our conference, it was agreed to conclude the meeting by a short review of each of the main trends in order to summarise and emphasise the major principles of our debates.

We are going to have three days of hard work with a particularly heavy programme. I hope that we were not too ambitious in trying to organise such a large survey, but in order to get an adequate prospective view, we really had to cover all aspects of antibiotics: the clinical and biochemical, the fundamental and practical, the human and veterinary. Some of you will perhaps be somewhat disorientated by some of the lectures which do not relate to your everyday activities. But our objectives was precisely to create a contact on a very broad basis and we hope that the quality of the lectures will give everybody the opportunity to find some interest in the different approaches to this problem.

I wish now to thank all of you for having agreed to spend some of your precious time working with us, all those who helped and advised us in organising this meeting, and all those who have come from distant places to join us today. One of our most distinguished guests however is not here with us. Many of you already know that Professor Perlman died a few days ago in Madison after fighting for a long time with enormous courage against a cruel disease, and it is with a great sadness that we face his absence from our meeting.

I wish furthermore to thank Dr. Ninet who has taken charge of organising the meeting from a practical and scientific point of view and I can assure you that he did his best to make the conference instructive and rewarding for all of us.

Many of the lectures and communications will be in English, some will be in French but we have provided simultaneous translation to avoid linguistic problems.

I really hope, therefore, that everything has been provided for the meeting to be successful.

Rhône-Poulenc devoted considerable attention to antibiotics when they first appeared many years ago. It was in our own laboratories that, after the second World War, the first milligrams of penicillin were prepared on this continent. In our factories, antibiotics from almost all the families were fermented. The Group's R & D budget for Human and Animal Health amounted to almost $100 Million in 1979 and antibiotics accounted for 10% of this budget.

Thus we feel very concerned about the new generation of antibiotics which is approaching and we trust that, with your help, our meeting will provide a substantial contribution to therapeutic progress by preparing in different ways the ground for developing the antibiotics of the future.

Contents

Part 1   Analysis of the Present Situation: Needs, Constraints and Objectives for the Antibiotics of the Future

Part 1

*Analysis of the Present Situation:
Needs, Constraints and Objectives
for the Antibiotics of the Future*

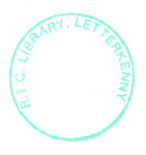

Introduction

R. BASTIN

Clinique des Maladies Infectieuses,
Hôpital Claude Bernard, Paris, France

Before proceeding to that which, in our opinion, is the aim of this symposium, to draw a sketch of the future of antibiotic therapy, we must first consider the present position of antibiotics, the eminent place they now occupy in the treatment of human and animal pathology, their often deplored use as animal feed additives and the requirements and restrictions on their use.

To this end, we will outline the present situation, an excellent introduction to the main body of our discussions.

The Present Situation in Antibiotic Therapy

The Phenomena of Bacterial Resistance

Whilst some microbial species have not developed substantial resistance (group A streptococci to penicillin G for example), the majority have acquired a fairly marked degree of resistance to antibiotics to which they were originally sensitive. Certain species (enterobacteria, *Pseudomonas*, staphylococci, etc.) acquired resistance some time ago; in others it is relatively new. The isolation of *Streptococcus pneumoniae*, resistant to beta-lactams and/or to chloramphenicol, and of gonococci and *Haemophilus influenzae* that produce penicillinase, may lead to reconsideration of some established therapeutic schemes if such findings increase from year to year.

Any microbial species is thus capable of acquiring resistance to an antibiotic, and the fact that for several years, a species has remained sensitive does not imply that this will always be the case. Resistance is usually enzyme-mediated and coded by a plasmid. This evidence alone justifies research into new molecules.

Comments on Pharmacokinetics

The clinician is entitled to expect that he will continually be provided with compounds with improved pharmacokinetic properties. As examples we can cite bacampicillin and amoxicillin which are as active as ampicillin but at lower doses and josamycin, the tissue concentrations of which exceed those of the earlier macrolides and which requires also twice daily dosing.

Incidents and Accidents in Antibiotic Therapy

These have received attention ever since the beginning of the great advance in anti-infective therapy. In particular we have the ototoxicity and nephrotoxicity of even the most recent aminoglycosides, which limit their use in the elderly and in the renally insufficient patient. There are also cases of sensitisation to beta-lactams, which are occasionally the cause of serious side-effects and therapeutic problems.

The Future

In the future, it would be desirable to concentrate attention on various goals.

Introduction of Molecules with Greater Antibacterial Activity

It is unlikely that compounds more active than present antibiotics against all organisms can be introduced. However, against certain organisms, especially those which have acquired plasmid mediated resistance, enterobacteria, *Pseudomonas* and staphylococci, that should be possible. Examples of these are the second generation cephalosporins, the cephamycins, which are especially stable to the beta-lactamases of Gram-negative bacteria and the acylureido-penicillins (azlocillin, mezlocillin, piperacillin). Very recently, cefsulodine was presented as the first cephalosporin active against *Pseudomonas aeruginosa.*

One can reasonably foresee that the hospital environment, the many applications of immunosuppression and the increased fitting of prostheses will only serve to magnify the risks of appearance of organisms very resistant to present-day antibiotics. This threat is particularly great in the case of *Pseudomonas* and related organisms, coagulase positive and negative staphylococci (cardiac prostheses and ventricular shunt valves), enterobacteria (*Klebsiella, Serratia, Enterobacter, Providencia*, indole-positive *Proteus*, etc.). We have already said that the evolution of certain organisms, such as the gonococcus or *Haemophilus influenzae* towards resistance was also foreseeable.

A better knowledge of bacterial enzymes might allow us to develop antibiotics increasingly stable towards these enzymes. Could we go as far as contemplating the inhibition of bacterial enzymic activity *in situ*?

But we must never forget one danger, that of overprescription of the new drugs and neglect of the earlier antibiotics. Let us stress therefore the everyday usefulness of penicillin G, the macrolides, etc. at present and probably for a long time to come. Thus, it would be helpful to reserve the newest cephalosporins and the acylureido-penicillins for urgent and appropriate indications. This general comment is vital in that it is directed at the problem of controlling the prescription of new compounds.

Development of Compounds with Improved Pharmacokinetic Properties

The development of compounds with improved pharmacokinetic properties compared to existing members of a given family of antibiotics is also a desirable goal. Improved properties may lead to:

1) less frequent dosing or injections,
2) better penetration into certain tissues (e.g. for treatment of purulent meningitis due to multiresistant organisms such as *Pseudomonas aeruginosa* or enterobacteria).

In this respect the interest of second generation cephalosporins being absorbed into the CSF at therapeutic levels must be emphasized. However more rapid assay methods, for example automatic tests, are requested to study diffusibility *in vivo*.

Development of Better Tolerated Molecules

The development of better tolerated molecules with more limited side-effects is a very difficult problem. An example is the nephro-toxicity of aminoglycosides. Greater knowledge of the mechanism of these toxic effects at the cellular level and even at the molecular level is required.

Theoretical research has to consider how to limit:

1) the accumulation and persistence of aminoglycosides in the renal cortex without interfering with their antibacterial effects;
2) the toxic changes in the lysosomal respiratory and metabolic systems of the cortical cells.

Practical research has to:

1) develop tests capable of giving an early indication of nephrotoxicity, e.g. the work of Mondorf on enzymuria (assay of urinary excretion of alanine aminopeptidase),
2) determine the most favourable strategy to adopt for the administration of aminoglycosides, e.g. continuous venous infusion, repeated intramuscular injections, intermittent treatment (a single daily injection, etc.),
3) consider the role of antibiotic associations or of drug interference in renal toxicity, etc.

Development of Molecules with Reasonable Cost

It is necessary to develop molecules the cost of which is not inconsistent with their usage in practice. The high cost of new antibiotics must be taken into consideration.

Conclusions

The development of new antibiotics is desirable. This involves complex fundamental research in biology and molecular biochemistry. The importance is stressed of standardised animal models, assays of tissue drug levels (e.g. by simple and reproducible radioimmunoassays), electron microscopy studies, etc.

One must not forget the other antibacterial agents, closely related to the antibiotics themselves. It is worth pursuing studies on certain chemotherapeutic agents related to antiseptics, but which have little toxicity and may be administered by several routes. An example is tauroline, a chemical derivative of taurine, initial clinical studies of which seem promising.

Antibiotics and Infections due to Enterobacteriaceae: Experience of a French University Hospital Centre

G. HUMBERT*, J. F. LEMELAND[+], J. LEROY[††], J. P. ROGEZ*
and G. BONMARCHAND[††]

* Département des Maladies Infectieuses, Hôpital Charles Nicolle, Rouen, France
+ Département de Bactériologie, Hôpital de l'Hôtel-Dieu, Rouen, France
†† Service de Réanimation, Hôpital Charles Nicolle, Rouen, France

Introduction

Infections due to Enterobacteriaceae are a major problem in the pathology of infection owing to their frequency, their potential severity linked with septic shock and/or underlying diseases and the difficulty of therapy owing to bacterial resistance, which is often unpredictable and is constantly increasing (Altemeier *et al.*, 1967, Dupont and Spink, 1969; Klastersky, 1972; McCabe and Jackson, 1962a, b).

Finland (1970), and later, McGowan *et al.* (1975), emphasized the predominant role played by Enterobacteriaceae in the pathology of infection in hospitals. The aim of this paper is to indicate the current prevalence of infections due to Enterobacteriaceae and the methods of treatment, by referring to data gathered in a French University Hospital Centre (U.H.C.).

The U.H.C. in Rouen has 2,688 beds (2,041 beds for acute cases and 647 beds for chronic cases) in 3 main hospitals (Charles Nicolle Hospital, 1,196 beds; Hotel Dieu Hospital, 519 beds; Bois Guillaume Hospital, 577 beds) and 46 wards covering all specialities.

We will be considering the following: (1) The number and the distribution of different Enterobacteriaceae isolated in the U.H.C. in Rouen over a 6-year period (1974–1979). (2) The usage of anti-microbial agents active against Enterobacteriaceae by the U.H.C. in Rouen. (3) The treatment of septicaemias due to Enterobacteriaceae in the Department of Infectious Diseases and the Intensive Care Unit.

Enterobacteriaceae Isolated at the U.H.C. in Rouen

We have only considered strains thought responsible for an infection and which had been subjected to antibiotic sensitivity testing.

Number of Strains Isolated by the Laboratory of Bacteriology Between 1974 and 1979

Table 1 shows that the total number of isolated organisms increased progressively until 1978 from 7,809 to 12,353, but decreased slightly

TABLE 1

Distribution of Aerobic Pathogens Isolated at Rouen University Hospital
during 6 Selected Years, 1974–1979

	1974	1975	1976	1977	1978	1979
Total number of isolates	7809	9250	9865	10643	12353	11041
Gram-positive cocci	2799	2892	3281	3829	4624	4070
% of total isolates	(35.9)	(31.3)	(33.3)	(36.0)	(37.4)	(36.9)
Staphylococcus aureus	1228	1360	1784	2302	2716	2348
Staphylococcus epidermidis	130	173	228	243	279	277
Pneumococcus spp.	210	208	133	174	166	161
Streptococcus spp.	1231	1151	1136	1110	1460	1334
Enterobacteriaceae	4039	5116	5382	5327	6216	5786
% of total isolates	(51.7)	(55.3)	(54.5)	(50.0)	(50.3)	(52.4)
Escherichia coli	1654	2118	2378	2392	2927	2858
Salmonella	68	75	92	118	125	85
Shigella	9	5	6	8	21	15
Klebsiella	512	787	721	745	842	688
Enterobacter	489	490	582	354	284	235
Serratia	299	331	315	464	393	406
Citrobacter	66	80	109	140	166	121
Proteus-Providencia	942	1230	1179	1106	1458	1378
Other Gram-negative bacteria	971	1242	1202	1487	1513	1185
%of total isolates	(12.4)	(13.4)	(12.2)	(14.0)	(12.3)	(10.7)
Moraxella − Acinetobacter	162	197	218	212	234	184
Pseudomonas aeruginosa	809	1045	984	1109	1087	867
Pseudomonas spp.	–	–	–	166	192	134

in 1979. However, the respective percentages of Enterobacteriaceae, Gram-positive cocci (staphylococci, streptococci, pneumococci) and other Gram-negative aerobic bacilli (*Pseudomonas, Moraxella*) remained almost constant throughout this period. On average, Enterobacteriaceae represented 52.4% of the isolated organisms, Gram-positive cocci 35.1% and other Gram-negative bacilli 12.5%.

This constancy was also found when we considered the annual variations in the different species of Enterobacteriaceae. *E. coli* was the most frequent species (44.6%), followed by the *Proteus-Providencia* group (22.9%), then *Klebsiella* (13.5%), *Serratia* (6.6%) and *Enterobacter* (7.9%) whose percentages fell slightly, and finally by *Citrobacter* (2.1%). *Salmonella* (1.7%) and *Shigella* (0.2%) were the least frequently isolated.

As these percentages were constant over the 6 years, we used those for 1979 alone in making a more detailed analysis of the prevalence of Enterobacteriaceae in the hospital setting.

Distribution of Enterobacteriaceae among Hospital Wards

We allocated the different wards of the U.H.C. in Rouen to six categories: medicine, surgery, urology, intensive care, paediatrics and gynaecology and obstetrics. Study of the ratios of the number of isolated strains to the number of beds shows that (Table 2):

TABLE 2

Distribution of Enterobacteriaceae Isolated in Different Departments of Rouen
University Hospital (1979)

	Medicine	Surgery	Urology	I.C.U.*	Paediatrics	Gynaecology	Total
Bed number	1607	576	40	46	326	93	2688
Enterobacteriaceae Total number	3298	991	250	250	818	179	5786
Salmonella	28	1	–	–	56	–	85
Shigella	2	–	–	–	13	–	15
E.coli	1671	483	94	72	383	155	2858
Klebsiella	423	107	29	33	94	2	688
Enterobacter	87	70	12	12	48	6	235
Serratia	194	78	67	34	28	5	406
Citrobacter	81	19	4	5	9	3	121
Proteus mirabilis	528	163	22	63	143	8	927
Proteus (indole-positive)	123	59	15	18	44	–	259
Providencia	161	11	7	13	–	–	192

* I.C.U. = Intensive Care Units

1) the largest proportion of Enterobacteriaceae were isolated in the urology ward and intensive care unit (undoubtedly due to the frequency of urinary tract infections);
2) all species were isolated in the medical wards;
3) *Salmonella* and *Shigella* were only encountered in medical and paediatric wards (except for 1 strain in a surgical ward);
4) indole-positive *Proteus* was not found in gynaecology wards and *Providencia* was not found in paediatric and gynaecology wards.

Distribution of Enterobacteriaceae According to the Origin of Specimens

We allocated specimens to 7 categories: blood, urine, specimens from the respiratory tract (sputum, transtracheal punctures), intravenous and intra-arterial catheters, stools, cerebrospinal fluid, and others (pus, specimens of fluids or mucosa, etc.).

TABLE 3

Distribution of Enterobacteriaceae at Rouen University Hospital According to the Origin of Samples (1979)

	Blood	Urine	Sputum	Catheter	Stools	C.S.F.	Others	Total
Total number	369	4455	249	19	114	5	575	5786
Salmonella	10	–	–	–	70	1	4	85
Shigella	–	–	–	–	15	–	–	15
E.coli	184	2355	45	3	27	3	241	2858
Klebsiella	45	538	46	2	–	–	57	688
Enterobacter	19	134	19	4	2	1	56	235
Serratia	27	278	58	3	–	–	40	406
Citrobacter	7	102	4	–	–	–	8	121
Proteus mirabilis	56	696	51	5	–	–	119	927
Proteus (indole-positive)	15	180	18	1	–	–	45	259
Providencia	6	172	8	1	–	–	5	192

Analysis of Table 3 shows that:

1) urinary tract infections were the largest source of Enterobacteriaceae, followed by various suppurations, bacteraemia and bronchopulmonary infections;
2) *E. coli* was the species most often isolated in cases of bacteraemia and urinary tract infections (close to 53%);
3) Enterobacteriaceae of the K–E–S group were the most frequently isolated species from bronchopulmonary infections (51%); (K: *Klebsiella*; E: *Enterobacter*; S: *Serratia*)

4) finally, urinary tract infections were almost the only source of *Providencia.*

Distribution of Positive Blood Cultures in 1979

TABLE 4

Occurrence of Bacteraemic Infections Due to Enterobacteriaceae at Rouen University Hospital in 1979

	Medicine	Surgery	Urology	I.C.U.	Paediatrics	Gynaecology	Total
Total number	199	70	9	37	50	4	369
Number of positive blood cultures per bed	0.12	0.12	0.22	0.80	0.15	0.04	–
Salmonella	5	–	–	–	5	–	10
Shigella	–	–	–	–	–	–	–
E. coli	109	29	5	18	19	4	184
Klebsiella	15	10	1	6	13	–	45
Enterobacter	10	5	1	–	3	–	19
Serratia	11	7	–	7	2	–	27
Citrobacter	5	–	1	1	–	–	7
Proteus mirabilis	30	13	1	5	7	–	56
Proteus (indole-positive)	10	4	–	–	1	–	15
Providencia	4	2	–	–	–	–	6

Analysis of Table 4 shows that:

1) the ratio of positive blood cultures to the number of beds was highest in the intensive care unit. The ratios for medical, surgical and paediatric wards were quite similar, they were slightly higher in urology wards and much lower in gynaecology wards;
2) whatever the ward, *E. coli* was the species most often isolated, followed by two groups with almost equal frequencies: the K–E–S group [in decreasing order of frequency: *Klebsiella* (K), *Serratia* (S) and *Enterobacter* (E)] and the *Proteus-Providencia* group (*Proteus mirabilis* in particular);
3) bacteraemia due to *Salmonella* was found in medical and surgical wards only.

Treatment of Infections Due to Enterobacteriaceae

The U.H.C. in Rouen is so complex that two approaches were used to study methods of treating infections due to Enterobacteriaceae. One was a global approach, based on the use of antibiotics over a given period of time. Although the conclusions are somewhat lacking, such a study allows the rough assessment of the prescribing physicians' habits and, indirectly, the evolution of bacterial resistance. The other approach is selective, being limited to the study of bacteraemia due to Enterobacteriaceae in given wards. These data, although more limited, can be used to analyse more precisely the factors of prognosis, the validity of initial treatment and the role of different community- or hospital-acquired bacteria.

Use of Antibiotics in the U.H.C. in Rouen from 1976 to 1979

This study was based on figures obtained from the Central Pharmacy of the U.H.C. Figure 1 gives a summary of the use of each family of antimicrobial agents active against Enterobacteriaceae for the four years.

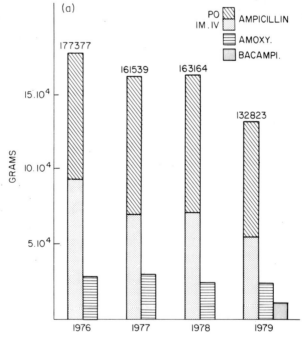

FIG. 1 (a–i)   Antimicrobial drug usage at Rouen University Hospital (1976–1979). (a) – Ampicillin.   (b) – Carbenicillin.   (c) – Cephalosporins.   (d) – Aminoglycosides. (e) – Colistin [i.m., i.v.].   (f) – Tetracyclines.   (g) – Chloramphenicol family.   (h) – Co-trimoxazole.   (i) – Quinolones.

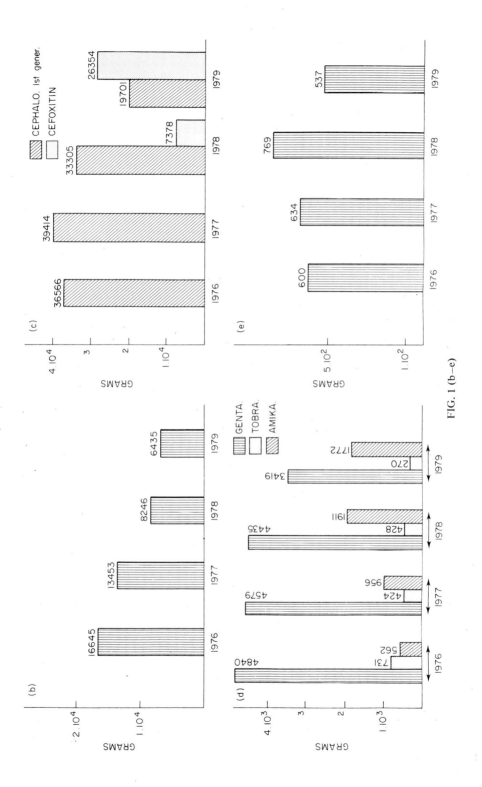

FIG. 1 (b–e)

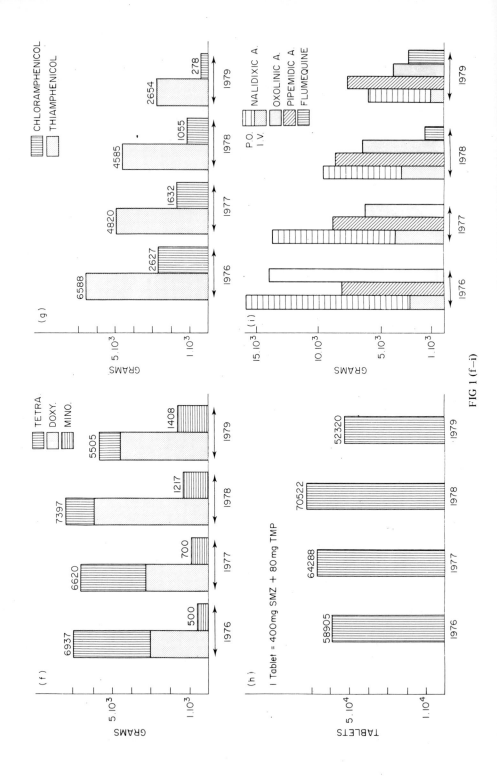

FIG 1 (f–i)

Ampicillin and its derivatives head the prescriptions whatever the route of administration. However, there was a marked fall (19%) in use from 1978 to 1979, testifying to the increasing resistance of hospital micro-organisms and to the progressive withdrawal of so-called "antibiotic cover". Reduction in the use of carbenicillin over the whole period was even more marked, owing to restriction of its use to *Pseudomonas* infections only and owing to the growing resistance of bacteria to this antibiotic. Use of cephalosporins remained high and was fairly stable from year to year. Nevertheless, since 1978, there has been a large fall in the use of cephalosporins of the so-called first generation (cephalothin, cephradine, cephapirin, cefazolin) resulting in increased use of cefoxitin (other second generation cephalosporins, cefamandole and cefuroxime, were not available from the Central Pharmacy until the last quarter of 1979). The dramatic increase in prescriptions for cefoxitin is certainly not explained by a parallel increase in bacterial resistance to other antibiotics; it is no doubt the result of "excessive" infatuation with this new product by physicians who were somewhat disappointed with the clinical results obtained with the older cephalosporins.

The use of aminoglycosides fell slightly from 1978. In contrast to cefoxitin, it was possible to limit usage of amikacin, a "reserve" aminoglycoside, by supplying the product on specific prescription only (like cefoxitin) and above all by restricting the antibiotic application to gentamicin-resistant and/or tobramycin-resistant Enterobacteriaceae. Prescriptions for parenteral colistin methane-sulphonate were steady from 1976 to 1978, then fell sharply in 1979, perhaps because of disappointing clinical results.

After ampicillin, cotrimoxazole took second place in medical prescriptions. Its use decreased markedly in 1979 for no clear reason. The same was true for the quinolones, in spite of the progressive introduction of new derivatives. This reduction was particularly evident for i.v. nalidixic acid, and coincided with the introduction of handier second generation cephalosporins.

It was difficult to assess the use of tetracyclines in the treatment of non-bacteraemic infections due to Enterobacteriaceae. In fact, apart from rare occasions when a precise indication had been obtained from antibiotic sensitivity tests, these products were most often prescribed for infections, ENT and bronchopulmonary in particular, the bacterial cause of which remained unknown since bacteriological specimens had not been collected. We should also mention that there was a very clear decline in use of the older tetracyclines (tetracycline hydrochloride, oxytetracycline) in favour of the new second generation products – doxycycline and minocycline – owing to their improved pharmacological properties and their ease of administration. The decline of the phenicols (chloramphenicol and thiamphenicol), which had begun 10 years earlier, continued. Their well-known haematological side-effects have made physicians more cautious in prescribing these products, which are increasingly reserved for specific therapeutic indications, in particular typhoid fever and certain types of bacterial meningitis.

Bacteraemia Due to Enterobacteriaceae

This study was conducted in the Department of Infectious Diseases and the Medical Intensive Care Unit; these wards, because of their role, had the largest proportion of severe infections in relation to the number of beds.

From the bacteriological, therapeutic and the prognostic points of view, the following cases should be distinguished (McGowan *et al.*, 1975): community-acquired bacteraemia (all cases in which the first culture with a significant bacterial pathogen was obtained before the third day of hospitalisation), and hospital-acquired bacteraemia (cases in which blood for the first culture positive for a significant pathogen was obtained on or after the third day of hospitalisation).

Analysis of 108 cases of bacteraemia due to Enterobacteriaceae (54 community-acquired and 54 hospital-acquired cases) treated in the two wards in 1978 and 1979 revealed the following:

Community-acquired bacteraemia   This included bacteraemia due to *Salmonella* (in practice these were all typhoid-paratyphoid infections) and bacteraemia due to other Enterobacteriaceae, which were by far the most frequent.

1) Typhoid-paratyphoid infections are constantly decreasing. Only 8 cases have been observed in the last two years: 5 typhoid and 3 paratyphoid B infections. The 8 strains isolated were all sensitive to chloramphenicol, ampicillin and cotrimoxazole *in vitro*. Treatment, currently well defined, consisted of chloramphenicol on 6 occasions and ampicillin on 2 occasions, at progressively increasing doses. The outcome was rapidly favourable in 7 cases; in the other case, the patient died on the 8th day, not from the typhoid infection, but from underlying myelocytic leukaemia.
2) Cases of bacteraemia due to other Enterobacteriaceae amounted to 46, five cases involving several microorganisms (Table 5). The most frequent cause was *E. coli* (73.5%) and the urinary tract was the principal portal of entry (60%). Initial treatment, pending the

TABLE 5

Community-Acquired Bacteraemia (1978–1979). I: Species and Portal of Entry

Species		Portal of entry	
E. coli	36	Urinary	29
Klebsiella	5	Biliary	8
Enterobacter	1	Digestive	4
Proteus mirabilis	3	Pulmonary	3
Proteus (indole-positive)	2	Bone	1
"Alkalescens"	1	Unknown	3
Other	1		

49 Enterobacteriaceae from 46 cases (5 polymicrobial).

results of blood cultures and antibiotic sensitivity tests, included either an antibiotic combination in 30 cases, usually a beta-lactam in combination with aminoglycoside, gentamicin or tobramycin (ampicillin + aminoglycosides, 16 cases; cephalosporins + amino-glycosides, 7 cases) or a single agent therapy in 13 cases (ampicillin or cephalosporins). Moreover in 3 cases the outcome was fatal within a few hours, because of overwhelming septic shock. Thirteen patients died (28%); in 7 cases death occurred from bacteraemia (including 6 cases of septic shock), and in 6 cases in relation to the underlying diseases (Table 6).

TABLE 6

Community-Acquired Bacteraemia (1978–1979). II: Outcome

Initial Antibiotic Regimen		Immediate Results		Outcome	
Combination	30	Cure	22	Cure	18
				Death (underlying disease)	4
		Death	4		
		Failure	4	Cure (surgery)	4
Single antibiotic	13	Cure	13	Cure	11
				Death (underlying disease)	2
None or inappropriate	3	Death	3		

Number of cases: 46.   Case fatality rate: 13/46 → 28.3%.

Obviously, we cannot compare the results obtained with antibiotic combinations to those obtained with single agents, as the latter involved cases which were neither clinically serious nor were they accompanied by severe underlying visceral disorders or septic shock.

Cases of hospital-acquired bacteraemia   These numbered 54, of which 9 were mixed infections. Here, the range of causative agents was much larger; the *Klebsiella–Enterobacter–Serratia* group is the most frequent, found with *E. coli* taking second place. The primary portals of entry were the urinary and digestive/biliary tracts (Table 7).

TABLE 7

Hospital-Acquired Bacteraemia (1978–1979). I: Species and Portal of Entry

Species			Portal of entry	
E. coli	23		Urinary	31
Klebsiella	13		Digestive	11
Enterobacter	6	29	Biliary	4
Serratia	10		Pulmonary	4
Proteus mirabilis	3		Catheter	4
Proteus (indole-positive)	1	8	Contamined infusion	2
Providencia	4		Peritoneal dialysis	2
Citrobacter	1		Decubitus ulcers	3
Other	1		Unknown	1

62 Enterobacteriaceae from 54 cases (9 polymicrobial).

TABLE 8

Hospital-Acquired Bacteraemia (1978–1979). II: Outcome

Initial Antibiotic Regimen		Immediate Results		Outcome	
Combination	41	Cure	32	Cure	27
				Death	5
				(underlying disease)	
		Death	6		
		Failure	3	Cure	3
Single antibiotic	5	Cure	3	Cure	3
		Death	2		
None or inappropriate	8	Death	8		

Number of cases: 54.   Case fatality rate: 21/54 → 38.9%.

Initial treatment (Table 8), in the majority of cases, consisted of an antibiotic combination: i.v. nalidixic acid + aminoglycoside, 16 cases; ampicillin + aminoglycoside, 12 cases; cephalosporin + aminoglycoside, 8 cases.

In 8 cases, the course was so rapidly fatal that antibiotics could not be prescribed in due time or were inoperant. Twenty-one patients died (38.9%); in 16 cases death occurred from bacteraemia (including 14 cases of septic shock), and in 5 cases was the result of underlying disease.

In all, 11 patients died of severe septic shock in the few hours following hospitalisation; immediate mortality was more frequently observed in cases of hospital-acquired bacteraemia. In 5 cases, the antibiotic therapy which had been active *in vitro* did not have enough time to act. In 4 patients, septic shock occurred while they were being treated by an antibiotic which was inactive against the causative microorganisms. Finally, in 2 patients, the clinical symptoms of shock did not suggest infections and antibiotics were not prescribed at the outset.

Recommendations for Therapy

Following this study, our personal experience compared with published data allows us to propose the following recommendations for therapy:

Community-acquired bacteraemia   Such cases are primarily due to *E. coli*, which usually gains entry via the urinary tract. Ampicillin seems to be the antibiotic of choice for initial treatment pending bacteriological results. In fact, this product, which is easily administered and cheap, is active against the majority of *E. coli* and *Proteus mirabilis* strains.

Combination with another antibiotic is not compulsory. However, in cases of severe infection, septic shock and/or severe underlying disease, it is justified to prescribe an ampicillin–aminoglycoside (gentamicin or tobramycin) combination at the outset due to the possible presence of some strains of ampicillin-resistant *E. coli* or of other generally resistant microorganisms (*Klebsiella*, indole-positive *Proteus*), against which aminoglycosides are usually active.

Hospital-acquired bacteraemia   In these cases the therapeutic approach will be different. In this setting, 3 essential findings guide the physician: the large variety of microorganisms which may be responsible, headed by the *Klebsiella–Enterobacter–Serratia* group; the multiple resistance patterns of microorganisms, which vary from ward to ward and are often unpredictable pending the results of antibiotic sensitivity tests; then the severity of the underlying disease, which may be the origin of the bacteraemia.

We therefore feel that an antibiotic combination is justified as initial treatment once bacteriological specimens have been collected, *provided that the adopted treatment regimen be revised appropriately once the blood culture and results of sensitivity tests are known.* The current patterns of bacterial resistance, the many possible portals of entry in such patients (urinary tract, tracheal and/or other types of catheters, drains, surgical wounds, etc.), the severity of the underlying disease and the ever present danger of septic shock are such that, *in aiming for immediate effect*, we suggest that initial antibiotic therapy consists of a second generation cephalosporin plus aminoglycoside. The new generation cephalosporins, which can better withstand the action of beta-lactamases from Gram-negative bacilli, have the advantage of being active against microbes (*E. coli, Klebsiella*) which have developed resistance to the first generation cephalosporins, against those organisms (indole-positive *Proteus, Serratia, Enterobacter*) which do not fall into the usual spectrum of activity of first generation cephalosporins and also against several anaerobic bacteria (*Bacteroides* spp., in particular) (Courtieu and Drugeon, 1979, Nightingale *et al.*, 1975; O'Callaghan, 1979; Washington, 1976).

In the hospital setting, about 20% of Enterobacteriaceae are currently resistant to aminoglycosides (e.g. in the Intensive Care Unit, 38% of klebsiellae, the predominant germs, are resistant to gentamicin and 15% resistant to tobramycin); in initial treatment, aminoglycosides such as amikacin are preferable (Meyer *et al.*, 1975; Tally *et al.*, 1975), even if it entails replacement of this "reserve" product by gentamicin or tobramycin when the results of sensitivity testing are known.

Miscellaneous cases   Several therapeutic regimens may be considered. Since there are a large number of nosocomial strains in the hospital setting, administration of ampicillin should be avoided. Carbenicillin and its analogues (ticarcillin) should, in principle, be reserved for *Pseudomonas* or indole-positive *Proteus* infections. Prescription of this product is only justified in cases of severe infections in neutropenic and/or immunodepressed patients for fear of bacteraemia due to *Pseudomonas*, the risk of which is statistically significant.

Colistin has the theoretical advantage of not being subject to transferable plasmid-mediated resistance and therefore of being remarkably active *in vitro* against many Enterobacteriaceae. But the frequently disappointing clinical results due to its usual lack of efficacy against *Proteus, Serratia* and *Providencia*, its potential nephrotoxicity and perhaps its poor tissue diffusion, have led us to stop using colistin as initial treatment. Our opinion concurs with the recommendations of the Veterans Administration Ad Hoc Interdisciplinary Advisory Committee on Antimicrobial Drug Usage (Kunin, 1977) which stated that:

> Polymyxin B sulphate and colistimethate have now been virtually replaced with more effective, less toxic drugs. The only indication for their use is serious infections caused by Gram-negative organisms (usually *Pseudomonas*) that are resistant to the preferred agents.

Enterobacteriaceae which carry multiple resistance to the usual antibiotics are often still sensitive to nalidixic acid, sometimes by virtue of synergy with polymyxins or aminoglycosides. The i.v. form is doubly advantageous since it can be administered to patients who do not tolerate any medication by the digestive route and since high serum levels can be obtained (Goulon *et al.*, 1975; Zinsser, 1970). We have always administered nalidixic acid in combination with an aminoglycoside, or more rarely with colistin, owing to the theoretical risk of mutant selection; our satisfactory results with this product have led us to apply it to initial treatment. Given very careful monitoring (particularly in respect to the acid-base balance) and provided that the product is administered as a continuous or intermittent slow drip, tolerance is usually very good.

Does cotrimoxazole, a major antibiotic along with the phenicols and aminopenicillins in *Salmonella* and *Shigella* infections, have a place in treating bacteraemia due to other Enterobacteriaceae, particularly since a parenteral form is available? It is difficult to answer this question because relatively few patients with serious systemic infections have been treated with trimethoprim-sulphamethoxazole (Grose *et al.*, 1979; Olcen and Eriksson, 1976). In one report from Scandinavia, 14 out of 18 patients with Gram-negative sepsis due to *E. coli, Proteus* sp., *Klebsiella* sp., *Bacteroides* sp., *H. influenzae* and *Salmonella typhi* responded satisfactorily to the intravenous preparation (Franzen and Brandberg, 1976). In our opinion, cotrimoxazole should only be prescribed as a second measure when strains resistant to other antibiotics of proven efficacy are present.

Although it is in principle reserved for the treatment of tuberculosis, rifampicin at concentrations which can be reached in the body is effective against many Gram-negative bacilli; it is freely diffusible and is excreted in urine and bile. When used alone, rifampicin has the disadvantage of rapidly leading to a high level of resistance by one-step mutation. For this reason, a number of *in vitro* studies have been carried out using rifampicin in combination with some other antibiotics. Thus, the combination rifampicin–polymyxin B (Traub and Kleber, 1975) or rifampicin–trimethoprim (Hamilton-Miller *et al.*, 1977) is synergic against *Serratia marcescens. In vitro* synergy between rifampicin and novobiocin has been demonstrated against *Salmonella typhi* (Shanson and Leung, 1976); it may be possible to use this combination for the treatment of typhoid due to strains resistant to chloramphenicol, cotrimoxazole and ampicillin. But the value of such combinations remains to be checked by appropriate clinical trials and, in any case, they must be a last resort for infections due to microorganisms with multiple resistance.

The ever increasing emergence of resistant strains, particularly in hospitals, has led to the development of new molecules belonging to very different antibiotic families; a non-exhaustive list appears in Table 9. All these products have proved highly active *in vitro* against

TABLE 9

Antibiotics in the Future

Ureido–penicillins: mezlocillin, azlocillin
Piperacillin, Apalcillin
Mecillinam
Newer cephalosporins: cefotaxime, cefoperazone, cefotiam, LY 127935, cefsulodin ...
Thienamycin
Newer aminoglycosides: epi–sisomicin, SCH 21420
Fosfomycin
Clavulanic acid

Enterobacteriaceae, and particularly against strains resistant to the "classical" beta-lactam antibiotics, but clinical trials are still too limited to determine preferential indications for each product and their exact place in the treatment of infections, bacteraemic or other, due to Enterobacteriaceae.

Conclusions

Antibiotic therapy, how appropriate it may be, is not the only factor intervening in the outcome of bacteraemia due to Enterobacteriaceae. Three factors play an essential part in the prognosis: the presence of septic shock, the nature and the severity of the underlying conditions and the treatment of the portal of entry.

The occurrence of septic shock is always an element for poor prognosis. In fact, whatever the nature and the origin of the micro-organism (community- or hospital-acquired), overall mortality rises from 14.2% when shock is absent to 59% when it is present (Table 10). It should be noticed that shock was considered directly responsible for 20 out of 24 fatal issues.

TABLE 10

Relationship of Septic Shock to Mortality

	Number	Deaths	%
Without shock	56	8	14.2
With shock	44	26*	59
Total	100	34	

* Mortality was directly related to septic shock in 20 patients.

The underlying condition is also an important element of prognosis (Freid and Vosti, 1968). As shown in Table 11, the percentage of

TABLE 11

Relationship of General Host Factors to Mortality in Adults with Bacteraemia

Underlying disease	Number	Cure	Deaths	
			Number	%
Non fatal or No disease	64	52	12	18.75
Ultimately fatal	20	11	9	45
Rapidly fatal	16	3	13	81.25
Total	100	66	34	34

deaths increases from 18% when severe visceral disorders are absent to more than 80% in cases of "rapidly fatal" underlying diseases. In this table, it can be seen that, compared to figures from other sources, relatively few diseases were "rapidly fatal". This is explained by the fact that, in our city, neoplasic diseases (haematological or solid tumours) are treated in a Cancer Institute which is independent of the U.H.C. in Rouen.

Finally, the importance of treating the portal of entry must be emphasized. Often neglected or misunderstood, this treatment, whenever it can be carried out, is nevertheless a primary necessity. Table 12, based on statistics for 120 cases of bacteraemia due to Gram-negative bacilli observed between 1968 and 1974 in the Infectious Diseases Ward and the Medical Intensive Care Unit, illustrates this recommendation.

TABLE 12

Relationship of Antibiotic Therapy and Treatment of the Portal of Entry to Mortality

Antibiotic therapy	Treatment of the portal of entry	
	Effective	Not effective
Appropriate	13%* (7/53)[+]	64% (25/39)
Not appropriate	30% (3/10)	100% (18/18)

* Case fatality rate
+ (No of Deaths/No of patients)

Acknowledgements

We wish to thank Mrs. N. Hantute, Pharm. D. and Mr. G. Maurey, Pharm. D., who kindly gave us the information concerning anti-microbial drug usage in Rouen University Hospital.

References

Altemeier, W.A., Todd, J.C. and Inge, W.W. (1967). *Ann. Surg.* **166**, 530—542.
Courtieu, A.L. and Drugeon, H.B. (1979). *Méd. Mal. Infect.* **9**, 199—205.
Dupont, H.L. and Spink, W.W. (1969). *Medicine* **48**, 307—332.
Finland, M. (1970). *J. Infect. Dis.* **122**, 419—431.
Franzen, Ch. and Brandberg, A. (1976). *Scand. J. Infect. Dis.* suppl. **8**, 96—100.
Freid, M.A. and Vosti, K.L. (1968). *Arch. Intern. Med.* **121**, 418—423.
Goulon, M., Schortgen, G., Tancrede, C., Nouailhat, F., Babinet, P. and Raphael, J.C. (1975). *Nouv. Presse Méd.* **4**, 13—16.
Grose, W.E., Bodey, G.P. and Ti Li Loo (1979). *Antimicrob. Agents Chemother.* **15**, 447—451.
Hamilton-Miller, J.M.T., Kerry, D.W. and Brumfitt, W. (1977). *J. Antimicrob. Chemother.* **3**, 193—194.
Klastersky, J. (1972). *Nouv. Presse Méd.* **1**, 183—187.
Kunin, C.M. (1977). *J. Am. Med. Assoc.* **237**, 1481—1482.
McCabe, W.R. and Jackson, G.G. (1962a). *Arch. Intern. Med.* **110**, 847—855.
McCabe, W.R. and Jackson, G.G. (1962b). *Arch. Intern. Med.* **110**, 856—864.
McGowan, J.E., Barnes, M.W. and Finland, M. (1975). *J. Infect. Dis.* **132**, 316—335.
Meyer, R.D., Lewis, R.P., Duane Carmalt, E. and Finegold, S.M. (1975). *Ann. Intern. Med.* **83**, 790—800.
Nightingale, C.H., Green, D.S. and Quintiliani, R. (1975). *J. Pharm. Sci.* **64**, 1899—1927.
O'Callaghan, C.H. (1979). *J. Antimicrob. Chemother.* **5**, 635—671.
Olcen, P. and Eriksson, M. (1976). *Scand. J. Infect. Dis.* suppl. **8**, 91—94.
Shanson, D.C. and Leung, T. (1976). *J. Antimicrob. Chemother.* **2**, 81 85.
Tally, F.P., Louie, T.J., Weinstein, W.M., Bartlett, J.G. and Gorbach, S.L. (1975). *Ann. Intern. Med.* **83**, 484—488.
Traub, W.H. and Kleber, I. (1975). *Antimicrob. Agents Chemother.* **7**, 874—876.
Washington, J.A. (1976). *Mayo Clin. Proceed.* **51**, 237—250.
Zinsser, H.H. (1970). *Med. Clin. North America* **54**, 1347—1350.

Discussion

Professor Acar: We really get to the heart of the matter here. Your therapeutic approach raises a number of questions. First of all, you suggest a revision of treatment after initial therapy with a second generation cephalosporin combined with an aminoglycoside (a new aminoglycoside, for which there is less chance of finding resistant bacteria). What is the rationale for revising this treatment and what is your time interval? Furthermore, what is the choice of antibiotics? Can you also maintain the same initial choice when the patient is in a state of shock?

Professor Humbert: I always base my recommendations on bacteriological data. At the present time, in the case of hospital-acquired bacteraemia, the most effective combination against Enterobacteriaceae in my hospital is a second generation cephalosporin and amikacin. Depending on the results of blood cultures and antibiotic sensitivity tests, obtained in 2 or 4 days at most, I might shift the treatment to a less expensive but efficient drug, for instance cephalotin, gentamicin or tobramycin.

This allows me to limit the use of new molecules. I personally believe their indiscriminate use should be absolutely avoided. Unfortunately, in my hospital, like in many French hospitals, we do not have, as in the U.S., an effective method for controlling antibiotic prescription.

Concerning septic shock, the treatment is essentially a symptomatic treatment, a resuscitation, and, you can give all the antibiotics you want. What is essential is to restore haemodynamics, and the choice of the antibiotic is secondary. *A priori*, I do not see any reason to change the usual choice.

Professor Kunin: I would like to make some comments on Professor Humbert's presentation, which I enjoyed very much. I want to speak for the clinician, because there are only a few clinicians at this meeting, most people being "scientists". It is very difficult to describe *in vacuo* how one would manage a patient with an infectious process. Clinicians are often asked how they would treat a patient who came into hospital with a temperature of 40°C and sepsis. There is no such entity as "sepsis of unknown origin". The individual patient must be examined and the epidemiological circumstances studied. Every individual is different, and many of them do not even have an infectious process.

I find Professor Humbert's position extremely difficult to present because, as an overview, every point he has made is correct, but for any individual human being seen clinically, the clinician has to start from the beginning and can use these statements only as the very broadest guidelines. The examination by Gram-stain of the pus and the nature of the underlying process are so critical and so variable that it is not possible to generalise further. We must talk about individual disease processes.

Professor Sabath: Concerning the fate of the bacteraemic patients, patients with bacteraemia of community origin in particular, I noticed that Professor Humbert's results were better in those patients who received only one drug than in those receiving multiple therapy. Is this perhaps because the most severely ill patients received two drugs, and the less severely ill patients were given the single drug?

Professor Humbert: Yes, this was the case. I made the point in my presentation that, by definition, a patient who has received only ampicillin or only a cephalosporin is one who did not show up a serious condition. An example is pyelonephritis, the patient has a temperature of $40°C$ and pyuria, and is treated with gentamicin; 48 hours later, 2 blood cultures are positive when the patient is already apyrexial. This is typical.

Professor Kernbaum: What are your criteria to interrupt the treatment in bacteraemia?

Professor Humbert: It is an obvious and frequently asked question. It all depends on the patient and on his clinical evolution. We refer essentially to the temperature curve and the regression of leucocytosis. In France, a Gram-negative infection is treated for about 3 weeks, in the absence of complications, but there is no rigid scientific basis for this 3 week period.

Professor Williams: With regard to the epidemiology of Professor Humbert's hospital, I gained the impression that *Pseudomonas aeruginosa* was not a very prominent organism. This is different from the situation in the United States, but similar to the position in the United Kingdom. One feature of therapy in the United Kingdom is that far more penicillins are used than cephalosporins, which may be the reason why *Pseudomonas* is less prevalent. What was the relationship between the use of the penicillins and the cephalosporins, in Professor Humbert's hospital?

Professor Humbert: On the first point I fully agree with you: in France we see very few severe infections with *Pseudomonas.* In the Intensive Care Unit at least, we succeeded, although with many difficulties, to strictly eliminate any protective antibiotherapy. In other words, formerly patients with a tracheotomy or a catheter always received ampicillin or cephalosporins. However, simply with good nursing and use of penicillin G only as prophylactic antibiotic, we decreased the number of our cases of sepsis. It was difficult to analyse the respective consumptions of penicillins and cephalosporins in the 3 different hospitals of the town, and their 45 departments. So I cannot give any specific figure.

Professor Chabbert: You told us that the first line treatment in bacteraemia, is ampicillin. I would like to know whether all *E. coli* are sensitive to ampicillin. Also what is the percentage of patients that should not have received ampicillin?

Professor Humbert: In 54 cases of community-acquired sepsis, there were only 2 strains of *E. coli* resistant to ampicillin. By chance these strains were found in patients who eventually received a combination of antibiotics, including gentamicin to which their strains of *E. coli* were ultimately sensitive. So, possibly in sepsis acquired outside hospital, it is wise to combine an aminoglycoside with ampicillin. Besides, there is an occasional *Klebsiella* that is sensitive to aminoglycosides.

Professor Labia: You mentioned that rifampicin is effective against the Enterobacteriaceae. Did you actually suggest the use of rifampicin in the treatment of infections by Enterobacteriaceae?

Professor Humbert: As a matter of fact the literature has shown many studies *in vitro* on combinations of rifampicin and trimethoprim. Personally, I have no experience with rifampicin in the treatment of serious infections due to Enterobacteriaceae, but rifampicin in combination with other antibiotics seems very useful in a certain number of serious infections due to *Staphylococcus aureus*, in particular in endocarditis.

Professor Modai: First, I wish to tell Professor Chabbert that we see an increasing number of subjects coming from the community with *E. coli* resistant to ampicillin, and probably Professor Humbert faced a favourable situation. Secondly, when dealing with sepsis with Enterobacteriaceae, how do you treat an immunodepressed patient or any emergency case of serious bacteraemia? How do you know whether this serious infection is due to *Staphylococcus aureus* or Enterobacteriaceae? As you do, I personally consider the problem as solved for a Gram-negative infection and I eventually change the treatment. It is obviously wiser to wait for the bacteriological diagnosis, but unfortunately you cannot always wait especially with cancer patients. What is your personal experience?

Professor Humbert: As you know, I have a limited experience with cancer patients. From the patient's history and clinical situation, you know in the vast majority of cases whether you are dealing with *Staphylococcus aureus* or a Gram-negative organism. With this last organism, keeping in mind the problem of bacterial resistance and waiting for the results of antibiotic sensitivity test, I prescribe what seems to me the most effective second generation cephalosporin and aminoglycoside. If you think of the more pessimistic hypothesis of a serious Gram-negative infection with the possibility of septic shock, you must try as much as possible to sterilize the focus of infection.

Professor Sabath: In his presentation, Professor Humbert mentioned a number of patients who had polymicrobial bacteraemia. Did any of those include anaerobic organisms?

Professor Humbert: Relatively few of them, there were only 3 patients with anaerobes. But I wish to add that only in recent years has the search for anaerobes been conducted validly and effectively. Furthermore, when we are dealing with a bacteriaemia in a patient who has had digestive tract surgery or pelvic surgery, we frequently add an i.v. nitroimidazole because the risk of anaerobic infection should not be neglected.

Antibiotics for Use Against *Pseudomonas aeruginosa* and other "Non-Fermenters"

L.D. SABATH

*Section of Infectious Diseases, University of
Minnesota School of Medicine, Minneapolis,
Minnesota, U.S.A.*

Introduction

The purpose of this chapter is to call attention to the antibiotics
that are active against *Pseudomonas aeruginosa* and other "non-
fermenters", describe some of the major problems with the use of
currently available antimicrobial agents, and make some comments
about agents which might be developed in the future, especially the
near future.

The "non-fermenters" are a heterogeneous group of Gram-negative
bacilli characterized by their inability to ferment carbohydrates. This
may be determined in OF basal medium (oxidation-fermentation test
medium) (Hugh and Leifson, 1953). The clinical importance of this
group of organisms has been commented upon by others (Gardner *et
al.*, 1970).

Pseudomonas aeruginosa, *Pseudomonas maltophilia*, and *Acinetobacter anitratum* appear to be the most frequently isolated glucose-
nonfermenting Gram-negative bacilli in clinical medicine (Hugh and
Gilardi, 1974). Although frequently considered to be saprophytes,
many of the other members of the genus *Pseudomonas* clearly cause
serious, sometimes fatal, infections.

General Problem of Antibiotics for *P. aeruginosa* and Other Nonfermentative Gram-negative Bacilli

P. aeruginosa, and many of the other nonfermentative Gram-negative
bacilli, are resistant to most of the commonly used, less toxic

antibiotics. Thus, the initial selection is mainly from a relatively short list of less desirable antimicrobial agents. In practice, the list of potential choices is further restricted by bacterial resistance to individual or groups of antibiotics.

Although *P. aeruginosa* is, without question, the most important pathogen of the nonfermentative Gram-negative bacilli, many of the others are also important pathogens. The antibiotic susceptibilities of these "other organisms" are often quite different from that of *P. aeruginosa*. One striking example is *P. cepacia* which is usually also quite sensitive to chloramphenicol and trimethoprim/sulphamethoxazole, and these are generally considered preferable to aminoglycosides for therapy.

Antibiotic susceptibility testing systems are numerous, and are the major routine means of determining which strain is susceptible to which antibiotic. There are four major deficiencies, however, with these systems (Sabath, 1978):

1) Absence of Correlation

The laboratory test results may not correlate with the clinical results which may be better or worse than would be expected on the basis of such tests. The virtual elimination of polymyxin B and colistin from consideration as possible therapeutic agents for systemic infections due to *P. aeruginosa*, even though the organism is invariably susceptible, is an example of how clinical experience (of ineffectiveness) will modulate the application of results from sensitivity tests.

2) Influence of Specific Host Factors

They may create local environments in which the antibiotic is much more or much less effective than would have been anticipated on the basis of *in vitro* sensitivity tests. These may be summarized as: (a) enhancement of activity due to antibiotic concentration in a particular body compartment (e.g. urine or bile), (b) diminished activity due to exclusion from, or poor penetration into a body compartment (i.e. the eye or cerebrospinal fluid), (c) enhancement of activity due to specific local factors that favour their action (e.g. favourable pH), (d) antagonism of antibacterial activity by products of inflammation, such as pH, low oxidation–reduction potential, pus, and various cations (Sabath, 1978), and (e) decreased normal host defences (e.g. granulocytopenia).

3) Antibiotic Effects at Subinhibitory Concentration

The general operational concept is that the minimum inhibitory concentration (m.i.c.) of antibiotic determined in the laboratory must be exceeded in the patient's blood. This concept fails to take into account the facts that: (a) most tissue levels of antibiotic are lower than blood levels, (b) there are few data indicating how much higher than the m.i.c. the blood level should be (Klastersky *et al.*, 1974), and (c) the effect of antibiotics on bacteria that occur at concentrations lower than the m.i.c. may be of importance (Lorian *et al.*, 1980).

4) Post-Antibiotic Effects on Bacteria

There are few data indicating how long after antibiotic concentrations have been lowered, either artificially *in vitro*, or by normal pharmacological excretory or bioconverting mechanisms, antibacterial activity continues. Eagle and his colleagues reported on very definite post-antibiotic effects of penicillin observed with Gram-positive cocci; the duration of the effect varied with the organism (Eagle *et al.*, 1950). More recently, Craig and his associates have conducted similar studies on currently available β–lactam antibiotics and aminoglycosides (Craig *et al.*, 1980). They found there was no post-antibiotic effect of β–lactam antibiotics against Gram-negative bacilli whereas the aminoglycosides had an effect that lasted for a number of hours. In contrast, both aminoglycoside and β–lactam antibiotics had post-antibiotic effects against Gram-positive cocci.

These four major deficiencies with *in vitro* susceptibility testing systems clearly demonstrate special problems, not only in differences in composition between laboratory tests and the patient's site of infection (including the interplay with the host inflammatory response and immune systems), but also with the temporal relationship of the duration and concentration of antibiotic at the infected focus. Murakawa and Sabath (unpub. data) have established a "kinetic ·model" showing that changing the antibiotic concentration in liquid media — to reflect changing concentrations of drug found in humans, resulting from normal drug absorption and excretion — will bring out clear differences in antibiotic effect that could not be demonstrated in the conventional "static" test system in which a specific concentration of antibiotic is added to a medium, but not varied during the incubation period.

Summary of the Major Antibiotic Groups Active Against Gram-negative Bacilli

There are seven major groups of antimicrobial agents with some activity against Gram-negative bacilli, and sometimes also *P. aeruginosa*. Each group has one or more major defects. The special problems of aminoglycosides and β–lactam antibiotics against *P. aeruginosa* will be discussed more elaborately in a later section of this chapter. The summary of the problems is as follows below.

Aminoglycoside Antibiotics

Their action is probably much less striking in the host than *in vitro* because of problems of antibiotic penetration, and antagonism of their action by products of inflammation [acid pH and low Eh (oxidation–reduction potential)] and by certain divalent cations. Some antibiotic resistance also exists.

Table 1 indicates the geometric mean $m.i.c._{50}$ and $m.i.c._{90}$ of 7 different aminoglycosides with good activity against *P. aeruginosa* (Zak, 1980).

TABLE 1

Inhibitory Activity of Different Aminoglycoside Antibiotics against *P. aeruginosa*

Antibiotic	Geometric mean of	
	$m.i.c._{50}$* (μg/ml)	$m.i.c._{90}$* (μg/ml)
Amikacin	2.0	6.3
Dibekacin	1.1	2.3
Gentamicin	1.4	3.6
Sisomicin	0.69	2.44
Tobramycin	0.45	2.2
Netilmicin	1.5	5.1
5–episisomicin	0.45**	12.5**

 * Mean of minimum concentrations found to inhibit 50% ($m.i.c._{50}$) and 90% ($m.i.c._{90}$) of isolates of *P. aeruginosa*. Data from examinations of selected resistant isolates were omitted.
** only few data available
(From Zak, 1980, with permission of Hans Huber Publishers and Ciba Geigy.)

β–lactam Antibiotics

Most of these have poor *in vitro* activity against *P. aeruginosa*. In addition the apparent m.i.c. by conventional *in vitro* testing is often lower (more favourable) than when determined with heavier inocula. The activities of newer and older β–lactam antibiotics are summarized in Table 2 (Zak, 1980).

TABLE 2

Inhibitory Activity of Different β–lactam Antibiotics against *P. aeruginosa*

Antibiotic	Geometric mean of	
	m.i.c.$_{50}$ * (μg/ml)	m.i.c.$_{90}$ * (μg/ml)
Carbenicillin	52	150
Sulbenicillin	22	54
Ticarcillin	21	88
Azlocillin	8.4	37
Apalcillin	1.1	ca. 14
Furazlocillin	5.3	21
Piperacillin	5.0	20
Thienamycin	8.0**	8–12.5**
Nocardicin A	25**	100**
Cefsulodin	3.1	12
Cefotaxime	19	49
SCE 1365	25**	n.a.
6059–S	14**	64**
Cefoperazone	3.6**	16–125**

* Mean of minimum concentrations found to inhibit 50% (m.i.c.$_{50}$) or 90% (m.i.c.$_{90}$) of isolates of *P. aeruginosa*. Data from examinations of selected resistant isolates were omitted.
** only few data available
n.a. data not available
(From Zak, 1980, with permission of Hans Huber Publishers and Ciba Geigy.)

Polymyxins

Polymyxin B and polymyxin E (colistin) are active against virtually all strains of *P. aeruginosa* and also most of the nonfermentative Gram-negative bacilli, but their clinical results have not been very impressive, probably mainly due to tissue binding of antibiotic. In addition, there is some evidence that colistin sulphomethate had much less activity than did colistin by itself, probably because of sulphomethyl groups "covering" free amino groups on the antibiotic; the free amino groups appear to be necessary for both activity and toxicity (Barnett *et al.*, 1964).

Chloramphenicol

Most strains of *P. aeruginosa* are resistant, by *in vitro* testing, but many of the nonfermentative Gram-negative bacilli are susceptible. The rare case of irreversible aplastic anaemia is a deterrent to the use of chloramphenicol, but the apprehension and fear of prosecution for "malpractice" — should there be adverse effects — are even greater deterrents.

Tetracyclines

There are currently seven different tetracyclines available for clinical use in the United States: tetracycline, chlortetracycline, oxytetracycline, demeclocycline, methacycline, doxycycline and minocycline. None of these, by conventional testing, appear to be active against *P. aeruginosa*, although these compounds are frequently "active" against many other Gram-negative bacilli. However, the actual concentrations of tetracyclines required to inhibit *P. aeruginosa in vitro* is (median value) 12.5 to 25 μg/ml (50 μg/ml for chlortetracycline) (Finland *et al.*, 1976), but these concentrations are easily achieved in the urine, and tetracyclines have been successfully used in treating infections due to *P. aeruginosa*, where the site is limited to the urinary tract (Stamey *et al.*, 1974; Musher *et al.*, 1975).

Sulphonamides (With or Without Trimethoprim)

Although many of the non-fermentative Gram-negative bacilli are sensitive to the combination of trimethoprim plus sulphamethoxazole, most strains of *P. aeruginosa* are resistant. Therefore, resistance limits the use of this category.

Miscellaneous Urinary Tract Antiseptics

Most, if not all, of these are not active against *P. aeruginosa*, and, therefore, are rarely used in urinary tract infections due to that organism. This group of antimicrobial agents includes nalidixic acid, nitrofurantoin, methenamine mandelate and assorted organic acids.

Specific Problems Inherent to the Use of Aminoglycoside Antibiotics

Some of the major problems inherent to the use of aminoglycosides have been noted in preceding sections, but the most important ones are assembled below.

Pharmacological Properties

Although aminoglycosides penetrate many tissues well, they have very poor penetration into the cerebrospinal fluid, do not penetrate the eye at all, do not enter cells, and have rather poor penetration into the biliary tree.

Toxicity

The major toxicities of aminoglycosides are on the eighth cranial nerve (both vestibular and acoustic branches), the kidney (producing a proximal tubular toxicity), the neuromuscular synapses (mainly seen if instilled into the peritoneal cavity of patients undergoing abdominal surgery who are receiving curare-like drugs), and allergy. The eighth nerve and nephrotoxicities are the most important toxicities both occurring much more frequently in elderly patients than in children. A recent study (Smith *et al.*, 1980) reported ototoxicity at 10% and 11% and nephrotoxicity at 26% and 12%, respectively, for gentamicin and tobramycin, even though there had been relatively close monitoring of blood levels. There has generally been an "understanding" that the nephrotoxicity of aminoglycosides is "completely reversible", but no detailed study documenting this is known to this author. Acute renal failure from a variety of causes was found to be relatively fully reversible in a study by Hall *et al.* (1970) in patients less than 40 years old, but not in older patients; this may have implications for the nephrotoxicity of aminoglycoside antibiotics.

Cost

Although the actual cost of aminoglycoside antibiotics, superficially, does not seem to be grossly different from alternatives, to "properly" administer them requires close monitoring of blood levels, either as the "peak", the "peak and trough", or even more than two determinations after a given dose to more accurately calculate the pharmacokinetics in an individual patient. Numerous workers in the field, including this author, believe all patients with serious infections for which aminoglycosides are given should have close monitoring of blood levels, to insure adequate therapy, and possibly to help avoid toxicity (Sabath, 1973). Furthermore, monitoring for toxicity is also required, i.e., measurement of renal function and hearing. These also have a cost. Especially in patients with rapidly fluctuating renal function, the cost of monitoring adequacy of therapy and possible toxicity far exceeds the cost of the drug itself.

Narrow Toxic: Therapeutic Ratios

The fact that "toxic" levels of aminoglycosides are often small multiples of the m.i.c. (e.g. gentamicin m.i.c. for *P. aeruginosa* is frequently 1.6 to 6.0, yet "toxic" levels are thought to be about 12 μg/ml), sometimes as low as 2, it is easy to see why even moderate variations in blood levels after given dose might lead to inappropriate therapy. This is the reason why many specialists in antibiotic therapy, including this one, advocate appropriate monitoring of serum aminoglycoside levels (Sabath, 1977b).

Resistance

Bacterial resistance to aminoglycoside antibiotics does exist, although this is much less common than is resistance to other currently available antimicrobial agents with the exception of the polymyxins (Finland *et al.*, 1976). The basis of aminoglycoside resistance of bacteria, in general, is one of the three mechanisms listed here:

1) *inactivating enzymes*, which convert active aminoglycoside into inactive conjugated products by one of three reactions: phosphorylation, acetylation, adenylylation;
2) *decreased ribosomal binding* of aminoglycoside to the 30S subunit of bacterial ribosomes (not yet described in *P. aeruginosa*);
3) *permeability barrier*, which excludes the aminoglycoside, preventing it from reaching the binding site (on the 30S ribosome which is necessary for antibacterial action to occur).

Most recent research on aminoglycoside resistance has been directed to problems and mechanisms concerning the aminoglycoside inactivating enzymes. These confer specificity of resistance, and probably account for the fact that tobramycin (which is inactivated by fewer of these) is active against many strains resistant to gentamicin, and the fact that amikacin (which resists even more of these enzymes) is active against many strains resistant to both gentamicin and tobramycin (Zak, 1980).

There is increasing interest in "permeability mutants" that have broad resistance to many aminoglycosides, due to their inability to be transported across the bacterial membrane.

Microcolony and Mucoid "Capsule" Formation

These special traits of *P. aeruginosa* are currently subjects of intense research, and probably account for much resistance of *P. aeruginosa* to aminoglycoside antibiotics, and also to other antibiotics (Govan and Fyfe, 1978; Lam *et al.*, 1980). In each of these instances, the elaboration of an extracellular polysaccharide barrier appears to be responsible for treatment failure and apparent resistance.

Antagonism by Products of Inflammation

There is very clear evidence that aminoglycosides are much less active at low pH (Abraham and Duthie, 1946; Sabath, 1968), under anaerobic conditions or where the oxidation–reduction potential is lowered (Kogut and Lightbown, 1963), in the presence of certain divalent cations, especially magnesium (Medeiros *et al.*, 1971) and of pus itself (Sabath, 1977a).

Major Problems with β–lactam Antibiotics

The shortcoming of the β–lactam antibiotics (the penicillins and cephalosporins) as therapeutic agents for infections due to *P. aeruginosa* are summarized below.

Bacterial Resistance via Drug Inactivation

This is mediated by three types of enzymes:

1) β–lactamase, the most common, by which the carbon–nitrogen bond in the β–lactam ring of penicillins or cephalosporins is hydrolysed, yielding the corresponding penicilloic or cephalosporoic acid;
2) amidase, or acylase, by which the side chain on the 6-amino group of penicillins is hydrolysed (a reaction that is mediated by many intestinal organisms, but which is highly pH dependent, and probably of little clinical significance), and
3) acetyl esterases, tissue enzymes that may cleave the acetyl group off the dihydrothiazine ring of cephalosporins (such as cephalothin) that have such side chains, yielding the desacetyl derivatives which are uniformly less active than their acetoxy precursors (Abraham and Sabath, 1965; Abraham, 1974).

Bacterial Resistance without Drug Inactivation

Relatively little is known of the basis for this. This may be due in large part to differences in permeability factors (Richmond *et al.*, 1976) which exclude drug from key binding sites (Table 3), or to other factors which were found to be highly environment dependent, when studied in *S. aureus* (Sabath, 1977a), or possibly due to mutations of

TABLE 3

In vitro Activity of Various Antibiotics against *P. aeruginosa* K 799/WT and its Mutant
K 799/61 (222) with Reduced Permeation Barrier

Antibiotic	m.i.c. (μg/ml)*		A/B**
	P. aeruginosa K 799/WT (A)	*P. aeruginosa* K 799/61 (B)	
Carbenicillin	16	0.02	800
Sulbenicillin	8	0.02	400
Ticarcillin	4	0.002	2000
Piperacillin	1	0.005	200
Azlocillin	2	0.005	400
Nocardicin A	16	1	16
Cefsulodin	0.2	0.02	10
Cefotaxime	8	0.01	800
Cefoperazone	1	0.002	500
SCE 1365	4	0.01	400
Gentamicin	0.2	0.1	2
Tobramycin	0.1	0.1	1
Amikacin	1	0.5	2
Sisomicin	0.1	0.05	2
Netilmicin	0.5	0.2	2.5
Dibekacin	0.2	0.2	1
Colistin	4	4	1

 * indicative of activity at target determined by agar diffusion test in OST agar OXOID
   using an inoculum of 10^6 organisms per ml
** indicative of penetrability (value 1 = very good penetration)
(From Zak, 1980, with permission of Hans Huber Publishers and Ciba Geigy.)

specific penicillin binding proteins (Spratt, 1980). Resistance, at least
to carbenicillin, has been observed to occur during a single course of
treatment, even when an aminoglycoside is also present (Smith *et al.*,
1970).

Inter—β—lactam Antagonism

This phenomenon was originally thought to be relatively uncommon
(Acar *et al.*, 1975) but it has been noted by at least four groups. In
this phenomenon, the co-presence of one β—lactam (especially a
cephalosporin, or 6—aminopenicillanic acid) will strikingly antagonize
the other β—lactam antibiotic, especially carbenicillin. More recently,
Bittner *et al.* (unpub. data) have noted that piperacillin is especially
prone to be antagonized. This antagonism is probably due to
blockade of access of critical binding sites (Acar *et al.*, 1975).

The Inoculum Effect

It has been known for over 30 years that a highly resistant organism (a penicillinase-producing *Staphylococcus aureus*) will appear to be quite sensitive if tested on solid medium with a dilute inoculum that would lead to the formation of widely separated colonies, if no drug were present (Luria, 1946). Conventional sensitivity tests of β-lactam antibiotics tend to call for relatively light inocula; when tested with heavy inocula the m.i.c. may increase from several hundred-fold to several thousand-fold (Sabath *et al.*, 1973 and 1975), with Gram-negative and Gram-positive organisms, respectively. The evidence suggests that many Gram-negative bacillary infections, including those due to *P. aeruginosa*, in which a dense concentration of organisms are seen on Gram stains of material from lesions, require higher concentrations of drug for inhibition than are seen in routine testing. This also suggests that such infections may not be treated successfully with β-lactam antibiotics except those that are highly resistant to hydrolysis by β-lactamases.

"Tolerance" to the Killing Action of β-lactam Antibiotics

The recent emphasis has been on staphylococci that are inhibited, but not killed by β-lactam antibiotics (Sabath *et al.*, 1977; Sabath, 1979), but there is evidence that at least two semisynthetic penicillins, BRL 1654 (Price *et al.*, 1971) and piperacillin (Sathe *et al.*, unpub. data), with impressive anti-pseudomonal activity failed to kill this organism. The clinical significance of this remains to be determined.

Penicillin Allergy

Estimates of the incidence of penicillin allergy in the general public vary from 2–5% to 3–10% (Parker, 1963), but a factor that should be of concern is the observation of Green *et al.* (1967) that about 17% of patients with bacterial endocarditis had a history of one or more adverse reactions to penicillin. This suggests penicillin allergy may be highest in those patients who need it most.

Permeability Problems

The comparative *in vitro* activities of β-lactam antibiotics are summarized in Table 3, emphasizing the enormous effect permeability has on activity (Zak, 1980; Richmond *et al.*, 1976).

Newer Concepts for Drugs with Activity against *P. aeruginosa*

Two recent books summarize the major problems encountered with *P. aeruginosa*, including its treatment (Brown, 1975; Sabath, 1980). Chapters in those volumes discuss some of the newer work on immunological approaches. The overall category of "newer" approaches might be listed as follows:

1) Active immunization;
2) Passive immunization;
3) Inhibitors of cell attachment to host,
4) β–lactamase inhibitors (to be used in conjunction with other β–lactam antibiotics);
5) Use of chelators (such as ethylenediaminetetraacetic acid, EDTA);
6) Gyrase inhibitors;
7) Inhibitors of metal transport systems (e.g. of pyochelins).

Summary

P. aeruginosa and other non-fermentative Gram-negative bacilli are among the more difficult infections to treat because these organisms, when they do cause infections, are most likely to cause those infections in debilitated and immunosuppressed patients, and also because many of them are "resistant" to many or all of the antimicrobial agents currently in use. The "resistance" may be due to inactivation of the drug, obstacle in access of the drug to its binding sites, primary insensitivity of the organism to the drug, special problems within the host or combinations of one or more of the above. It is fair to say that none of the antibiotics currently in use is ideal. Numerous exciting new avenues of therapy are currently under investigation.

Acknowledgements

The assistance of Jane E. Anderson in the preparation of this chapter is greatly appreciated.

References

Abraham, E.P. (1974). "Biosynthesis and Enzymic Hydrolysis of Penicillins and Cephalosporins". University of Tokyo Press.
Abraham, E. and Duthie, E.S. (1946). *Lancet* I, 455–459.
Abraham, E.P. and Sabath, L.D. (1965). *Enzymology* 29, 221–232.
Acar, J.F., Sabath, L.D. and Ruch, P.A. (1975). *J. Clin. Invest.* 55, 446–453.

Barnett, M., Bushby, S.R.M. and Wilkinson, S. (1964). *Br. J. Pharmacol.* **23**, 552–574.

Brown, M.R.W. (1975). "Resistance of *Pseudomonas aeruginosa*". John Wiley and Sons, London.

Craig, W. *et al.* (1980). *Rev. Infect. Dis.* (In press).

Eagle, H. *et al.* (1950). *Ann. Intern. Med.* **33**, 544–571.

Finland, M., Garner, C., Wilcox, C. and Sabath, L.D. (1976). *J. Infect. Dis.* **134** (Suppl.), S75–S96.

Gardner, P., Griffin, W.B., Swartz, M.N. and Kunz, L.F. (1970). *Amer. J. Med.* **48**, 735–749.

Govan, J.R.W. and Fyfe, J.A.M. (1978). *J. Antimicrob. Chemother.* **4**, 233–240.

Green, G.R., Peters, G.A. and Geraci, J.E. (1967). *Ann. Intern. Med.* **67**, 235–249.

Hall, J.W., Johnson, W.F., Maher, F.T. and Hunt, J.C. (1970). *Ann. Intern. Med.* **73**, 515–521.

Hugh, R. and Gilardi, G.L. (1974). *In* "Manual of Clinical Microbiology", 2nd edn. (E.H. Lennette, E.H. Spaulding and J.P. Truant, eds), pp. 250–269. American Society for Microbiology, Washington, D.C.

Hugh, R. and Leifson, E. (1953). *J. Bacteriol.* **66**, 24–26.

Klastersky, J., Daneau, D., Swings, G. and Weerts, D. (1974). *J. Infect. Dis.* **129**, 187–193.

Kogut, M. and Lightbown, J.W. (1963). *Biochem. J.* **89**, 18P–19P.

Lam, J., Chan, R., Lam, K. and Costerton, J.W. (1980). *Infect. Immun.* **28**, 546–556.

Lorian, V., Atkinson, B.A. and Amaral, L. (1980). *In* "*Pseudomonas aeruginosa:* The Organism, Diseases it Causes and their Treatment". (L.D. Sabath, ed.), pp. 193–205. Hans Huber Publishers, Bern, Stuttgart and Wien.

Luria, S.E. (1946). *Proc. Soc. Exp. Biol. Med.* **61**, 46–51.

Medeiros, A., O'Brien, T.F., Wacker, W.E.C. and Yulug, N.F. (1971). *J. Infect. Dis.* **124** (Suppl.), S59–S64.

Musher, D.M., Minuth, J.N., Thorsteinsson, S.B. and Holmes, T. (1975). *J. Infect. Dis.* **131** (Suppl.), S40–S44.

Parker, C.W. (1963). *Am. J. Med.* **34**, 747–752.

Price, K.E., Leitner, F., Misiek, M., Chisholm, D.R. and Pursiano, T.A. (1971). *Antimicrob. Agents Chemother.* – 1970, 17–29.

Richmond, M.D., Clark, D.C. and Wotton, S. (1976). *Antimicrob. Agents Chemother.* **10**, 215–218.

Sabath, L.D. (1968). *Antimicrob. Agents Chemother.* – 1967, 210–217.

Sabath, L.D. (1973). *In* "Proc. 9th Ann. Inf. Dis. Conf. – Infectious Disease Reviews Vol. 2, pp. 17–44. Futura Publishing Co., Mount Kisco, New York.

Sabath, L.D. (1977a). *J. Antimicrob. Chemother.* **3** (Suppl. C), 47–51.

Sabath, L.D. (1977b). *In* "Significance of Medical Microbiology in the Care of Patients". (V. Lorian, ed.), pp. 198–202. Williams and Wilkins, Baltimore.

Sabath, L.D. (1978). *Infection* **6** (Suppl. 1)., S67–S71.

Sabath, L.D. (1979). *In* "Microbiology – 1979". (D. Schlessinger, ed.), pp. 299–303. American Society for Microbiology, Washington, D.C.

Sabath, L.D. (1980). "*Pseudomonas aeruginosa:* The Organism, Diseases it Causes and their Treatment". Hans Huber Publishers, Bern, Stuttgart and Wien.

Sabath, L.D., Garner, C., Wilcox, C. and Finland, M. (1975). *Antimicrob. Agents Chemother.* **8**, 344–349.

Sabath, L.D., Wheeler, N., Laverdiere, M., Blazevic, D. and Wilkinson, B.F. (1977). *Lancet* **I**, 443–447.

Sabath, L.D., Wilcox, C., Garner, C. and Finland, M. (1973). *J. Infect. Dis.* **128**, (Suppl.), S320–S326.

Smith, C.B., Lipsky, J.J., Laskin, O.L., Hellmann, D.B., Mellits, E.D., Longstreth, J.F. and Lietman, P.S. (1980). *New Engl. J. Med.* **302**, 1106–1109.

Smith, C.B., Wilfert, J.N., Dans, P.E., Kurrus, T.A. and Finland, M. (1970). *J. Infect. Dis.* **122** (Suppl.), S14–S25.

Spratt, B.D. (1980). *Phil. Trans. R. Soc. London Ser. B* **289**, 273–283.

Stamey, T.A., Fair, W.R., Timothy, M.M., Millar, M.A., Mihara, G. and Lowery, Y.C. (1974). *New Engl. J. Med.* **291**, 1159–1163.

Zak, O. (1980). *In "Pseudomonas aeruginosa:* The Organism, Diseases it Causes and their Treatment". (L.D. Sabath, ed.), pp. 133–159. Hans Huber Publishers, Bern, Stuttgart and Wien.

Discussion

Professor Williams: After Professor Humbert's paper, Professor Kunin offered some mild criticism in that Professor Humbert gave specific recommendation about enterobacteria, whereas every patient is different. I agree to a certain extent and Professor Sabath has pointed out all the difficult problems, but has not given any specific recommendations. I have three questions.

Firstly, the question of gentamicin versus tobramycin for *Pseudomonas aeruginosa.* We believe that tobramycin has more intrinsic activity against *Pseudomonas.* There is one group of enzymes which are prevalent in *Pseudomonas*, which are unable to inactivate tobramycin which is therefore perhaps to be preferred?

Secondly, the problem of the different antipseudomonal cephalosporins. There are now at least six of these which Professor Sabath showed on his list. We have also done some studies with these. I would like to know what Professor Sabath thinks about them.

Thirdly, the question of combined therapy, whether two antibiotics should be used rather than one. There is marked synergy between carbenicillin and the aminoglycosides, and it is possible to reduce quite markedly the toxic:therapeutic ratio. The m.i.c.'s of aminoglycosides in combination with carbenicillin against gentamicin-resistant rods fall to relatively low levels in many laboratory tests.

Professor Sabath: Concerning the first point, I agree with Professor Williams. Purely on the basis of greater activity of tobramycin over gentamicin *in vitro*, I would choose tobramycin every time even though the laboratory may report that the organism is sensitive to both drugs. In our hands, tobramycin is always the more active of the two drugs whether the laboratory report says that the organism is sensitive or resistant. That is why I would always choose tobramycin – because of the narrow toxic:therapeutic ratio.

Concerning the second point about the newer β–lactams, we have only *in vitro* results so far. From what I have read of their clinical use, I think that it is premature to reach any conclusions. May I point out, however, one important difference – related to the second question versus the first – that, because of the wide toxic:therapeutic ratio with most β–lactam antibiotics, some of these smaller differences with the β–lactam drugs may not be as important as the difference between tobramycin and gentamicin about which we have just spoken. Certainly *in vitro* cefsulodin is the most active, having the lowest m.i.c.'s of that list.

On the other hand, it would be premature to say that will hold in the future because some of the other β–lactam antibiotics, which have slightly higher or even considerably higher m.i.c. values, may finally prove very useful, and also because there is such a wide toxic:therapeutic ratio among other factors. I cannot answer firmly that question because of inadequate data in the medical and microbiological community in general about this problem.

Professor Williams' third question is exciting. I dealt only briefly with multiple drug therapy for pseudomonal infections. It is rather interesting that Balche, from Albany, New York, in surveying recently some results with *Pseudomonas* bacteraemia, had some data showing that survival was greatly improved when there had been multiple drug therapy in which synergy had been demonstrated, as compared to the use of only one drug. This was in serious pseudomonal infection resulting in bacteraemia. There has been some editorial comment in the same journal from Vincent Andriole from Yale, more or less commenting in a wider range. Those are some hard clinical data, which suggest that the use of multiple drugs, with synergy, is clinically useful in *Pseudomonas* bacteraemia – although the data are still on the small side.

A related aspect is the possible adverse effects – that is, antagonism. With the drugs now being used, antagonism is of two sorts. First, I know of a few anecdotal cases in which the use of an aminoglycoside plus a β–lactam resulted in poor activity in *Pseudomonas* endocarditis. Reverting to only one drug resulted in a better result. I can think of one very dramatic instance of this from California. Secondly, I referred to the work reported by Acar and myself of antagonism of carbenicillin by other β–lactam antibiotics. I know of no other comments reported in the press on this, but I have received information of increasing observations of that kind from a number of laboratories in the United States. It may be an important problem with some of the newer cephalosporins which seem much more able to antagonise some of the antipseudomonal β–lactams. To say that it is almost an uncharted sea would be nearly correct. I am grateful to Professor Acar for having the interest to explore that problem at a time about 10 years ago when he and I were possibly the only people to have observed it in our own laboratories.

Professor Acar: Is combined therapy really the best choice now in any case of *Pseudomonas* infection, with the possibility of synergy – using a drug like carbenicillin plus tobramycin, for instance, even if the strain is resistant to carbenicillin?

Professor Sabath: If the strain is shown to be resistant to carbenicillin, I would not add that drug. There is no point in adding a drug for which resistance has been demonstrated. In the acute situation, alluded to by Professor Kunin, when each patient is different, and all the facts are not known, it is my practice – and I would certainly recommend this – to use the best of the aminoglycosides for the suspected organism, with the best of the β–lactams. This is what I would do until the facts are known.

I recommend this practice because of the shortcomings of aminoglycosides which I enumerated in my presentation. Even though they look marvellous when tested separately in the laboratory, all the factors which mitigate against aminoglycosides operating are certainly present, also those that mitigate against the operation of the β–lactams. Since each has so many problems I would play all my favourable cards immediately – preferably before the death of the patient!

Professor Kunin: Once again, we have to return to the clinical example. I do not think that such a global approach is very helpful. I will give an example. There are a number of different situations that I can visualise when an individual might have a pseudomonal infection. Perhaps it might be in the urinary tract in the presence or absence of a catheter; in someone with chronic bronchitis who has been treated with multiple antibiotics and who has *Pseudomonas* in the sputum, perhaps accompanied with a little pneumonia; it might be a patient in the intensive care unit with a tracheostomy in place, when there are huge amounts of *Pseudomonas* grown; it might be the immunocompromised host with leukaemia, the patient with severe burns, or even the patient on peritoneal dialysis who has *Pseudomonas* colonising the peritoneal cavity.

I submit that each of the above situations is distinctly different, requiring different approaches to their management. Of course, it sometimes does warrant combined therapy, for example, in the leukaemic patient or the patient with severe burns. However, the clinical experience is superb with one drug, say, an aminoglycoside, in patients with urinary infections and it gives very high urinary concentrations of the drug. These patients do very well, and the host factor is the determinant, not the susceptibility of the organism. The same is true in the patient with tracheostomy in whom the best action to take very often is to have good tracheal care – in this case, the only reason for giving an antibiotic is to treat the physician not the patient.

I think that it is not appropriate to make the global statement that two drugs would be used against all *Pseudomonas* infections.

Professor Sabath: I am certainly grateful to Professor Kunin for making those comments. May I point out, however, to him and to everyone else that there is such an entity as recovery without any treatment being given. In the pre-antibiotic era people did not invariably die from all infections. The fact that it is possible to survive without any therapy applies to the colonisation situations as well as some of the less severe situations. When I suggested starting treatment with two antibiotics I was referring to the severely ill patients.

I did not mention it in the main part of my presentation – because it is slightly away from the main theme – but patients with urinary tract infections due to *Pseudomonas aeruginosa* may be treated also with drugs other than those three major groups – for example, erythromycin, with alkalisation of the urine, or with tetracycline, with acidification of urine. That can be done, even though those drugs are considered inactive by *in vitro* testing. It is related to their concentration in the urine and the fact that their activity can be optimised.

The individual approach to treatment is very important, and I thank Professor Kunin for helping to emphasise that today.

Dr. Waldvogel: Coming back to the 2 previous authors' presentation, I wish to emphasise a point which is of great importance to me: emergence of totally resistant organisms towards present antibiotics seems to be a minor therapeutic problem; most infections with an unfavourable outcome were treated with antibiotics to which the pathogen was sensitive, at least *in vitro.*

I would be interested to have Professor Sabath's comment on two aspects of this problem: first, shouldn't we invest more time and effort to analyse and delineate possible host factors which are operational in the outcome of an infection? Secondly, another possibility to be investigated would consist in exploring the composition of bacteriological media used to test antibiotics: sensitivities obtained with conventional media might show different results, if incubation were carried out in more physiological media, reproducing interstitial fluid, for example. Does Professor Sabath think that our present microbiological approach is adequate?

Professor Sabath: Each of Dr. Waldvogel's points is very important. The fact that there is such a high mortality with *Pseudomonas* pneumonia, for example — it is a very good example — indicates the discrepancy between the laboratory results and what happens in patients. *Pseudomonas* pneumonia may carry a mortality rate of 50 to 80 per cent, even though the laboratory tests show that the drugs which are being used to treat it are active, that the organism is sensitive to those drugs. I agree completely that there should be much more emphasis on the physiological conditions. I hope that Professor Sebald will comment in her presentation on the anaerobic conditions — although she has been asked specifically about the treatment of anaerobes — which certainly antagonise the activity of aminoglycosides even against facultative aerobes.

With regard to laboratory testing, this is another matter which needs to be raised. A number of people whose primary profession is the supervision of medical microbiological laboratories have frequently raised the matter of pH and concentration factors which could easily be implemented in the laboratory tests to evaluate drugs for the treatment of urinary tract infections. This is something that might also be done in the consideration of tissue infections.

A related point, looking to the future, would be the development of some test — although I do not know what it might be at the moment — that might shed some light on the degree of anaerobiosis at the focus of infection, thus enabling the person selecting which drugs to choose to know whether an aminoglycoside might be able to operate, under the conditions of the focus of infection, even though it cannot be tested directly. That is a rather futuristic suggestion, but relates to Dr. Waldvogel's second question.

Anaerobes and Antibiotics

M. SEBALD, M. MAGOT and G. PRIVITERA

Laboratoire des Anaérobies, Institut Pasteur,
Paris, France

Introduction

Anaerobic bacteria are characterised by their anaerobic mode of metabolism and by their hypersensitivity to oxygen, which varies from group to group, but is such that they can never grow in the presence of oxygen at atmospheric pressure. Being deficient in oxygenase(s), they are unable to incorporate molecular oxygen directly for their biosynthetic reactions, and lacking a complete cytochrome chain, they do not use molecular oxygen as a terminal electron acceptor. The oxidoreduction reactions which they carry out involve the activity of electron transport proteins functioning only at low redox potentials. Their sensitivity to oxygen appears to be connected with a fairly general absence of catalases, peroxidases and superoxide dismutases.

Anaerobic bacteria are present throughout the environment in the exogenous flora of the ground and atmosphere, and in the endogenous flora of the various body cavities of man and animals. Certain toxigenic clostridia are especially dangerous owing to the serious intoxication and toxigenic infections that they can cause. The non-sporulating organisms, which in certain areas considerably outnumber the aerobes, are also capable of leading to serious infections. The majority of these organisms belong to about ten genera listed in Table 1, which also shows the frequency with which they are isolated.

Because of the particular technology essential to the study of these bacteria, their role in various infections has been, and is, often neglected.

TABLE 1

Isolation Frequency of Principal Pathogenic Anaerobes

	Bacilli	%		Cocci	%
Gram-negative non-sporulating	*Bacteroides fragilis*	22	Gram-negative	*Veillonella*	0.5
	Other species of *Bacteroides*	4	Gram-positive	*Diplococcus*	3
	Fusobacterium	7		*Streptococcus*	3.5
				Staphylococcus	2
Gram-positive sporulating	*Clostridium perfringens*	28			
	Other species of *Clostridium*	15			
Gram-positive non-sporulating	*Eubacterium*	1			
	Bifidobacterium	1			
	Corynebacterium	12			
	Actinomyces	1			

Activity of Antibiotics against Anaerobic Bacteria

A study of the activity of antibiotics against anaerobic bacteria over several years has led to a number of conclusions which may be summarized as follows:

(1) Anaerobic bacteria have until very recently remained sensitive to the majority of antibiotics. In addition, given the length of time required to isolate them, it used to be thought unnecessary in routine practice to confirm *in vitro* the sensitivity to antibiotics of the isolated organisms. However during the last 5–10 years the situation has changed, for resistance has appeared in the majority of groups which were formerly sensitive. First there was resistance to tetracyclines, then to macrolides and lincosamides, then to β–lactams and just occasionally to chloramphenicol.

(2) Phenomena of resistance first appeared in *Clostridium perfringens* and *Bacteroides fragilis*, perhaps due to their higher frequencies of distribution. At present, the distribution of resistance within these two species ranks at its highest level. In these two cases at least, and they are the only ones well studied in this respect, resistance determinants are extrachromosomal and often transferable. *Clostridium difficile* is another species showing multiple resistance to antibiotics (George *et al.*, 1978). The determinants have not yet been studied extensively, but the resistance is undoubtedly connected with the occurrence of pseudomembranous colitis during and after antibiotic therapy.

(3) Independently of this general and recent evolution some special situations have remained almost unchanged since the earlier

observations. They are: (a) the consistent resistance of anaerobic bacteria towards aminoglycosides; (b) their sensitivity to metronidazole; (c) the resistance of the *fragilis* group of *Bacteroides* to β—lactam antibiotics.

These general or more specific conclusions deserve further comment.

Resistance to Aminoglycosides

Anaerobes are always resistant *in vitro* to aminoglycosides at least at concentrations attainable therapeutically. They are especially resistant to (in order of increasing resistance): gentamicin, framycetin, neomycin, paromomycin and kanamycin (Finegold and Sutter, 1971).

Slight variations can occur but are without practical significance (gentamicin is a little more active than kanamycin against *B. fragilis* and *B. melaninogenicus*, while the reverse is true for *Fusobacterium fusiformis*).

It has been shown in aerobes that the penetration of aminoglycosides involves oxygen through an oxidative phosphorylation process — hence the hypothesis that the universal resistance of anaerobes to aminoglycosides is due to their lack of a mechanism for oxidative phosphorylation. This was recently confirmed (Bryan *et al.*, 1979) by the demonstration that in *B. fragilis* and *C. perfringens* aminoglycosides do not accumulate in the cell, although ribosomes from these organisms bind the aminoglycosides as effectively as those from *E. coli*, and the aminoglycosides are not inactivated by cell-free extracts of the anaerobes tested. It may therefore be concluded that the aminoglycosides are inactive against the anaerobes through lack of penetration. The presence of aminoglycoside-inactivating enzymes has to our knowledge never been shown in anaerobes.

No study of the activity of these antibiotics *in vivo* has been carried out, but it is generally accepted that: (1) they are ineffective; (2) the administration of aminoglycosides ranks high in the list of factors that can lead to an eventual anaerobic infection.

Sensitivity to Nitroimidazoles

This subject has recently been extensively reviewed (May and Baker, 1979; Finegold, 1977) and we shall only note the basic information.

As strong oxidants, nitroimidazoles accept electrons preferentially and irreversibly, so well that they behave as an electron sink. They interfere with the action of electron transport proteins which operate at comparable redox potentials, such as the ferredoxins (E_0' of metronidazole = -0.470 V, E_0' of ferredoxin = -0.460 V). Reduced metronidazole derivatives can combine with DNA and inhibit the biosynthesis of nucleic acids. The nature of the intermediate derivatives is not clearly established, but they are probably free-radical derivatives ($R-NO_2$:) which are toxic either directly, or by leading to the production of superoxide (O_2 :) or other free radicals (Willson and Searle, 1975).

All strictly anaerobic bacteria are sensitive to metronidazole and its analogues (m.i.c. $\leqslant$ 1 μg/ml) and the activity is bactericidal. Some groups are always resistant (*Corynebacterium*) or usually resistant (*Actinobacterium*, cocci) and that is certainly connected with various little known metabolic characteristics of these groups for which the description "strict anaerobe" is debatable.

At present there is only one strain of *B. fragilis* unambiguously resistant to metronidazole (m.i.c. = 32 μg/ml). It was isolated by Ingham *et al.*, (1978) from a patient receiving long-term treatment with metronidazole for Crohn's disease (more than 2 kg in 3½ years). It has been shown (Tally, 1980) that this strain has an impaired ability to reduce the molecule (from a measure of its nitroreductase activity), and that the intracellular penetration of metronidazole is also decreased in this strain. It is also resistant to tetracycline and all β—lactams, including moxalactam (Sebald, unpub. data). This resistance is non-transferable and is not mediated by extra-chromosomal DNA (Tally, 1980; Sebald, unpub. data). It could therefore be a permeability mutant.

Resistance of Bacteroides fragilis to β—lactams

Bacteroides fragilis and related species (*B. distasonis, B. thetaiotaomicron, B. ovatus, B. vulgatus*) have long been noted for their resistance to penicillin, while, for example, another Gram-negative group, *Fusobacterium*, is sensitive to this antibiotic. This character is sufficiently consistent to have been used by us for diagnostic purposes since 1962. *Bacteroides* are also often resistant to ampicillin and carbenicillin. *Bacteroides fragilis* strains are also resistant to the first generation cephalosporins: cephaloridine, cephalothin, etc., but they are more sensitive to the new cephalosporins: cefuroxime > cefamandole > cefoxitin, in order of decreasing sensitivity.

β—lactamase activity was demonstrated in *B. fragilis* by Pinkus *et al.* (1966). In some of the initial studies a disparity appeared between the observed resistance to β—lactams and β—lactamase activity. Then it was shown that this discrepancy was only apparent as the enzyme is not located on the surface but is usually intracellular and bound to membranes; it is only released by ultrasonication, osmotic shock and lysis by phages or enzymes. There is a direct relationship between the m.i.c. value and the level of β-lactamase activity. The enzyme is constitutive and shows a greater activity towards the cephalosporins than to penicillins, i.e. it is more a cephalosporinase. Its substrate profile is: cephaloridine > cefazolin > cefamandole > cefoxitin, in order of decreasing affinity. The enzyme is inactivated by cloxacillin, pCMB (p—chloromercuribenzoate), cefoxitin and carbenicillin (Weinrich and Del Bene, 1976; Britz and Wilkinson, 1978a).

The β-lactamases have a molecular weight of 29–31,000 (estimated by gel filtration) to 40–43,000 daltons (estimated by gel electrophoresis) (Nord, 1980). They have an isoelectric point at an acid pH, mainly around 4.9 and 5.3–5.6, which clearly distinguishes them from the corresponding enzymes from enterobacteria (*E. coli*, *Klebsiella*), *Pseudomonas* and *Haemophilus*. They also differ through the absence of common antigens. They are sensitive to inhibitors of β-lactamases, e.g. clavulanic acid and CP 45899 at 1 μg/ml, which lower the m.i.c. of cephaloridine against resistant strains (Olsson *et al.*, 1979).

Several studies (Stiffler *et al.*, 1974; Tinell and Macrina, 1976; Sebald, unpub. data) have not been able to demonstrate extra-chromosomal determinism of this resistance or its transmissibility. It would nevertheless appear that the resistance genes are usually located extrachromosomally (Frank Young, cited by Sykes, 1979).

That the β-lactamase of *B. fragilis* is also active *in vivo* can be shown in the rabbit by intraperitoneal injection with capsules containing *B. fragilis* and parenteral administration of [14]C—penicillin. The radioactivity is then estimated in the capsule. It is 15% of the serum level in infected animals and 25% of the serum level in control animals (O'Keefe *et al.*, 1978).

The presence of β-lactamase is not always responsible for the resistance of this group of organisms to β-lactams. There are also strains resistant to all β-lactams including cefoxitin. However, the β-lactamase isolated from these strains is inactive against cefoxitin (Nord, 1980), which leads one to suspect the existence of a diffusion barrier impeding access of the antibiotic to its target site.

One single publication (Burt and Woods, 1976) suggests that transfer of ampicillin resistance from *E. coli* to *Bacteroides* or *Fusobacterium* can take place provided the recipient strain is heated in order to inactivate the restriction enzymes, but the exconjugants are usually unstable and do not further transfer their resistance to *Bacteroides* or back to *E. coli.* In general, the anaerobic strains used have not been characterised, but some of them are *B. fragilis.*

Resistance to several antibiotics (ampicillin, amoxicillin, chloramphenicol, tetracycline and minocycline) has been transferred from *Bacteroides fragilis* to *E. coli.* Multiple resistance transfer took place but the transcipients later segregated. Some extrachromosomal material, not in the form of covalently closed circles, was identified in this multiresistant strain (Mancini and Behme, 1977). In conclusion, resistance of *B. fragilis* to β–lactams is due to the presence of β–lactamases with properties different from those in aerobic bacteria. Resistance is not transferable in *B. fragilis* and could be plasmid-mediated.

β–*lactam Resistance in Anaerobes other than B. fragilis*

Whilst resistance to β–lactams was found some years ago in clostridia and *B. fragilis*, its appearance has recently been observed in all other groups, particularly among *Fusobacterium* and *Bacteroides* other than *B. fragilis* (*B. melaninogenicus, B. oralis*, etc.) and we are currently witnessing its emergence.

In *Clostridium ramosum*, there is an intermediate level of resistance due to an inducible β–lactamase (Weinrich and Del Bene, 1976) which hydrolyses penicillin G, ampicillin and carbenicillin but not cefoxitin. Penicillin G has the effect of inducing resistance to: ampicillin (x 200), cefamandole (x 40), penicillin G (x 25) and cephaloridine (x 10), the induction factor given in parentheses being the ratio of the rates of hydrolysis after and before induction. The substrate profile for the enzyme is: ampicillin > penicillin G = cephalosporin C > carbenicillin > cephaloridine > cefazolin > cefamandole > cefoxitin. The enzyme is inhibited by pCMB and cefoxitin.

Certain strains of *Clostridium clostridiiforme* are highly resistant to β–lactams (Weinrich and Del Bene, 1976) and also possess an inducible β–lactamase with the following substrate profile: ampicillin = penicillin G > carbenicillin, and cephaloridine > cefazolin > cefamandole > cefoxitin, which is identical to that for the *B. fragilis* and *C. ramosum* enzymes. However, unlike the latter two enzymes, that from *C. clostridiiforme* is not inhibited by pCMB, cloxacillin or cefoxitin.

The β–lactam resistance of *Capnocytophaga ochracea*, which is due to a penicillinase, does not appear to be borne by the 70 Md plasmid (Cm Tc Kana Sm) or the 25 Md plasmid (cryptic) harboured by this organism and transferable to *E. coli* (Guiney and Davis, 1978).

Tetracycline Resistance

Resistance to tetracyclines currently occurs at a fairly high frequency among various anaerobes, in particular *Clostridium perfringens* and *Bacteroides fragilis* (Martin *et al.*, 1972).

In *C. perfringens*, resistance to tetracycline has been observed in England since 1968 (Johnstone and Cockcraft, 1968). It is either solitary (Sebald, unpub. data; Rood *et al.*, 1978) or associated with chloramphenicol (Cm) resistance. It has been shown that this resistance is plasmid-mediated and that it is transferable, probably through conjugation (Brefort *et al.*, 1977 and 1978; Sebald and Brefort, 1975; Sebald *et al.*, 1975).

In the case of the strain studied in our laboratory, the plasmid Tc Cm (pIP 401) contains 54 Kb. Whilst resistances to both antibiotics are eliminated in a single treatment of the organism with curing agents and are jointly transferable, frequent segregation of these characters is observed with loss of resistance to Cm, either during or after transfer. This involves a deletion of 6 Kb. Resistance to Tc is transferable *in vivo* (Brefort *et al.*, 1977). The expression of tetracycline resistance conferred by plasmid pIP 401 is inducible. Plasmid pIP 401 from *C. perfringens* is transferable to *C. difficile*, where it is also expressed by induction. It is noteworthy that this same *C. difficile* is also capable of intraspecies transfer of constitutive resistance to tetracyclines, which may be plasmid-mediated (Ionesco, 1980). In another strain of *C. perfringens*, tetracycline resistance is transferable and plasmid-mediated (a plasmid of 45 Kb) (Rood *et al.*, 1978).

In *Bacteroides* of the *fragilis* group, resistance to tetracyclines was encountered in 30% of the strains isolated in U.S.A. in 1972. Its emergence in France is more recent but it now affects more than 50% of the strains (Sebald *et al.*, 1980). The m.i.c. values for these strains range from 4 to 64 μg/ml. Expression of this resistance is usually inducible by tetracycline and minocycline, but it is constitutive in some strains isolated from man or in mutants isolated by culture in the presence of Tc at a sub-inhibitory concentration (Privitera *et al.*, 1979b; Sebald *et al.*, 1980).

A study of the uptake of radioactive tetracycline by a sensitive strain of *B. fragilis*, by an inducibly resistant transcipient either induced or noninduced, and by a constitutively resistant transcipient has shown (Fayolle *et al.*, 1980) that accumulation of tetracycline occurs in 2 phases: a rapid passive phase lasting 5 minutes which is independent of the expression of the genes for Tc resistance and a slow active phase inhibited by rotenone (energy uncoupler). This latter phase lasts at least 15 minutes and is subject to negative control by the tetracycline resistance genes. This biphasic accumulation is analogous to that observed in *E. coli*, but unlike the latter (Levy and McMurry, 1978) only the second phase involves active uptake and is negatively controlled by the tetracycline resistance genes. It is likely that, as in *E. coli*, the antibiotic induces in *B. fragilis* a membrane protein necessary for the expression of resistance.

Tetracycline resistance in *Bacteroides* of the *fragilis* group is usually transferable to a sensitive strain of *B. fragilis* lacking a plasmid (Privitera *et al.*, 1979a). Transfer is either inducible by tetracycline (tra_i) or is constitutive (tra_c) according to whether the organism is inducible or constitutive for the expression of tetracycline resistance. This fact, shown initially with two inducible strains and their constitutive mutants (Privitera *et al.*, 1979b), has been confirmed recently in a large number of strains (Sebald *et al.*, 1980). These results suggest that the expression of resistance and its transfer are subject to the same mechanism of regulatory control, and the genes responsible for both functions may be situated on the same operon which is subject to negative control. This is confirmed by the inability in one of the strains studied in detail to isolate mutants with these functions dissociated. The expression of tetracycline resistance and its transfer are also induced *in vivo* (Privitera *et al.*, 1980). This can be shown in monoxenic mice, populated with a Tc_i^r strain, to which tetracycline is administered at a low concentration in the drinking water. The organism found in the faeces is induced for the Tc^r character and for the transfer of this property.

In *Capnocytophaga ochracea*, a 70 Md plasmid, coding for resistance to tetracycline, chloramphenicol, kanamycin and streptomycin has been demonstrated (George *et al.*, 1978). This plasmid is transferable to *E. coli*, probably by conjugation.

Chloramphenicol Resistance

A small number of *B. fragilis* strains are resistant to chloramphenicol (Cm). In one strain (Britz and Wilkinson, 1978b), this resistance is due to a chloramphenicol acetyl transferase (CAT), the activity of which should be distinguished from that of a non-specific thioesterase. The enzyme has an optimum pH of 7.8 and a molecular weight of $89,000 \pm 3,000$ daltons. It is inhibited by pCMB and DTNB [5,5'−dithiobis(2−nitrobenzoic acid)]. Its Km and heat sensitivity are comparable to those of the staphylococcal enzymes, whilst in its sensitivity to DTNB, it resembles the type II enzyme from *E. coli*. The *B. fragilis* enzyme therefore belongs to a new class of CAT. The localisation of the genetic determinant of this CAT has not been established. It is not possible to isolate organisms resistant to this antibiotic by mutagenesis of Cm sensitive strains. This might just be an evidence for the extrachromosomal localisation of the gene if the chloramphenicol molecule has two active sites in anaerobes, as suggested by Tally's results (Tally, 1980).

We noted above the plasmid involvement in the chloramphenicol resistance of a strain of *C. perfringens*, its transmissibility and the fact that the plasmid also codes for resistance to Tc (Brefort *et al.*, 1977 and 1978). This resistance is connected with the production of a CAT (Bouanchaud, unpub. data). In another strain of *C. perfringens*, also resistant to Tc and Cm and with plasmid-mediated and transferable Tc resistance, resistance to Cm is neither plasmid-mediated nor transferable (Rood *et al.*, 1978).

Macrolide and Lincosamide Resistance

Clindamycin inhibits protein synthesis by interfering with the binding of aminoacyl–tRNA to the A–site on the ribosome. It also affects peptide chain initiation at the P–site on the 70 S ribosome (Upjohn Co., pers. comm.).

Anaerobes were originally very sensitive to these antibiotics but resistance has appeared rapidly in various organisms, in particular *Clostridium* (Wilkins and Thiel, 1973) and *B. fragilis* (Salaki *et al.*, 1976). This resistance occasionally concerns only one of these groups of antibiotics, for example, either erythromycin or clindamycin. In the case of single resistance to erythromycin, this could be spurious resistance for it is known that pH is important for the activity of this antibiotic and it is possible that CO_2 inhibits its activity. Usually the resistance is multiple. The extrachromosomal mediation of the resistance and its transferability have been shown in *C. perfringens* (Brefort *et al.*, 1977 and 1978) and in *B. fragilis* and related species (Fayolle *et al.*, 1980; Privitera *et al.*, 1979a and b; Sebald *et al.*, 1980; Tally *et al.*, 1979; Welch *et al.*, 1979).

In *C. perfringens*, the same 61 Kb plasmid (pIP 402) carries the genetic determinants of resistance to erythromycin (Em) and clindamycin (Cl). These two resistance characters can be eliminated together. However they possess different structural genes, since a temperature-sensitive mutant for clindamycin resistance can express its erythromycin resistance at the non-permissive temperature (Sebald, unpub. data). This plasmid was not transferable *in vitro* from the wild-type strains originally studied (Brefort *et al.*, 1977; Rood *et al.*, 1978). However, it was transferable to a sensitive strain in experiments carried out in dixenic mice (Brefort *et al.*, 1977 and 1978) and the transcipients obtained which were resistant to tetra-cyclines, erythromycin, and clindamycin had the chromosomal characters of recombinants. A transcipient studied in detail had the ability to transfer further its Tc and Em Cl plasmids and to mobilise the chromosome (chromosome mobilising ability property or Cma$^+$). It harboured two plasmids, plasmid pIP 402 (Em Cl) and a 48 Kb plasmid, pIP 408, coding for tetracycline resistance and shown by the methods used to be similar to plasmid pIP 406, i.e. to the original pIP 401 with the Cm region deleted. The Cma$^+$ property is localised on plasmid pIP 408 and it can only be expressed when the transfer function of the plasmid itself is intact (Sebald, unpub. data). Two inverted repeated sequences of 1.4 Kb are present in this plasmid, but they have not been located with reference to the resistance genes.

In *Bacteroides fragilis* and related species, there is also evidence for plasmid-mediated resistance to Em Cl, and this resistance is occasionally transferable, but not always. In a strain studied independently in two laboratories (Privitera *et al.*, 1979a; Welch *et al.*, 1979), the Em Cl plasmid comprises 46 Kb. Often a region of 17.3 Kb is spontaneously deleted from it and it then loses its resistance character. By studying homoduplex formation it is possible to locate two pairs of inverted repeated sequences on this plasmid: one of 0.75 Kb marking a 17.3 Kb loop, and the other, of 0.20 Kb, marking a loop of 4.1 Kb. The two loops formed by these inverted repeated sequences by the homoduplex method are 4.5 Kb apart (Magot, unpub. data). The other plasmid studied contains 16 Kb (Tally *et al.*, 1979). In certain strains, transfer of the Em Cl plasmid is independent of that for Tc resistance. But usually (Sebald *et al.*, 1980) the Em Cl plasmid behaves as if it is incapable of autonomous transfer and is co-transferred by a Tc plasmid. Indeed, from the majority of strains resistant to Tc, Em and Cl, Em Cl transcipients are never isolated and only Tc Em Cl or Tc transcipients are recovered. The ratio of Tc Em Cl transcipients to Tc transcipients is remarkably constant for a given strain whatever the number of transcipients obtained whether the organism inducible for transfer of Tc is induced or not. In each case, resistance transfer involves contact between the donor and recipient cells, probably through a mechanism of conjugation.

Future Objectives

An examination of the present situation shows that from now the emergence of antibiotic resistance among anaerobes must receive consideration, particularly if this resistance is transferable. It will be essential in the future to monitor the antibiotic resistance of strains isolated in pathology laboratories, and to test systematically each new antibiotic against the anaerobes. It will also be necessary to follow meticulously the frequency of the appearance of pseudo-membranous colitis due to *C. difficile* during and after antibiotic therapy, and, if it increases, to include this species in any screening test for new antibiotics.

In the longer term, two objectives should be achieved. First, a greater knowledge of the "barrier effects" exerted mainly by the strictly anaerobic bacteria within the intestinal flora on pathogenic species will enable protection of this flora during antibiotic therapy, or its repopulation after antibiotic administration. Second, a better understanding of the mechanisms of oxygen toxicity will lead to a better understanding of the mode of action of antibiotics specific to anaerobes, such as the nitroimidazoles. It would also help to determine whether this antibiotic property could be related to other properties of these agents, such as radiosensitisation.

References

Brefort, G., Magot, M., Ionesco, H. and Sebald, M. (1977). *Plasmid* 1, 52–66.

Beefort, G., Magot, M., Ionesco, H. and Sebald, M. (1978). *In* "Microbiology – 1978". (D. Schlessinger, ed.) pp. 242–245. American Society for Microbiology, Washington, D.C.

Britz, M.L. and Wilkinson, R.G. (1978a). *Antimicrob. Agents Chemother.* 13, 373–382.

Britz, M.L. and Wilkinson, R.G. (1978b). *Antimicrob. Agents Chemother.* 14, 105–111.

Bryan, L.E., Kowand, S.K. and Ven Den Elzen, H.M. (1979). *Antimicrob. Agents Chemother.* 15, 7–13.

Burt, S.J. and Woods, D.R. (1976). *J. Gen. Microbiol.* 93, 405–409.

Fayolle, F., Privitera, G. and Sebald, M. (1980). *Antimicrob. Agents Chemother.* 18, 502–505.

Finegold, S.M. (1977). "Proceedings of the International Metronidazole Conference. Montreal 1976". Excerpta Medica, Amsterdam.

Finegold, S.M. and Sutter, V.L. (1971). *J. Infect. Dis.* 124 (suppl.), S56–S58.

George, W.L., Sutter, V.L. and Finegold, S.M. (1978). *Curr. Microbiol.* 1, 55–58.

Guiney, D.G. and Davis, C.E. (1978). *Nature* (London) 274, 181–182.

Ingham, H.R., Eaton, S., Venables, C.W. and Adams, P.C. (1978). *Lancet* I, 214.

Ionesco, H. (1980). *Ann. Microbiol.* (Inst. Pasteur) 131A, 171–179.

Johnstone, F.R. and Cockcraft, W.H. (1968). *Lancet* I, 660–661.

Levy, S.B. and McMurry, L. (1978). *Nature* (London) 276, 90–92.

Mancini, C. and Behme, R.J. (1977). *J. Infect. Dis.* 136, 597–600.

Martin, W.J., Gardner, M. and Washington, J.A. II. (1972). *Antimicrob. Agents Chemother.* 1, 148–158.

May and Baker, Ltd. (1979). "Flagyl (metronidazole) in Anaerobic Infections". The Priory Press. England.

Nord, C.E. (1980). *In* "Les Bactéries Anaérobies". Symposium International. Masson, Paris. (To be published).

O'Keefe, J.P., Tally, F.P., Barza, M. and Gorbach, S.L. (1978). *J. Infect. Dis.* 137, 437–442.

Olsson, B., Dornbusch, K. and Nord, C.E. (1979). *Antimicrob. Agents Chemother.* **15**, 263–268.

Pinkus, G., Veto, G. and Braude, A.I. (1966). *J. Bacteriol.* **96**, 1437–1438.

Privitera, G., Dublanchet, A. and Sebald, M. (1979a). *J. Infect. Dis.* **139**, 97–101.

Privitera, G., Fayolle, F. and Sebald, M. (1980). *Antimicrob. Agents Chemother.* (Submitted for publication).

Privitera, G., Sebald, M. and Fayolle, F. (1979b). *Nature* (London) **278**, 657–659.

Rood, J.I., Scott, V.N. and Duncan, C.L. (1978). *Plasmid* **1**, 563–570.

Salaki, J.S., Black, R., Tally, F.P. and Kislak, J.W. (1976). *Am. J. Med.* **60**, 426–428.

Sebald, M. and Brefort, G. (1975). *C.R. Hebd. Séances Acad. Sci., Sér. D* **281**, 317–319.

Sebald, M., Bouanchaud, D. and Bieth, G. (1975) *C.R. Hebd. Séances Acad. Sci., Sér. D* **280**, 2401–2404.

Sebald, M., Privitera, G. and Fayolle, F. (1980). *Antimicrob. Agents Chemother.* (Submitted for publication).

Stiffler, P.W., Keller, R. and Traub, N. (1974). *J. Infect. Dis.* **130**, 544–548.

Sykes, R.B. (1979). *In* "Genetics of Industrial Microorganisms". (O.K. Sebek and A.I. Laskin, eds), pp. 170–176. ASM, Washington.

Tally, F.P. (1980). *In* "Les Bactéries Anaérobies". Symposium International. Masson, Paris. (To be published).

Tally, F.P., Snydman, D.R., Gorbach, S.L. and Malamy, M.H. (1979). *J. Infect. Dis.* **139**, 83–89.

Tinell, W.H. and Macrina, F.L. (1976). *Infect. Immun.* **14**, 955–964.

Weinrich, A.E. and Del Bene, V.E. (1976). *Antimicrob. Agents Chemother.* **10**, 106–111.

Welch, R.A., Jones, K.R. and Macrina, F.L. (1979). *Plasmid* **2**, 261–268.

Wilkins, T.D. and Thiel, T. (1973). *Antimicrob. Agents Chemother.* **3**, 136–137.

Willson, R.L. and Searle, A.J.F. (1975). *Nature* (London) **255**, 498–500.

Discussion

Professor Acar: What do we know about the digestive flora of patients who received metronidazole for years, for instance people who have digestive diseases?

Professor Sebald: I do not think that there have been any comprehensive studies on the flora and what we see in the literature seems to be very diverging. We hear that corynebacteria, for instance, are selected, which would have been natural, but sometimes we also hear that they are destroyed, which is rather difficult to understand since they are metronidazole-resistant. Obviously, metronidazole-resistant strains are selected. At least one example is very well known.

The Ecology of Transferable Antibiotic Resistance

M.H. RICHMOND and V. PETROCHEILOU

*Department of Bacteriology, University of Bristol,
Bristol, England*

Introduction

It is an almost universal experience that the introduction of a novel antibiotic into clinical use is followed by the emergence of resistant populations of bacteria which render the agent markedly less effective for therapeutic purposes. Probably the first example of this was the emergence of sulphonamide resistant isolates of the pneumococcus following the introduction of the first sulphonamides in the years immediately before and during the last world war (Garrod and O'Grady, 1971). Similar examples are all too familiar with novel aminoglycosides and β–lactams (Benveniste and Davies, 1973; Richmond and Sykes, 1973). Provided that a gene capable of specifying the appropriate type of inactivating enzyme is present somewhere in the microbial population, the use of the agent will select resistant populations.

The presence of an appropriate resistance gene is probably the essence of the matter. In certain cases – the absence of resistance of Group A streptococci to β–lactams is a case in point – such genes do not seem to be present, and it seems hard for this evolutionary step to occur. This implies that the evolution of a mechanism of resistance to some antibiotic *de novo* is a statistically unlikely event. Consistent with this view is the fact that most of the resistance traits we know were there even before the time when the antibiotics in question were first used for human therapy (Ambler, 1980).

If it is agreed that the evolution of novel resistance mechanisms is a rare event, it follows that the appearance of resistance traits in an ever wider range of bacterial species and genera must be the consequence of gene transfer. Thus an understanding of the transmissibility of antibiotic resistance genes becomes crucial if one is to understand the evolution of antibiotic resistant populations; correspondingly, the evolution of the resistance proteins themselves is qualitatively of less importance (Bennett and Richmond, 1978).

Mechanisms of Gene Transfer

Until recently it was assumed that antibiotic resistance genes could only move between different bacterial cells by one of three distinct transfer mechanisms: *transduction* (where the gene is transmitted from one bacterial cell to another as part of a bacterial virus genome), *transformation* (where the gene is transmitted as a fragment of unprotected DNA) and *conjugation* (where the gene is transmitted as part of a highly evolved transmissible extrachromosomal element, or plasmid). Now we know that one has to add a fourth mechanism of transfer: *fusion* — the situation where two cells, perhaps of different species, merge to make a single structure which is viable and which can give rise to daughter forms which contain DNA derived from both participants in the fusion (Hopwood, 1977).

Of these four mechanisms of gene transfer, transduction and conjugation have been shown to occur under natural conditions. Transfer by transformation is more problematic since naked DNA is very susceptible to destruction by nucleases; and so far no one has clearly shown gene exchange by fusion except under some highly artificial laboratory conditions.

Unquestionably, the ability of resistance genes to be transferred between bacterial cells, and consequently the potential of such genes to spearhead the emergence of resistant populations, is greatly influenced by the genetic location of the genes in the bacteria. If they are carried as part of a bacterial plasmid, transfer is much more likely than is the case when they are chromosomal (Bennett and Richmond, 1978). This is probably for two reasons: first, the presence of a gene on a plasmid means that, in most cases, the replication of the gene does not require integration into the bacterial chromosome. Thus a resistance gene newly transferred from some other bacterial cell does not have to recombine in the new host cell to survive. The second reason why plasmid linked genes are transferred more effectively is because of their size. Plasmid genomes are often about the same size as those of bacteriophages, and as a result plasmids seem to be able to replace phage genomes in the course of phage maturation relatively efficiently. The result is a transducing phage —

a virus in which the normal DNA content has been replaced by one of bacterial plasmid origin.

Gene Transposition

The evolutionary potential of many resistance genes is greatly enhanced by the fact that they are often carried in bacterial plasmids as part of a so-called "transposon" (Bennett and Richmond, 1978). Some examples are given in Table 1. A transposon is a structured unit

TABLE 1

Patterns of Antibiotic Resistance Known to be Transposable to Date

Pattern	Organism	Transposon
penicillin + cephalosporin (TEM β–lactamase)	Many Gram-negatives	TnA types
tetracycline (two distinct types)	Many Gram-negatives	Tn10, Tn1721
kanamycin	*Escherichia coli, Pseudomonas aeruginosa*	Tn5
mercuric ions	*Escherichia coli, Pseudomonas aeruginosa*	Tn501
trimethoprim + streptomycin + spectinomycin	*Escherichia coli*	Tn7
gentamicin	*Escherichia coli, Pseudomonas aeruginosa*	–
trimethoprim	*Escherichia coli*	Tn10
chloramphenicol	*Escherichia coli*	Tn9
penicillin + cephalosporin + streptomycin + sulphonamide	*Escherichia coli*	Tn4
neomycin + kanamycin	*Escherichia coli*	Tn6
erythromycin	*Staphylococcus aureus*	–

of DNA which has the ability of being able to move "en bloc" from one self-replicating piece of DNA in a bacterial cell to another. Figure 1 shows a typical example of such a transposon – in this case one capable of specifying resistance to β–lactam antibiotics, a so-called TnA unit, because of the presence of a β–lactamase (*bla*) gene. The total length of the transposon corresponds to about 4500 base pairs, of which the *bla* gene contributes about 1000. The element is bounded by so-called "inverted repeats" – sequences of 38 base pairs which are rotationally symmetrical, that is, the sequence at one end of the transposon is identical with the sequence at the other when it is read in the opposite direction (Richmond *et al.*, 1980).

At the moment it is still not precisely certain how a transposon

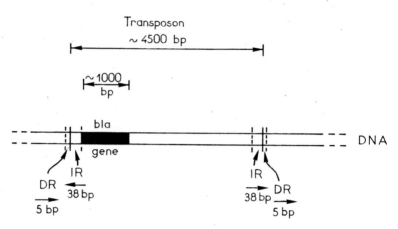

FIG. 1   Organisation of a typical ampicillin resistance transposon. Abbreviations: IR, inverted repeat; DR, direct repeat; b.p. nucleotide pair; *bla* gene, β–lactamase gene. Reprinted from Richmond *et al.* (1980) with permission.

moves from one bacterial replicating unit (replicon) to another. What is certain is that the whole structure including the inverted repeats moves, and that the *bla* gene (in cases where this is the resistance gene carried by the transposon) moves too. The result is an enhanced flexibility of the genetic organisation underlying resistance to β–lactams. For example, if the β–lactamase gene is part of a transposon located in the bacterial chromosome, transposition can allow this gene group to leave that site and become part of a plasmid; and from there cell-to-cell transfer can effect its transmission to another bacterial species. Transposons therefore tend to facilitate the emergence of resistant populations, and together with the mechanism of inter-cell gene transfer can be said to be one of the key mechanisms which give rise to antibiotic resistant populations.

Up to this point we have stressed two types of transfer which facilitate the emergence of such resistant bacterial populations; the transposition of genes from one replicon to another and the transfer of the replicons from one bacterial cell to another. In the context of infectious disease we have, of course, a third element; the infection of one multicellular organism by another by a process of cross-infection. Thus the spread of antibiotic resistance can be studied at three key levels of organisation: the transposon, the extrachromosomal element and the infectious bacterium. It is the interplay of these three organisational units which we will now examine to see how each plays its part in the evolution of resistant bacterial populations under natural conditions.

Gene Transfer 'in vivo'

The various methods of gene transfer discussed here have been studied most intensively in the laboratory, and the question arises as to whether these processes also occur *in vivo*, and whether the frequency with which they take place is high. Basically this has been studied in two main ways: first, by feeding appropriate resistant strains to volunteers and examining the effect that they have on the resident flora (Anderson, 1975; Williams-Smith, 1975); and secondly, by monitoring the situation as it develops in a limited number of individuals in which resistant bacteria are known to be prevalent, but in which no organisms have deliberately been fed (Richmond, 1977). Of the two approaches, the second seems by far the most satisfactory. It is rare for individuals to receive single loads of bacteria in the way that occurs when bacteria are fed; and the fact that the fed bacteria are often administered in milk, or some buffer, to minimise the killing effect of the acid trap in the stomach, makes feeding procedures of even more dubious value. In contrast, to monitor a natural situation seems much more relevant and representative. The disadvantages of this approach are that much more detailed work is involved and that the experiments continue for much longer periods.

In our department we have made a major effort to follow the *E. coli* flora of a married couple, one of whom (the wife) at various times received substantial amounts of tetracycline for the treatment of acne (Petrocheilou *et al.*, 1977, 1979). The development of this situation revealed that all the mechanisms of gene transfer found to occur *in vitro* also seemed to occur *in vivo*. On several occasions in the course of the survey, cross-infection of resistant *E. coli* strains was observed to occur between the married couple. R—plasmid transfer also occurred from the abundant resident strains to other *E. coli*. On the majority of occasions, however, the novel resistant strains established in this way proved less able to survive in the people under study, than the resident strains from which the resistance plasmids seemed to come.

This particular study did not show definitive evidence for the transposon transposition *in vivo*. It did, however, show clearly that the analogous phenomenon of insertion sequence transfer did take place (Bennett *et al.*, 1980). The phenotypic evidence for this was the appearance of tetracycline sensitive derivatives of the tetracycline resistant *E. coli* which were prevalent in the people under observation. The initial interpretation of this observation was that these *E. coli* strains had lost their R—plasmid, thus making them sensitive. However, a detailed examination showed that the change of phenotype was due to the duplication of one of the "inverted repeats" of the tetracycline resistance transposon present on the plasmids, and its insertion into the middle of the tetracycline resistance genes of the transposon. The inverted repeat of the transposon in question is an insertion sequence of the type studied by Saedler; and the fact that this unit can manifest its insertional properties *in vitro* argues strongly that transposition *in vivo* is also possible.

This suggestion that transposition must be able to occur *in vivo* is also supported by the analysis of a number of situations where the emergence of populations of resistant bacteria has occurred under circumstances where previously all strains had been sensitive. Perhaps the best documented example is that of the emergence in humans of separate tetracycline and ampicillin resistant clones in *Haemophilus influenzae* (Elwell *et al.*, 1977). Both resistant clones owed their resistance to plasmids, and in both cases the resistance genes were carried as part of an appropriate transposon. The fact that both the ampicillin resistance plasmid and the tetracycline resistance plasmid involved in this situation were identical except for the individual resistance transposon they carried argues strongly that, in this situation, the emergence of the ampicillin resistant strains, on the one hand, and the tetracycline resistant ones, on the other, was the result of transposition of the appropriate transposons to a *Haemophilus* plasmid which, up to that time, carried no antibiotic resistance genes.

In summary, then, it seems clear that cross-infection, conjugation and transposition all occur *in vivo* to give rise to the potential spread of resistance in situations where it had not been prevalent before. How far the resistance actually spreads is determined by the impact of selection pressure.

Frequency of Resistance Transfer

It is hard to make any firm statements about the frequency with which transfer occurs *in vivo*. In the early days of the study of this topic it was often assumed that transfer occurred during the course of treatment, with the resulting resistant organisms seriously undermining therapy. In practice such a situation seems to be the exception rather than the rule. Where therapy is prolonged, as was the case in the original outbreaks of dysentery which alerted the Japanese to the antibiotic resistance transfer problem itself (Watanabe, 1963) or in the treatment of burns (Lowbury *et al.*, 1969), resistant strains may indeed emerge during treatment; but in the majority of short-duration clinical conditions, it seems more likely that the infectious organism is itself either resistant or not at the start of the infection and this situation persists during the course of the episode. Much will depend, therefore, on the incidence of resistant pathogens in the particular place at the particular time. If the pathogens are commonly resistant, this will be reflected in the nature of the infections themselves. It follows from this that some idea of the prevalence of resistance among the potential pathogens in a given place is useful as a predictor of the probability of resistant infections.

The observation that infecting pathogens do not commonly acquire resistance during the course of an infection, unless it is very prolonged, is supported to some extent by observations made during monitoring studies of the type described in the previous section of this article. Even where a potential source of transferable resistance is present in a person for long periods, transfer of the plasmids in question to sensitive bacteria occurs relatively infrequently. As a result one can conclude that resistance gene transfer by conjugation is likely to have a strategic rather than a tactical role in the response of potentially pathogenic bacteria to the use of antibiotics. This is in sharp contrast to the beliefs of several years back, where transfer was thought to have a much more immediate effect, only because "the wild-fire spread" of plasmids through susceptible populations could be shown to occur in the laboratory (Hayes, 1968). In practice, such experiments were probably misleading because they underestimated the dampening effect of highly heterogeneous populations of bacteria on the transfer process. Having said this, however, there is little doubt that, on occasion, resistance can spread extremely rapidly through a hitherto universally sensitive population (Lowbury *et al.*, 1969).

Distribution of Resistant Bacteria in the Human Environment

As far as humans are concerned, antibiotic resistant bacteria are broadly concentrated to two large reservoirs. The first is in the human population itself, primarily those who are under treatment with antibiotics, but also those who have acquired resistant bacteria by cross infection. The other is the farm animal and poultry populations, particularly where these are being raised under intensive husbandry conditions. There are also inanimate connections between these two large reservoirs as is outlined in Figure 2 (Linton, 1977).

Over the last ten to fifteen years it has been conventional to recognise the reservoir of resistant bacteria as a human health hazard. Certainly the incidence of resistant *E. coli* in the farm animal and poultry reservoir is high, and from time to time resistant *Salmonella* spp. are to be found in this reservoir as well. Currently over 70% of all *E. coli* from chickens reared under commercial conditions are resistant to tetracycline, and analogous figures for streptomycin and sulphonamide are about 80% and 90% respectively. For pigs and

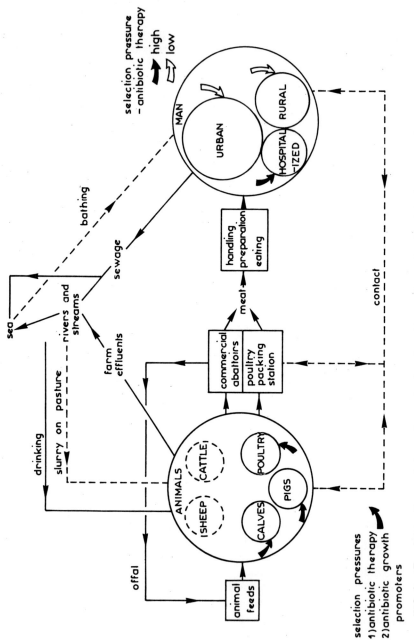

FIG. 2 *E. coli* flow diagram between farm animals and poultry on the one hand and the human population on the other. (Reprinted from Linton, 1977, with permission)

cattle reared under intensive conditions it is not uncommon to find more than 60% of the *E. coli* that are isolated to show resistance to at least one antibiotic. About 15% of the strains are multiply resistant in that they show resistance to at least three antibacterial agents. Undoubtedly these resistant organisms can reach the human population and give rise to a potential threat of disease; and in the case of *Salmonella* spp. there is no doubt that disease has actually been caused (Anderson, 1968). The route of infections is two fold. On the one hand, those handling the animals daily can become infected directly from the animals (Levy, 1978); on the other, bacteria may pass along the food chain, contamination of meat for consumption occurring most commonly at slaughter (Linton *et al.*, 1977a). With poultry, in particular, this is impossible to prevent (Linton *et al.*, 1977b).

Although the reservoir of resistant bacteria in farm animals and poultry is large, and although organisms do pass from these reservoirs to reach the human population, it has always been difficult to decide whether this source of infection is clinically significant. If one looks at the situation in quantitative terms, it seems hard to believe that it can be against the effect of the human therapeutic use of antibiotics. It is known that the administration of a standard course of tetracycline to a human patient results in the conversion of the alimentary flora of the person concerned to the resistant state within 24 hours of the start of the course (Richmond, 1975). This is the result of the selection by the tetracycline of the small number of tetracycline resistant bacteria which are present in the gut contents of all individuals whether they have recently received this antibiotic or not. It is also known that in England in an average year (1977 is the last year for which statistics are available from the Government Statistical Survey) about 20% of the whole population receives a therapeutic course of tetracycline each year (Table 2). If one accepts that each of these courses will effectively convert the gut content of the person taking the course to a tetracycline resistant state, and if one assumes (as the evidence undoubtedly suggests) that this state of affairs will last for at least 13 days following the beginning of the therapeutic course, one can calculate that about 1% of the population of England is carrying a rich tetracycline resistant flora in his or her alimentary tract on any one day, which is the direct result of the use of tetracycline for human therapy. And moreover this does not take into account any resistant organisms which may be prevalent because of the cross-infection or because of the use of other antibiotics. The existence of this enormous load of tetracycline resistant bacteria in the human population which can be attributed directly to the

TABLE 2

Distribution of the Number of Prescriptions for Tetracycline for Human Use in Various Regions of England in 1977

| | England | Northern | Yorkshire | Trent | East anglia | Thames | | | | Wessex | Oxford | South West | West Midlands | Mersey | North West |
						NW	NE	SE	SW						
Prescriptions*	8237	660	705	773	197	643	660	623	482	390	296	446	963	537	862
Population*	46435	3125	3582	4545	1981	3470	3714	3599	2883	2640	2198	3148	5176	2501	4074
Prescription per head per year	0.17	0.21	0.20	0.17	0.10	0.19	0.18	0.17	0.17	0.15	0.13	0.14	0.19	0.21	0.21

* All values in thousands

Data taken from Department of Health and Social Security Statistical Survey for 1977, kindly provided by Mrs. M.J. Roberts.

therapeutic use of tetracycline in humans, argues that the quantitative impact of resistant organisms from farm animals must be negligible in comparison with that generated in the human population itself.

If there is no quantitative impact, is there any qualitative effect? Are any of the types of bacteria emanating from the animal population a particular hazard to man? It has been proved that *Salmonella* spp. of farm origin have caused disease and even deaths in man (Anderson, 1968). So, as far as this group of organisms is concerned, cross-infection of resistant bacteria can be observed in practice (Petrocheilou *et al.*, 1977, 1979) and it is indeed probable that many of these salmonellae originally acquired their resistance plasmids from *E. coli* in the reservoir. Certainly the incidence of plasmid-carriage in salmonellae species is tending to increase as time goes by.

Among *E. coli* the situation is far less clear cut. Although it is probable that *E. coli* of animal origin can survive in man (Williams-Smith, 1975), it is by no means clear that they can cause overt disease. Indeed human pathogenic *E. coli* seem to be rather specific for their human host. In practice therefore the situation with resistant *E. coli* of animal source is likely to be similar to that with salmonellae. An occasional strain may reach the human population from the animal reservoir and prove to have undesirable properties. On balance, however, it seems rather likely that the main source for resistant bacterial populations in humans is the humans themselves, with cross-infection, plasmid transfer and transposon transposition each playing their part.

Outside hospitals, the main threats of resistant bacteria to humans are posed by *E. coli*, with a few specialist pathogens (e.g. *Haemophilus influenzae, Neisseria gonorrhoeae*) causing additional problems under some limited circumstances. In hospitals, however, the situation is sharply different; and where there are particularly vulnerable patients at risk (e.g. intensive care units, transplant units, terminal cancer wards and urology clinics) one finds a much richer and more diverse resistant flora. It is here, where many are chronically sick, and where given organisms are found to persist for long periods in relays of patients passing through the wards, that R—plasmid transfer is probably at its most important for human beings. It is in these circumstances, for example, that the plasmid carrying isolates of *Klebsiella aerogenes*, of *Pseudomonas aeruginosa*, of *Enterobacter* and of other Enterobacteriaceae are common, and it is here that there is good evidence that their resistance plasmids have arisen, often relatively recently, from *E. coli* strains.

Conclusions

It is certain that populations of resistant bacteria emerge by the operation of selection pressure on resistant bacteria. These in turn may arise by the acquisition by sensitive bacteria of resistance plasmids. This step seems certain to be caused by one of the means of inter-cell gene transfer which we have discussed above, but all the probabilities point to its occurring in the absence of antibiotic selection pressure. It is also probably a rare event. In their turn the plasmids which confer resistance will have acquired their resistance genes by the acquisition of a resistance transposon (transposition). Once again this is likely to have occurred in the absence of direct antibiotic selection pressure, and to have been a rare event. All the evidence suggests that the "invention" of antibiotic resistance genes themselves is extremely rare, and that the great majority of genes which cause clinical problems were "invented" long before antibiotics were used by man as therapeutic agents, at least if by this we mean the use of antibiotics in modern medicine (Richmond, 1980).

As would seem likely *a priori*, the chance of transfer making a major impact on the emergence of resistant populations is much higher when the general background is sensitive. This occurs either when the antibiotic in question has a novel mode of action, something which may, for example, include a widened spectrum of activity, or when there seems to have been no resistance prevalent in a particular species up to that time (Medeiros and O'Brien, 1975). The first situation is examplified, for example, by the invention and widespread use of ampicillin; the second by the prolonged sensitivity of *Haemophilus influenzae* to β–lactam antibiotics, a situation which came to a sudden end about 5 years ago. A similar pattern of events has more recently involved species of pneumococci; but we have yet to see the appearance of penicillin resistance among Group A streptococci.

Once resistance is prevalent, it seems that the emergence of important novel strains is more difficult. This is probably because selection pressure operates not just to encourage the evolution of antibiotic resistant bacteria; it also selects for bacteria well able to survive under a full range of environmental conditions, of which an ability to survive antibiotics is merely one. So it seems, as selection pressure of antibiotic use continues, that bacteria which are resistant but which are also very well able to survive in some particular ecological niche begin to emerge. This step has much importance for the evolution of resistant populations, since adaptation to survive well in a given niche may well lead to the survival of antibiotic resistance in the absence of antibiotic selection pressure; as such a state of affairs has been reached, steps such as banning the use of antibiotics may not necessarily lead to the disappearance of the resistant populations, particularly if they become genetically linked to the genes which specify survival.

References

Ambler, R.P (1980). *Proc. R. Soc. London, Ser. B.* **289**, 321–331.
Anderson, E.S. (1968). *Annu. Rev. Microbiol.* **22**, 131–180.
Anderson, E.S. (1975). *Nature* (London) **255**, 500–502.
Bennett, P.M. and Richmond, M.H. (1978). *In* "The Bacteria", Vol. 6. (L.N. Ornston and J.R. Sokatch, eds) pp. 1–69. Academic Press, New York and London.
Bennett, P.M., Richmond, M.H. and Petrocheilou, V. (1980). *Plasmid* **3**, 135–149.
Benveniste, R. and Davies, J. (1973). *Annu. Rev. Biochem.* **42**, 471–506.
Elwell, L.P., Saunders, J.R., Richmond, M.H. and Falkow, S. (1977). *J. Bacteriol.* **131**, 356–362.
Garrod, L. and O'Grady, F. (1971). *In* "Antibiotic and Chemotherapy". 3rd edn., pp. 16–17. Livingstone, Edinburgh.
Hayes, W. (1968). *In* "The Genetics of Bacteria and their Viruses." Blackwell, Oxford.
Hopwood, D. (1977). *Dev. Ind. Microbiol.* **18**, 111–123.
Levy, S.B. (1978). *J. Infect. Dis.* **137**, 688–690.
Linton, A.H. (1977). *In* "Antibiotics and Antibiosis." (M. Woodbine, ed.), pp. 315–343. Butterworths, London and Boston.
Linton, A.H., Howe, K., Hartley, C.L., Clements, H.M., Richmond, M.H. and Osborne, A.D. (1977a). *J. Appl. Bacteriol.* **42**, 365–378.
Linton, A.H., Howe, K., Bennett, P.M., Richmond, M.H. and Whiteside, E.J. (1977b). *J. Appl. Bacteriol.* **43**, 465–469.
Lowbury, E.J.L., Kidson, A., Lilly, H.A., Ayliffe, G.A.J. and Jones, R.J. (1969). *Lancet* **II**, 448–452.
Medeiros, A.A. and O'Brien, T. (1975). *Lancet* **I**, 716–718.
Petrocheilou, V., Richmond, M.H. and Bennett, P.M. (1977). *Antimicrob. Agents Chemother.* **12**, 219–225.
Petrocheilou, V., Richmond, M.H. and Bennett, P.M. (1979). *Antimicrob. Agents Chemother.* **16**, 225–230.
Richmond, M.H. (1975). *In* "Microbiology – 1974". (J. Schlessinger, ed.), pp. 27–35. American Society for Microbiology, Washington.
Richmond, M.H. (1977). *In* "R-factors: Their Properties and Possible Control". (J. Drews and G. Högenauer, eds), pp. 61–78. Springer Verlag, Vienna and New York.
Richmond, M.H. (1980). *In* "The Molecular Basis of Antibiotic Action", 2nd edn. (E.F. Gale, E. Cundliffe, P.E. Reynolds, M.H. Richmond and M. Waring, eds). John Wiley, London and Chichester (In press).
Richmond, M.H. and Sykes, R.B. (1973). *Adv. Microb. Physiol.* **9**, 31–87.
Richmond, M.H., Bennett, P.M., Choi, C.-L., Brown, N., Brunton, J., Grinsted, J. and Wallace, L. (1980). *Proc. R. Soc. London, Ser. B.* **289**, 349–359.
Watanabe, T. (1963). *Bacteriol. Rev.* **27**, 87–115.
Williams-Smith, H. (1975). *Nature* (London) **255**, 500–502.

Discussion

Professor Tomasz: Professor Richmond has nicely documented the fact that one cannot assume that resistant organisms will disappear simply by stopping the antibiotic. Clearly, behind this, there must be some, as yet undetected, selective positive pressure – which is why these resistant organisms prevail. As Professor Richmond said, not only are they resistant but also markedly persistent. Are the effects to which he referred drug-specific? Is it known whether there is some connection, either genetic or physiological, between the mechanism of resistance to tetracyclines or sulphonamides for instance and the physiology of adhesion factors or their synthesis?

Professor Richmond: The evidence is beginning to accumulate. For instance, one can cite the presence of certain capsular antigens on *Escherichia coli* cells which certainly favour colonisation. I will bet – at this stage, no more than that – that what will emerge is that the intensive use of antibiotic, on one hand, and the husbandry of animals in intensive rearing conditions and in very uniform environment, on the other hand, will have selected for the carriage of genes on given pieces of DNA plasmids which relate to both those environmental circumstances. Some colonisation factors will probably be found to be present on resistance plasmids – or perhaps resistance factors on colonisation plasmids. This seems to me to be a major area for research, one in which not enough is known. The real problem at the moment is that there are still not really any good ways of determining the ability of an organism to persist in a real-life situation. Clearly, experiments cannot be done on whole animals in this regard.

In answer to Professor Tomasz' question, underlying this is probably a genetic linkage between characters which determine persistence and characters which determine resistance.

Dr. Salem: Returning to the question that was asked, has Professor Richmond been able to do in reverse his experiment with the colonisation of calves with the sensitive organism, using a resistant organism in the absence of a selective pressure with an antibiotic, to see whether that colonises calves more easily than the sensitive strain?

Professor Richmond: No, that has not been done. Our broad aim has been to try to decontaminate the gut contents of these animals prior to slaughter. This is not a very profitable way forward, of course. I did not include the data in my presentation, although I thought about doing so. It is certainly true that carcases become contaminated on slaughter. If it is possible to contaminate with sensitive organisms, that is at least one step in the right direction.

It is not possible to rely on any one group of *E. coli* to displace any others. It can be done on one occasion with spectacular results; when it is repeated, that does not happen. The underlying mechanisms involved are not understood.

Dr. Salem: Could Professor Richmond also comment on the relationship of duration of the persistence of the resistant organisms after therapy with the duration of the therapy? I notice that the examples chosen were with quite long therapy.

Professor Richmond: We have a certain amount of data on tetracycline use. In our experience, a single 250 mg-tablet of tetracycline will establish a tetracycline resistant gut flora in a human being, in 80 per cent of the cases within 36 hours. Having established it, that resistant population, on average, will last three or four days. With a standard course, which tends to be five days with 250 mg per day, or something similar, it can be more or less guaranteed that the individual's gut flora will contain a lot of tetracycline resistant *E. coli* for 10 days after the end of therapy.

Professor Tomasz: For the understanding of the persistence of resistant bacteria, it might be useful to understand the opposite phenomenon which is very frequently observed in the laboratory — namely, that continuous positive selection is necessary for the persistence of a plasmid-carrier strain. In gonococcus or *Haemophilus*, for instance, when the antibiotic resistant organism is isolated from a patient, unless positive selection by the antibiotic is continuously applied the plasmid is lost. Is the reason for that known?

Professor Richmond: No, I do not think so. The observation that strains carrying plasmids are invariably and automatically at a disadvantage in *in vitro* conditions — in laboratory conditions — can be challenged. Some studies have been published on plasmid-carrying bacteria grown in continuous culture. If the growth of the continuous culture is limited with phosphorus, in which, of course, the plasmid is rich since it is DNA, the population emerges rather rapidly as a sensitive population. To put it in homely terms, the organism will dispense with all the phosphorus-containing reactions that it is able to dispense with and yet still maintain its life.

Paradoxically, if the cultures are limited for carbon, the population becomes 100% plasmid-carrying. I do not think that this observation is at all clearly understood.

Although the literature states categorically that the carriage of a plasmid is a disadvantage, and in energetic terms ultimately this must be true, I do not think that the relationship between plasmid carriage and growth rate is invariably correct. It is hard to experimentally dissociate these two fundamental observations. Many people who have tried to cure *E. coli* strains which have R-factors find this is extremely difficult to do.

Dr. Labia: Does heavy metal pollution, for example, mercury or lead, have any influence on the ecology of plasmids?

Professor Richmond: It is always possible, is it not? Resistance to mercuric ions is a transposable character. Plasmids exist where there is resistance to mercuric ions and to penicillin, for example β–lactamase production, on the same plasmid. It has to be concluded that pollution with heavy metals would provide an environmental factor which would indirectly select for the persistence of the organism. What may be more at issue here, in fact, is the production of surface antigens, or perhaps the suppression of the production of surface antigens, that might camouflage the organism with respect to the immune response of the host, or something like that. It could be quite a non-specific factor. For the sake of argument, let us say that an organism often fails to colonise because an immune response is induced in the host. If the organism could camouflage itself in some way against that immune system, it might persist longer. Some of the influences, in fact, may therefore be negative influences.

Dr. Labia: It has been said that intensive use of mercurial antiseptics in hospitals may select resistant bacteria in water wastes.

Professor Richmond: That is possible. Another area that is quite interesting is that in the United Kingdom — I do not know about France — for many years cadmium compounds were used for treating cloth material, particularly for furnishings. Material to be used for covering furniture was treated with cadmium salts to suppress the persistence of staphylococci transferred from the back of the head on the furniture. Toxic heavy metals are used quite widely.

Evolution of Resistance Patterns

J. DUVAL

*Laboratoire de Bactériologie et de Virologie,
Hôpital Henri Mondor, Créteil, France*

Introduction

Numerous scientists, in different places, periodically study antibiotic resistance. Finland (1979) has recently devoted a general review to this problem. My purpose is not to present a new synthesis of these investigations but to bring to your attention some personal observations. I shall describe some facts established in my laboratory where we perform all the bacteriological tests for a general hospital devoted to adults and located in the suburbs of Paris. Most of the medical and surgical specialities are represented in this 1300 bed centre including an emergency unit and haematology and oncology departments. It has been operating for 10 years; the experience described below covers this whole period, since the opening in 1969.

Materials and Methods

All pathogenic or potentially pathogenic bacteria studied were clinical isolates and were submitted to an antibiotic sensitivity test; this was carried out using the agar diffusion method with Mueller-Hinton's medium and discs from the Institut Pasteur, Paris.

The following antibiotics were tested on *Staphylococcus aureus*: penicillin G (Pen), methicillin (Met), tetracycline (Tet), chloramphenicol (Cmp), erythromycin (Ery), spiramycin (Spi), lincomycin (Lin), pristinamycin (Pri), streptomycin (Str), kanamycin (Kan), gentamicin (Gen), tobramycin (Tob), lividomycin (Liv), amikacin (Akn), rifampicin (Rfa), sulphamides (Suf) and cotrimoxazole (Tsu). Against Gram-negative bacilli: ampicillin (Amp), carbenicillin (Car),

cefalotin (Ctn), a representative of all the first generation cephalosporins, colistin (Col), nitrofurantoin (Fur), nalidixic acid (Nal),
tetracycline, chloramphenicol, aminosides, rifampicin, sulphamides,
cotrimoxazole.

Interpretation of the inhibition areas was performed following
ICS's standards and the strain was classified as sensitive, semi–
sensitive or insensitive to the antibiotic under study. In drawing up
the graphs which are now to be shown, we have taken into account
semi–sensitive and insensitive strains.

Thus, except for the first two years corresponding to the progres-
sive opening of the different departments, 1200 to 1900 strains of
Staphylococcus aureus were tested as well as 6000 to 7000 strains of
Gram-negative bacilli every year.

We shall examine successively the results for both groups of
bacteria.

Staphylococci

In the 1950s–1960s staphylococci were the major bacteria responsible for hospital infections. Although now caught up by Gram-
negative bacilli, they still play an important part. The number of
isolated strains is increasing again; 1823 in 1978 among which 143
were haemocultures.

As soon as antibiotics were used, the first observations reported
were noteworthy: first the appearance of, then the rapid replication
of penicillin-resistant strains following the extensive use of this
antibacterial drug, an evolution closely followed in London by
Barber and Garrod (1963): 14% of resistant strains in 1946, 38% in
1947, 59% in 1948 and 80% in 1950. The further introduction of the
first of other types of antibiotics gave comparable results; drug-
resistant microorganisms appear for each antibiotic, their frequency
increases to reach a level which depends on the antibiotic and where
it seems to stabilize (Chabbert, 1972).

The evolution we have noted from 1969 to 1978 is shown in
Figure 1. Penicillin G resistance is maintained for 80 and 90% of the
isolates. The proportion of bacteria which exhibit heterogenous
resistance to semi-synthetic penicillins of the oxacillin–methicillin
group has decreased in our hospital from 40% in 1969 to 20% at
present, although generally high in France and diversely estimated in
different countries. Let us also note a decrease in tetracycline and
chloramphenicol resistance. The characteristics of macrolide resistance, constitutive or inductible, reveal a greater frequency of
erythromycin resistance compared with spiramycin and lincomycin.
The evolution shows a slight decrease in erythromycin resistance,

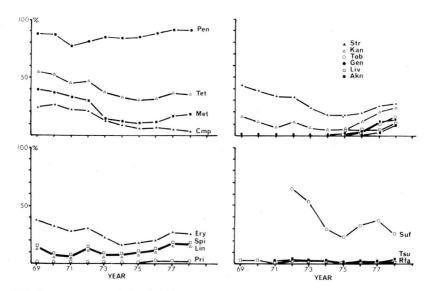

FIG. 1   Proportion of *Staphylococcus aureus* isolates resistant to various antibiotics (between 1969 and 1978).

whereas spiramycin and lincomycin resistance have slightly increased, indicating an increase in the ratio of constitutive patterns. Pristinamycin resistance, first detected in 1975 (Dublanchet *et al.*, 1977), is rare despite its plasmidic nature. Rifampicin resistance is exceptional, cotrimoxazole resistance is rare. Sulphamide resistance seems to be decreasing. Resistance occurs towards all aminosides and emerges most frequently with streptomycin and kanamycin. Having decreased relatively, it has been increasing since 1975; this is particularly true for kanamycin resistance. At the same time new plasmidic resistance appeared with gentamicin, tobramycin and, to a lesser degree, with amikacin; this resistance is of two types G.K.To and K.To; consequently, both concern kanamycin (Soussy *et al.*, 1975, 1976). The G.K.To type has undergone a very rapid extension and today its incidence has reached 20%, whereas the K.To type is not very frequent (less than 1%) (Soussy and Duval, 1979).

At present some staphylococci accumulate a high number of resistances. During the first six months of 1979, from 825 isolated strains, 19 (2.3%) were sensitive to 2 or 3 antibiotics only. Pristinamycin, rifampicin and cotrimoxazole are the compounds which are most often active, sometimes chloramphenicol, once only methicillin. Let us mention, however, that these strains are vancomycin sensitive.

Gram-Negative Bacilli

Hospital Gram-negative bacilli show a resistance very superior to that of staphylococci.

Species and Their Distribution

In the course of 1978, 5944 strains were isolated. Their distribution is shown in Table 1. One can see that the strains which have remained

TABLE 1

Distribution of 5944 Strains of Gram-Negative Bacilli Isolated in 1978

Escherichia coli	2118	Klebsiella pneumoniae	560	Miscellaneous	168
Proteus mirabilis	719	Enterobacter	641		
		Serratia	192		
		Indole-positive Proteus	279		
		Providencia	44		
		Citrobacter	145		
		Pseudomonas aeruginosa	665		
		Acinetobacter	413		
Total	2837		2939		168

relatively sensitive and which are not specifically linked with hospitals (*E. coli* and *P. mirabilis*) (column 1) represent a number of strains fairly equal to that of hospital bacteria (column 2). This ratio has been kept almost constant (about 0.9) since 1972.

Overall Appreciation

Overall, there has been a fairly marked stability during this 10-year spell (Fig. 2), except for a temporary increase in resistance between 1973 and 1974, the significance of which is difficult to assess: it may be an artefact linked to variations in the experimental techniques or an actual, transitory increase which may reflect the epidemiological situation at that time. As a matter of fact, *Enterobacter, Serratia* and *Providencia* isolates were more numerous at that time. If this increase in resistance were indeed valid, resistance could have been evolving until 1974 and we are now experiencing a certain decrease.

On this fairly stable background, various trends can, however, be pointed out, namely a slow but probably real increase in ampicillin, cotrimoxazole and nalidixic acid resistance; a decrease, since 1973, in sulphamide and nitrofuran resistance; and an obvious evolution of gentamicin resistance, with the appearance in 1969 of a plasmidic resistance to this antibiotic. We then observed a rapid rise in the frequency of resistant strains until 1974, followed by a decrease and a stabilization around 20% of the strains. Among the other

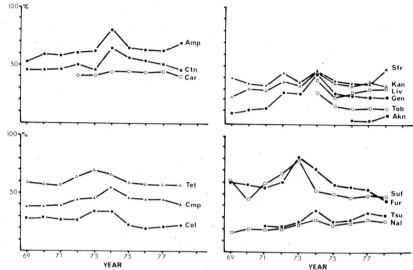

FIG. 2 Proportion of Gram-negative bacilli isolates resistant to various antibiotics (between 1969 and 1978).

aminosides, tobramycin resistance, often linked to that of gentamicin, was by the way established from the first use of the compound. It follows, at a slightly lower level, gentamicin resistance. Amikacin resistance, still not very important, is developing slightly.

In conclusion, the overall appreciation can be summarized in the following five statements.

1) None of the antibiotics eludes resistance.
2) Those for which resistant strains are the least numerous correspond to three groups: aminosides (gentamicin, tobramycin and amikacin especially), polymyxins and quinolones (nalidixic and pipemidic acids).
3) The frequency of ampicillin resistant strains is high: 60%.
4) Rifampicin was not plotted on the graph since most of the strains are not very sensitive to it. It would be indicated only in special cases, in associations, with regard to possible synergies.
5) With the other antibiotics, the frequency of resistant strains varies from 30 to 50% of isolates.

Analysis According to Species

Two species are much more sensitive and present a particularly stable behaviour, *E. coli* for which a slow increase of ampicillin resistance is noted (Fig. 3), and *Proteus mirabilis* for which tetracycline, polymyxin and nitrofuran resistance are natural (Fig. 4). The

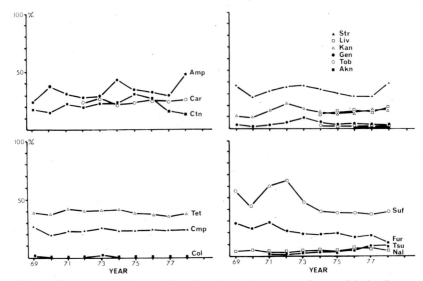

FIG. 3   Proportion of *Escherichia coli* isolates resistant to various antibiotics (between 1969 and 1978).

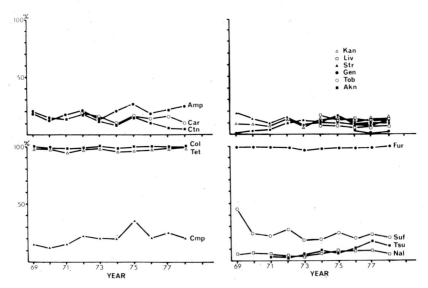

FIG. 4   Proportion of *Proteus mirabilis* isolates resistant to various antibiotics (between 1969 and 1978).

regularity of the graphs obtained for these two species gives perhaps some value to the biphasic evolution of the whole and of some other species.

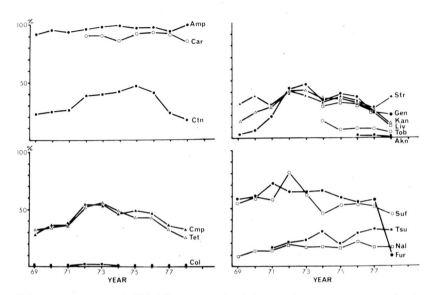

FIG. 5   Proportion of *Klebsiella pneumoniae* isolates resistant to various antibiotics (between 1969 and 1978).

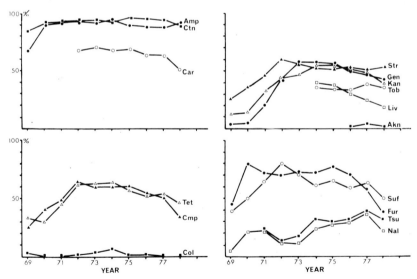

FIG. 6   Proportion of *Enterobacter* isolates resistant to various antibiotics (between 1969 and 1978).

This is notably the case for *Klebsiella pneumoniae* (Fig. 5) which is almost constantly resistant to ampicillin and to carbenicillin; on the contrary, *Enterobacter* (Fig. 6) are mostly resistant to ampicillin

and cefalotin but only half the time resistant to carbenicillin. Genta-
micin and tobramycin resistance occurs much more frequently in
Enterobacter than in *Klebsiella*. Resistance occurs still more in
Serratia (Fig. 7) which are bacteriologically close to the two

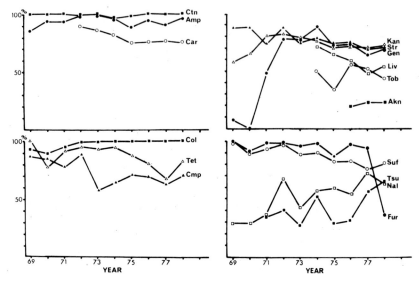

FIG. 7   Proportion of *Serratia* isolates resistant to various antibiotics (between 1969 and
1978).

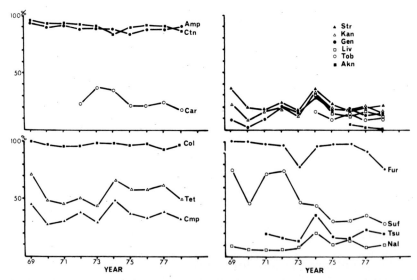

FIG. 8   Proportion of indole-positive *Proteus* isolates resistant to various antibiotics
(between 1969 and 1978).

preceding groups. Cotrimoxazole and nalidixic acid resistance regularly progresses; polymyxin resistance is a natural characteristic of this group.

Indole positive *Proteus* (Fig. 8), in addition to their natural and

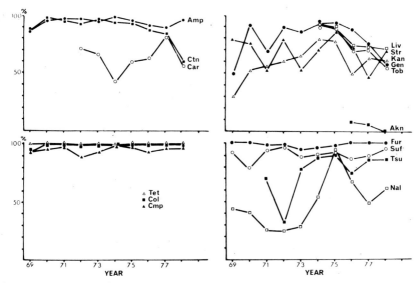

FIG. 9   Proportion of *Providencia* isolates resistant to various antibiotics (between 1969 and 1978).

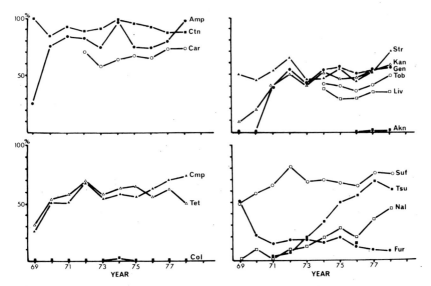

FIG. 10   Proportion of *Citrobacter* isolates resistant to various antibiotics (between 1969 and 1978).

very frequent resistance to tetracyclines, polymyxins and nitrofurans also exhibit ampicillin and cefalotin resistance; carbenicillin is often active. *Providencia* (*Proteus inconstans*) are particularly resistant (Fig. 9) but luckily more rarely isolated, except during epidemic crises. The evolution shows a fairly marked stability in the behaviour of indole positive *Proteus*; the behaviour of *Providencia* is more irregular.

Citrobacter (Fig. 10) are often polyresistant; cotrimoxazole and nalidixic acid resistance regularly increases. Only polymyxins and amikacin are, with certain exceptions, regularly active.

Pseudomonas aeruginosa (Fig. 11), very frequently isolated in hospital departments, shows a great stability in the high resistance frequencies for most of the antibiotics, except for carbenicillin, polymyxins and a few aminosides (gentamicin, amikacin, and tobramycin). Its resistance to aminosides has recently made great strides forwards.

Acinetobacter (Fig. 12) behave similarly. However, their resistance to carbenicillin ceaselessly increases, their resistance to gentamicin emerges frequently, but in contrast to *Pseudomonas*, they can be sensitive to tetracyclines, cotrimoxazole, sulphamides and nalidixic acid. But resistance to this latter has lately increased, after a long period of stability.

Frequency of Polyresistant Strains

Fifteen antibiotics have been retained to provide a basis for analysis. They can be used for treating general infections, excluding nitrofurans which are used for treating urinary or intestinal tract infections only. They are listed as follows: ampicillin, carbenicillin, cefalotin, streptomycin, kanamycin, lividomycin, gentamicin, tobramycin, amikacin, chloramphenicol, tetracyclines, colistin, rifampicin, nalidixic acid, cotrimoxazole. Polyresistant strains have been classified into 4 categories:

- category 0 = no active antibiotic
- category 1 = only one active antibiotic
- category 2 = two active antibiotics
- category 3 = three active antibiotics.

The analysis of the antibiograms performed on 2936 strains isolated in the first six months of 1979 (Table 2) reveals a frequency of 8.54% of the isolates for the four categories, with respectively: 1.53% for category 0, 0.54% for category 1, 3.34% for category 2, 3.13% for category 3. It should be noted that 3 groups come to the fore owing to the frequency of isolated polyresistant strains. These are *Pseudomonas aeruginosa, Enterobacter* and *Serratia.* Amongst

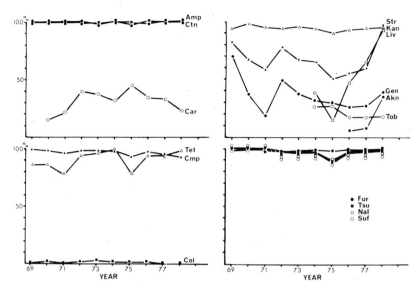

FIG. 11   Proportion of *Pseudomonas aeruginosa* isolates resistant to various antibiotics (between 1969 and 1978).

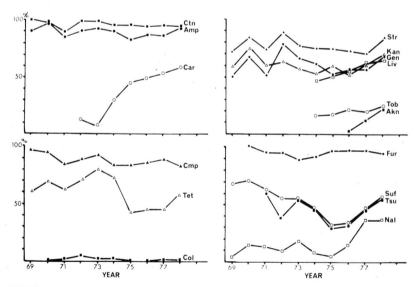

FIG. 12   Proportion of *Acinetobacter* isolates resistant to various antibiotics (between 1969 and 1978).

these latter, 35% are "completely resistant"; on the other hand, they are the only group to possess such strains. *Citrobacter, Acinetobacter* and *Providencia* are often polyresistant too.

TABLE 2

Distribution of Polyresistant Strains Among 2936 Gram-negative Bacilli Isolated in the
First Six Months of 1979

Bacterial species	No. of isolated strains	Categories				
		0	1	2	3	Total
Serratia	128	45	3	39	1	88
Pseudomonas aeruginosa	310		8	25	33	66
Enterobacter	372		1	18	29	48
Citrobacter	66		1	4	9	14
Acinetobacter	172			2	12	14
Providencia	15		1	5	3	9
Pseudomonas sp.	9			4		4
Indole-positive *Proteus*	138		1	1	1	3
Proteus mirabilis	334		1		3	4
Klebsiella	305				1	1
Escherichia coli	1087					0
Total	2936	45	16	98	92	251
%		1.53	0.54	3.34	3.13	8.54

No *E. coli* is found in any of these categories and, rather unexpectedly, only one strain of *Klebsiella pneumoniae* is present in category 3.

Some antibiotics are active on these polyresistant strains. In category 1, amikacin may be used against species having a natural polymyxin resistance (*Serratia, Proteus, Providencia*) and colistin in most cases against others (*Enterobacter, Citrobacter, Pseudomonas aeruginosa*). In category 2, the same observations are made. As regard to *Serratia, Proteus* and *Providencia*, amikacin sensitivity is almost always maintained; the second active antibiotic is most often tobramycin, another aminoside, which is therefore of little interest clinically. Concerning the other species, colistin remains active, most often associated to amikacin sensitivity. In category 3, the analysis is clearly more complex. Here again colistin and amikacin are the two products which are most often still active, and often, two out of these three active antibiotics are aminosides (50 times out of 89).

These polyresistant bacteria were isolated from miscellaneous samplings. The importance of their clinical meaning is therefore variable. The majority were isolated from urine and certain of them were nitrofuran sensitive, although very few among the most resistant. Others are taken from sputum and tracheal samplings, or various suppurations. However, some were isolated from haemocultures.

By comparing our results with those obtained from similar investigations conducted in our hospital in 1973 (Table 3), the evolution of the incidence of the multiresistant bacteria isolation can

TABLE 3

Frequency of Polyresistant Strains among Gram-negative Bacilli

Category	1973	1979
0	0.4	1.53
1	3.5	0.54
2	4.7	3.34
3	non evaluated	3.13
Total	8.6	8.54

be appreciated. At that time, 12 out of the 15 above-mentioned antibiotics were involved in this study since tobramycin, amikacin and lividomycin had not yet been put into use and only strains belonging to categories 0, 1, 2 had been numbered (Soussy *et al.*, 1974). Thus, the four 1979 categories correspond exactly to the three categories of 1973, but this gain, which is mainly linked to the new aminosides, is for the most part only an apparent gain. As a matter of fact, as has been demonstrated above, numerous strains belonging to categories 2 and 3 are sensitive to two aminosides. They should be classified in categories 1 and 2 respectively, increasing these latter and decreasing category 3 by the same amount.

Some Factors Involved in Evolution of Resistance

The evolution of a new resistance such as gentamicin resistance, which has increased very rapidly as a whole since its appearance in 1969, but irregularly according to bacterial species, shows the epidemic nature often exhibited by plasmidic resistance but also the unequal "receptivity" of bacterial species, so that these new resistances most often become associated with strains already possessing several resistances. Variations which can be established in resistance levels from one hospital to another (Soussy *et al.*, 1974), and even between different departments of a same hospital at a given period (Table 4) demonstrate that favourable local factors interfere with the diffusion of resistant strains. It has been widely demonstrated that the selection pressure exerted by a widespread use of antibiotics is a determining factor of this evolution, but also, of course, the epidemic diffusion of resistant strains may be partly linked to an epidemic nature inherent in certain strains and certainly to crossed transmission in the hospital environment.

Two personal remarks can be added to this report. We described a few years ago the impact of restriction measures, when prescribing antibiotics, on the frequency of Gram-negative bacilli septicaemia

TABLE 4

Percentage of Resistant Gram-negative Bacilli Isolated in Several Departments of
Henri Mondor Hospital in 1979

	Hospital overall	Urology	Haematology	General surgery	Intensive care	General medicine	Rhumatology
Carbenicillin	37	53	48	42	41	32	20
Gentamicin	21	39	28	20	17	18	7
Nalidixic acid	27	41	30	32	31	27	21

induced by additional infection in an intensive care unit; application
of this measure was rapidly followed by a quite significant decrease
in these dreadful complications (Rapin *et al.*, 1975). On the other
hand, we took up in our hospital an identical policy regarding the
use of antibiotics and this led to a real decrease in the use of broad-
spectrum antibiotics, namely of β-lactamines; has this fact contributed to limiting resistance increase?

Advantages Offered by New Products

This overall appreciation would not be complete, if newly marketed
products were not recalled. Others are under investigation. Some
of the β-lactamines are more active than the old ones against *Pseudomonas aeruginosa* (piperacillin, azlocillin, cefsulodin); others
present a broader spectrum of activity, i.e. the so-called second and
third generation cephalosporins and cephamycins (cefoxitin, cefamandole, cefuroxime, cefotaxime, moxalactam).

Various studies have already outlined the respective advantages of
these compounds. Within the limits of this appreciation regarding
clinical isolates, only fragmentary results can be given. For a few
months, cefoxitin and cefamandole activity (Table 5) have been
regularly tested. These compounds have proved to be active on a
very large proportion of not only *E. coli* but also *Klebsiella, Proteus*
and *Providencia*. Cefoxitin is active on 50% of *Serratia* but on a very
few *Enterobacter*; cefamandole behaves inversely and moreover, it is
much more often active on *Citrobacter* than cefoxitin. On the
contrary, most of *Pseudomonas* and *Acinetobacter* show resistance
to both compounds which therefore does not solve all the problems.

The latest compounds such as cefotaxime and moxalactam are
superior to the above-mentioned compounds but they have not been
regularly tested yet, in daily practice. The following observation can
be made: among 8 "completely resistant" *Serratia* strains, cefotaxime
was shown to be active on 7.

TABLE 5

Resistance of Gram-negative Bacilli to Cefamandole and Cefoxitin (in 1979)

	Cefoxitin		Cefamandole	
	No. of tested strains	% R	No. of tested strains	% R
Escherichia coli	1380	1	1009	1
Klebsiella pneumoniae	375	2	322	5
Enterobacter	465	86	422	40
Serratia	155	48	132	93
Proteus mirabilis	398	0	384	2
Indole-positive *Proteus*	152	3	132	8
Providencia	30	3	30	3
Citrobacter	104	78	84	11
Pseudomonas aeruginosa	496	99	443	99
Acinetobacter	156	92	141	94
Total	3711	33	3099	29.6

Conclusion

This is the present situation concerning the evolution of bacterial resistance in our hospital, which is no doubt a reflection of the general situation in French hospitals, in spite of certain variations. The clearest conclusion is that phenomena, previously observed with staphylococci when antibiotic therapy became established, still appear and now extend to Gram-negative bacilli. After a period of spread, resistance is proving to be stabilized at a certain level; this level varies according to the antibiotics, species and places, but also shows moderate oscillations.

A rational use of antibiotics, to fight against the epidemic transmission of resistant strains in hospital departments, should contribute to restricting the frequency level of the different resistance patterns.

References

Barber, M. and Garrod, L.P. (1963). "Antibiotic and Chemotherapy". Livingstone, Edinburgh.

Chabbert, Y.A. (1972). *In* "Techniques en Bactériologie", Vol. 3 (G.L. Daguet and Y.A. Chabbert, eds), p. 213. Flammarion Médecine-Sciences, Paris.

Dublanchet, A., Soussy, C.J., Squinazi, F. and Duval, J. (1977). *Ann. Microbiol.* (Inst. Pasteur) **128 A**, 277–287.

Finland, M. (1979). *Rev. Infect. Dis.* **1**, 4–21.

Rapin, M., Duval, J., Le Gall, J.R., Soussy, C.J., Lemaire, F. and Harari, A. (1975). *Nouv. Presse Méd.* **4**, 483–486.

Soussy, C.J. and Duval, J. (1979). *Nouv. Presse Méd.* **8**, 3413–3416.

Soussy, C.J., Bouanchaud, D.H., Fouace, J., Dublanchet, A. and Duval, J. (1975). *Ann. Microbiol.* (Inst. Pasteur) **126 B**, 91–94.

Soussy, C.J., Denoyer, M.C., Duval, J., Goldstein, F., Guibert, J.M., Acar, J.F. and Begue, P. (1974). *Méd. Mal. Infect.* **4**, 341–348.

Soussy, C.J., Dublanchet, A., Cormier, M., Bismuth, R., Mizon, F., Chardon, H., Duval, J. and Fabiani, G. (1976). *Nouv. Presse Méd.* **5**, 2599–2602.

Discussion

Professor Waldvogel:　You mentioned 45 strains of *Serratia* which were totally resistant to some products. Could you give us some epidemiological data on these strains? Were they specimens? Were they different strains? Were they found in the same place? Is there any kind of artificial increase due to a phenomenon of mini-epidemics in the hospital?

Professor Duval:　Yes, there are such mini-epidemics in the urology department. Some were also found by Professor Acar some years ago and new ones are quite possible. Most of these bacteria were isolated from urines.

Professor Waldvogel:　Which means that this figure of 45 may in fact be swollen up artificially?

Professor Duval:　It is right. For each patient we have one isolate but a strain that goes from one patient to another is inevitably counted several times. This is misleading of course.

Dr. Labia:　What is the place of cefoxitin and cefamandole against the poly-resistant strains of group 0, 1 and others?

Professor Duval:　We did not test this very regularly on these strains. However, on some of them, in particular for 15 *Serratia* tested with cefoxitin, we saw that cefoxitin is active two times out of three, which is not far from the 50% noted in a more comprehensive study. Cefamandole was quite better on other species we tested. And now on some 3000 strains tested (which of course are not all multi-resistant) about 30% of strains in these populations were resistant to either product: 33% to cefoxitin and 29% to cefamandole which is not much different. So, we rely very much on new products.

Professor Acar:　In the restriction policy that you have for antibiotics we are talking about a sort of overall restriction in the Henri Mondor Hospital. It is not a selective restriction as that has been proposed in other hospitals.

Professor Duval:　Yes, it was an overall reduction policy at that time. But now one uses penicillin G or metronidazole more likely in some pre- or post-operative infections, in digestive surgery, etc. So there are various factors to take into consideration but the figures that I have shown in fact concern the previous period.

Professor Acar:　Yes, this brings us to the problem of use of antibiotics in hospitals.

Antibiotic Therapy of Infections Caused by Common Bacterial Pathogens

J. FROTTIER and S. KERNBAUM

Clinique des Maladies Infectieuses B. (Prof. R. Bastin),
Hôpital Claude-Bernard et Université Paris VII.
Paris, France

Introduction

The choice of antibiotic therapy depends on the following:
- the sensitivity of the causative organism,
- the characteristics of the infection (severity, localisation, etc.),
- the host (susceptibility to allergy, renal and/or hepatic insufficiency, state of the immune defence system, pregnancy, etc.),
- the antibiotic itself (pharmacology, mode of administration, possible interference with other therapy, spectrum of activity, cost of treatment, etc.).

We shall examine systematically therapy of infections caused by six common bacterial pathogens: streptococci, pneumococci, staphylococci, meningococci, gonococci and *Haemophilus influenzae*. Several reviews dealing with this subject have already been published (Garrod *et al.*, 1973; Kagan, 1974; Kucers and McBennett, 1975; Neu, 1978; Weinstein, 1975).

We should first of all underscore two general points. Firstly, in current practice, one antibiotic only is prescribed as a rule, except for severe infections which justify a combination therapy which exerts a synergistic bactericidal effect. The question of antibiotic combinations was the subject of a recent international symposium (Bastin *et al.*, 1977). Secondly, a topical form of antibiotic should not be prescribed for skin infections. Antiseptics are at least as effective and risk neither sensitising the patient nor selecting the appearance of resistant microorganisms.

Infections Due to Streptococci

The streptococci are a heterogeneous family of microorganisms. Some are normally saprophytic, the others give rise to frequent, polymorphic and occasionally serious infections.

Group A streptococci, the type most often implicated in infections, are sensitive to benzylpenicillin (penicillin G) (Bastin *et al.*, 1977; Christol *et al.*, 1971). This antibiotic, usually bactericidal on its own, has a very low minimal inhibitory concentration (m.i.c.). Its bactericidal action is reinforced by combining it with an aminoglycoside (usually streptomycin). Penicillin G can only be administered parenterally. When small doses are sufficient, as for tonsilitis, scarlatina or any other mild infection, two equivalent penicillins are available for oral use: penicillin V and phenethicillin.

Ampicillin is a second choice antibiotic. Its m.i.c. is greater, its spectrum of activity is broader (with a greater risk of superinfection), the skin reactions to which it can give rise are more frequent, and its treatment cost is higher. Some clinicians use it to replace, by the oral route, high doses of penicillin G. The digestive tolerance of the aminopenicillins is indeed better than that of the oral equivalents of penicillin G. Furthermore, amoxicillin and bacampicillin give excellent blood levels and thereby represent for the clinician an appreciable therapeutic advance.

The antibiotic sensitivity of streptococci of groups B (Lerner *et al.*, 1977), C and G is scarcely different from that of microorganisms in group A, sensitivity to penicillin G (the first line antibiotic) being only slightly inferior.

Among the group D streptococci, it is advisable to distinguish between *Streptococcus bovis* and the enterococci (Bastin *et al.*, 1977; Christol *et al.*, 1971). We have studied the antibiotic sensitivity of 25 strains of *S. bovis* causing endocarditis. The antibiotic which was active in most cases was penicillin G. Examined alone at a concentration of 50 units/ml, it was bactericidal in this test to 16 out of 25 strains, this was increased to 23 out of 25 strains when associated with streptomycin and to 25 out of 25 strains by combination with gentamicin. The penicillin G—aminoglycoside combination is the treatment of choice which has given us the best clinical results. The enterococci are less sensitive than *S. bovis* to penicillin G (Bastin *et al.*, 1977). In cases of endocarditis which we have observed, this antibiotic was individually bactericidal *in vitro* to only 20% of the organisms, whilst ampicillin was bactericidal to 25%. On the other hand, the penicillin G—streptomycin combination was bactericidal to 94% of the strains, as against 60% for penicillin G—gentamicin, ampicillin—streptomycin and ampicillin—gentamicin combinations. There are exceptional strains of enterococci highly resistant to streptomycin, against which gentamicin, combined with penicillin G, is active.

The *S. viridans* strains giving rise to alpha-haemolysin are numerous: *Streptococcus* H, K, *mitis, sanguis, salivarius*, etc. (Pulliam and Handley, 1979). These microorganisms remain sensitive to penicillin G (Christol *et al.*, 1971), which is individually bactericidal at a concentration of 50 units/ml to 65% of the strains isolated from cases of endocarditis that we have treated. Pristinamycin is as often bactericidal in our experience (Bastin *et al.*, 1977). The combination which we always prescribe as a first line treatment is penicillin–streptomycin, but pristinamycin–penicillin and pristinamycin–ampicillin are universally active *in vitro* against our strains. However, these saprophytic streptococci of the buccal cavity can develop a degree of resistance to penicillin in patients receiving oral prophylaxis against relapse of rheumatic fever (Parillo *et al.*, 1979; Sprunt *et al.*, 1968). This resistance can give rise to therapeutic problems when these streptococci are the cause of bacterial endocarditis.

The factor which can hinder the use of penicillin G in streptococcal infections is the occurrence of sensitisation. When this happens, some clinicians, including ourselves, try nevertheless to prescribe it when it is essential, while employing a technique to aid tolerance. In practice, for a patient thought to be allergic, it is wiser to use an antibiotic from a family other than the cephalosporins, but it is still advisable to monitor its activity by sensitivity testing. As a rule, the choice is either a true macrolide, such as erythromycin (which gives the better serum levels) or spiramycin (for high tissue levels), or a related drug such as a lincosamide (lincomycin) or synergistin (pristinamycin). Some strains of streptococci resistant to macrolides and/or to lincomycin have however been described (Garrod *et al.*, 1973; Kagan, 1974; Kucers and McBennett, 1975; Dixon and Lipinski, 1974). These represent fewer than 5% of group A streptococci and about 30% of group D streptococci responsible for cases of endocarditis that we have treated (Bastin *et al.*, 1977). We have also recorded that 30% of group A streptococcal strains that we examined in 1976 were resistant to tetracyclines (Frottier, 1977). In our series of endocarditis cases, this resistance reached 45% of group D and *viridans* streptococci (Bastin *et al.*, 1977). For the treatment of a severe streptococcal infection in a patient sensitive to penicillins, vancomycin, alone or combined with an aminoglycoside, offers the most effective alternative, despite the side-effects that it can generate.

This treatment scheme for streptococcal infections should be preserved for pregnant women and infants, since neither penicillin nor the macrolides are contra-indicated in these patients. In renal insufficiency, very high doses of penicillin should not be prescribed and vancomycin should be used with care, by relating its dosage to the glomerular filtration rate and by monitoring the serum level.

For prophylactic treatment of streptococcal infections two forms are universally accepted. Prophylaxis against relapse of Bouillaud's disease is well defined. The choice would be benzathine—penicillin, one intramuscular injection every 15 to 21 days. This is preferable to oral dosage with penicillin V, since the latter could be forgotten in error, and it may induce resistance among the saprophytic streptococci of the buccal cavity (Parillo *et al.*, 1979; Pulliam and Hadley, 1979; Sprunt *et al.*, 1968). The duration of prophylaxis is less well determined, but should be at least 5 years.

Prevention of bacterial endocarditis in patients with cardiac valve disease is more complex. In such patients it is necessary to examine regularly for latent infectious foci, especially dental or pharyngeal, and these should be treated with antibiotics. Any operative procedure involving the buccal cavity must be accompanied by protective treatment of the subject against an infection by a saprophytic streptococcus. Various prescriptions have been proposed for this purpose. It seems to us reasonable to begin treatment 1 to 2 hours before the operation and to continue for 3 to 5 days. Streptomycin (1 g daily in 2 intramuscular injections) should be combined with a β—lactam, such as penicillin G (about 5 million units i.m. daily) or amoxicillin (3 g p.o. daily) or, in the allergic patient, pristinamycin (2 or 3 g daily).

To forestall an infection by group D streptococci following operation on the urinary or digestive tracts in a subject with cardiac valve disease, it is advisable to combine an aminoglycoside (such as gentamicin) with ampicillin or amoxicillin (3 to 4 g daily). This therapy, with the same duration as given above, is also active against a number of Gram-negative bacteria.

Pneumococcal Infections

Streptococcus pneumoniae is also a saprophytic organism that can become the agent of major infections.

Penicillin G is still the best antibiotic available with which to combat this encapsulated streptococcus (Kernbaum, 1979). It should be noted however that since 1967 strains of various serotypes have been isolated which require 10 to 100-fold higher concentrations of β—lactams to inhibit them (Acar *et al.*, 1974; Goldstein *et al.*, 1978). They have been isolated from healthy subjects and from patients in

New Guinea, Australia, United States, Canada, Great Britain and South Africa (Appelbaum *et al.*, 1977; Dixon, 1974; Hansman, 1975 and 1977; Hansman *et al.*, 1971; Howard *et al.*, 1978; Jacobs *et al.*, 1978; Naragi *et al.*, 1974; Paredes *et al.*, 1976; Suksuwan, 1975; Tempest *et al.*, 1974). In 1979, two multiresistant French strains, of serotype 23, were isolated (Dublanchet and Durieux, 1979; Peyrefitte *et al.*, 1979). When such organisms are responsible for infections other than meningeal ones, they can be controlled by the use of penicillin G at very high doses. When, on the other hand, they are the cause of meningitis, they can occasion therapeutic difficulties and even treatment failures. In this case the drug of choice is chloramphenicol. It should be prescribed at full dosage (3 g daily for adults and 50 to 100 mg/kg daily for children), starting with the injectable hemisuccinate form ('Solnicol') given in discontinuous fashion through an infusion line. However, chloramphenicol resistant strains have been known since 1972 in France, Poland, Japan, Australia and Great Britain. They produce an enzyme that inactivates the antibiotic and is probably plasmid-mediated (Appelbaum *et al.*, 1977; Cybulska *et al.*, 1970; Dublanchet and Durieux, 1979; Miyamura *et al.*, 1977; Jacobs *et al.*, 1978). Furthermore, pneumococcal strains simultaneously resistant to penicillin G and chloramphenicol and even to several other antibiotics have been reported (Harves and Mitchell, 1976). Thus treatment of meningitis can become much more difficult, and it is not surprising that the 3 cases described by Appelbaum *et al.* (1977) eventually died. It seems to us that vancomycin might be tried against these organisms (Hawley and Gump, 1973). It penetrates well into inflamed meninges and might be associated with some intrathecal treatment.

We should emphasise that the cephalosporins, although active *in vitro*, are usually devoid of clinical activity against pneumococcal infections.

Therapy of pneumococcal infections has not to be modified for the pregnant woman, the infant or the renal insufficient patient. The occurrence of sensitisation to β–lactams is an indication to use macrolides, and, in the case of a purulent meningitis, chloramphenicol.

Prophylaxis of pneumococcal infections (Anon., 1979a) is considered only for asplenic patients or for those whose spleen is non-functional (drepanocytic homozygotes). In these patients a systemic infection could take on the utmost severity. This prophylaxis is afforded either by vaccination, usually effective though not without failures and sometimes badly tolerated, or by benzathine–penicillin prescribed for life at the same doses used to prevent relapse in rheumatic fever. Prophylaxis can also be considered for patients liable to recurrent meningitis.

Staphylococcal Infections

Whether they be coagulase—positive staphylococci (which are usually pathogenic) or staphylococci which lack this enzyme, these organisms are characterised by their adaptability and their variable sensitivity to antibiotics. Treatment of an infection by staphylococci cannot be decided upon until the strain has been isolated and its antibiotic sensitivity determined. While awaiting this result, the infecting strain should be considered to be like the majority of "non-hospital" strains and more than 80% of "hospital" strains in being capable of secreting a penicillinase which inactivates penicillins G and V and ampicillin derivatives (Anon., 1979b; Buré et al., 1975; Fleurette, 1977; Noble and Naidoo, 1978). Thus the first line choice is either a penicillin of the methicillin group or else pristinamycin (the most active of the synergistins). These narrow spectrum antibiotics, which are generally (but not always) bactericidally active at normal therapeutic dosages, can for severe infections (e.g. septicaemia, endocarditis etc.) be combined with an aminoglycoside, such as gentamicin (Buré et al., 1975; Fleurette, 1977).

Among the methicillin group, methicillin binds only slightly (40%) to serum proteins. It has the disadvantage of giving rise occasionally to an immune tubulo-interstitial haematuric nephritis and so we are unable to recommend it. Oxacillin binds very strongly (90%) to protein, which offsets its lower m.i.c. value. Cloxacillin and dicloxacillin have been introduced more recently. They are administered orally. The therapeutic advantage which they offer seems limited. Nevertheless, for about 15 years coagulase—positive and even coagulase—negative (Laverdière et al., 1978) staphylococci resistant to methicillin and its derivatives have been isolated.

Pristinamycin is nowadays rather more likely to be active than the methicillin family against the staphylococci. It has the disadvantage of not being available in an injectable form and its bactericidal power cannot be assessed in serum. It does, however, have the advantage of being well tolerated.

Other antistaphylococcal agents are, in our opinion, of second choice for they are either less active or give rise to numerous side-effects. Penicillin G, if the organism is sensitive to it, has the lowest m.i.c. value and costs the least. The cephalosporins, the most active of which is cephalothin, have an activity corresponding to that of the methicillin group. They do have a broader spectrum and, where combined with an aminoglycoside, show greater renal toxicity. The lincosamides (lincomycin and clindamycin) are less frequently active and give rise to side-effects (mainly digestive) which cannot be discounted. The macrolides are a little less active but better tolerated.

Fusidic acid and rifampicin are effective against most staphylococci but their use often results in the appearance of resistant mutants, and they cannot therefore be prescribed alone. On the other hand rifampicin penetrates well within the cytoplasm of leucocytes, which is a useful property in the rare staphylococcal infections which resist treatment with an antibiotic of the methicillin group (Beam, 1979). The aminoglycosides (e.g. gentamicin) are bactericidal *in vitro*. Like other authors, we prescribe them only in association with one of the antibiotics described above or with vancomycin, with which they are normally synergistic. Finally, vancomycin is always active against staphylococci, is bactericidal and binds feebly (10%) to serum proteins. But its toxicity limits its use to systemic infections by staphylococci against which the other antibiotics exert an action which is bacteriologically or clinically inadequate.

In the patient who is allergic to penicillins, pristinamycin or rifampicin or vancomycin are used, eventually in combination with an aminoglycoside. In renal insufficiency, only the aminoglycosides and vancomycin should be administered carefully, observing the dosage indicated by tables relating it to blood creatinine, and monitoring their serum levels. In pregnancy the aminoglycosides are avoided since they can damage the eighth cranial nerve pair in the foetus. In the infant, no antistaphylococcal agent is *a priori* contra-indicated, but the aminoglycosides are reserved for severe infections.

Meningococcal Infections

Among infections due to meningococci, cerebrospinal meningitis poses the major therapeutic problem. Until 1969, these organisms were very sensitive to sulphonamides, and treatment by a single injection of a long-acting sulphonamide was successful during the African epidemics of meningococcal meningitis. Thirty to forty per cent of strains are currently resistant to sulphonamides, which should not therefore be selected for treatment without prior sensitivity testing (Brion *et al.*, 1979; Buogo, 1977).

The most active antibiotics are penicillin G and ampicillin and its derivatives. The daily dosage of penicillin G (which is our preference) is, for the adult, 20–30 million units given either as a continuous venous perfusion or by direct i.v. injection at a rate of 2 million units every 2 hours (in order to avoid reaching critical threshold of 10 u/ml in C.S.F., above which there is a risk of convulsions). The dosage of ampicillin is 150–200 mg/kg in 6 intravenous injections. In patients allergic to β–lactams, the usual alternatives are thiamphenicol or chloramphenicol hemisuccinate, by the venous route: 3 g for adults and 50–100 mg/kg for children. Cotrimoxazole (trimethoprim–sulphamethoxazole combination) could also be used if the organism is sulphonamide sensitive.

In complicated forms of meningococcaemia, the antibiotic regimen is the same as for the common form of the disease, and can be associated with the treatment of those complications.

In Africa, during the epidemics of cerebrospinal meningitis in rural areas, Rey and colleagues recommended treatment with a single intramuscular injection of an oily suspension of chloramphenicol (Saliou *et al.*, 1977). Excellent results were achieved (with only 7% mortality) from a dosage ranging from 1 to 3 g depending on weight. A second injection was administered two days later if the first had had no clinical effect.

Anti-meningococcal oral chemoprophylaxis of close contacts is effected by a 5 day course of antibiotic treatment. The choice of an antibiotic which does not diffuse into the meninges is recommended. The combination of minocycline with rifampicin gives the most consistent results (Munford *et al.*, 1974). However, vestibular side-effects from minocycline and the risk of emergence of rifampicin resistant strains, added to which is the high cost of treatment, deter most clinicians from using this combination in practice. It seems just as reasonable to us to choose a macrolide (such as spiramycin, which gives the best concentrations in saliva). Prophylaxis can also be accomplished with anti-meningococcal A or C vaccine, which can be used to check an epidemic or to limit the spread from a source of infection.

Gonococcal Infections

Against uncomplicated gonococcal urethritis most clinicians prescribe a single dose treatment (Anon., 1979c; Sparling and Lee, 1978). The penicillins remain the antibiotics of choice. Aqueous procaine penicillin G, given as an intramuscular injection of 4.8 million units preceded by a 1 g dose of probenecid, has the advantage of eliminating incipient syphilis. Ampicillin (3.5 g) or amoxicillin (3 g) may be given by mouth, each with 1 g of probenecid. Neither the long acting forms of penicillin (e.g. benzathine–penicillin) nor the oral preparations of penicillin (e.g. penicillin V) are recommended for treatment of gonococcal infections.

A special problem is posed by the recent appearance of penicillinase-producing gonococci, identified in the U.K., Australia, Far East, U.S.A., Norway, and lately in France. Their spread is naturally feared. However, their rarity is such that in France it is not yet justified to modify classical treatment regimens, but greater vigilance is all that is needed.

Other antibiotics can be prescribed for gonococcal urethritis. For single dose treatment, spectinomycin can be given as an intramuscular injection (2 g), and possibly thiamphenicol by the oral route (2.5 g). Alternatively, for 5 day treatment tetracyclines may be selected, 2 g daily being given in 4 divided doses one hour before or two hours after meals.

Whatever the antibiotic selected, the following additional considerations are basic to the treatment of gonococcal infections. First, the possible course of syphilis should be followed serologically; second, a complete bacteriological cure should be ensured at the end of treatment for urethritis; third, sexual partners should be treated. In practice the majority of infections recurring after the therapeutic regimens have been followed are the result of re-infection and require examination for a latent focus of infection (salpingo—oophoritis, bartholinitis, etc.), and an investigation of partners who may have gone unrecognised, with a view to treatment.

There are alternative treatments for other localised gonococcal infections (Anon., 1979c; Sparling and Lee, 1978). In ano-rectal infections, penicillins are apparently more effective than other antibiotics. Localised complications such as orchio—epididymitis and salpingo—oophoritis, and systemic manifestations, e.g. septicaemia, meningitis, arthritis, and cutaneous gonococcal infection, can be cured only by means of high doses of antibiotics prescribed for at least 10 days. Penicillin G (10—20 million units daily intravenously) and ampicillin or amoxicillin (one dose of 3—4 g followed by 2 g daily) are the most effective. The only indication for an alternative medication is allergy to penicillins, in which case a tetracycline is preferred (except during pregnancy) or else erythromycin and, for meningitis, chloramphenicol. Treatment of complications and systemic manifestations due to penicillinase-producing gonococci calls for cefoxitin, which has proven activity, or tetracyclines or thiamphenicol. Nevertheless, none of these antibiotics is clear of resistance and sensitivity testing must always be carried out.

Patients sensitised to penicillins or to probenecid can be treated with tetracyclines, thiamphenicol, erythromycin (2 g daily for 5 days) or spectinomycin. In pregnancy, when penicillins are the treatment of choice, spectinomycin can be used in the event of sensitisation to β—lactams. In the neonate, penicillins are also the best curative treatment. Ophthalmia can be prevented by application of an ointment or eye-drops containing tetracyclines or erythromycin, or of a 1% solution of silver nitrate.

Infections with Haemophilus Influenzae

Until 1973, ampicillin was consistently active against *H. influenzae*. Since then, penicillinase-producing (and thus aminopenicillin resistant) strains have been isolated in the U.S.A., Canada, the U.K. and France (Anon., 1976; Dabernat *et al.*, 1978; Elwell *et al.*, 1975; Goldstein *et al.*, 1977; Gunn, 1974; Katz, 1975; Lambert-Zechovsky and Bingen, 1979; Medeiros and O'Brien, 1975; Rossier *et al.*, 1977; Sorin and Mozziconacci, 1977; Stewart, 1974; Tometh *et al.*, 1974). These strains originated not only from cases of meningitis but also from pneumopathies and upper respiratory tract infections. In the meningitis cases, ampicillin, despite being used at high dosage (300 mg/kg daily), was ineffective and the cerebro-spinal fluid was not sterile even after 24–48 hours of treatment. The frequency of such observations increased and ranged from 3 to 10%.

Because of this new situation, the bacteriologist must examine any newly isolated strain for possible synthesis of β–lactamase, using rapid techniques (Kammer *et al.*, 1975). While awaiting the result of this test, we believe it reasonable to prescribe for meningitis either ampicillin at very high dosage (400 mg/kg daily) or, right from the start, chloramphenicol (which is bactericidal to sensitive strains) at normal dosage (50–100 mg/kg daily) (Brunel *et al.*, 1980). The macrolides and trimethoprim–sulphonamide combinations can be recommended as first line treatments for upper or lower respiratory tract infections. In the face of the inconsistent efficacy of macrolides when prescribed alone, Schwartz proposed combining erythromycin with a sulphonamide straight away.

The possibility of encountering strains of *H. influenzae* resistant to chloramphenicol deserves mention (Kattan, 1976). Their frequency, however, remains very low and should not cause the therapeutic regimens described above to be modified. Even more unusual are strains with multiple resistance towards ampicillin and chloramphenicol. They have been isolated from infections other than meningitis and generally remain sensitive to macrolides and trimethoprim–sulphonamide combinations. Resistance to tetracyclines, including minocycline, has become frequent (10–15% of strains) (Dabernat *et al.*, 1978). The isolation of a multi-resistant strain responsible for meningitis warrants a test of its sensitivity to trimethoprim–sulphonamide combinations as well as to the new cephalosporins and cephamycins. It would be most desirable to have at one's disposal for such a case cephalosporins or cephamycins which are at the same time stable to β–lactamases, and diffusible at therapeutic levels into the cerebro-spinal fluid. Thus cefamandole may be worth trying (Kammer *et al.*, 1975).

Conclusion

At the conclusion of this necessarily succinct account, we can infer that whilst certain common bacterial pathogens are still sensitive to β–lactams, the majority will gradually acquire some degree of resistance to these antibiotics. With this in prospect, the main line of research to be followed is the establishment of new antibiotic molecules which are not altered by bacterial enzymes. The stability of some of the newer cephalosporins and cephamycins to β–lactamases is an example. It might also be conceivable to restore the original sensitivity of the organism by neutralising the enzymes it secretes. Finally, substances other than antibiotics might be implicated, including immunostimulants or antiseptics which are injectable by one of the usual parenteral routes.

References

Anonymous authors (1976). *Morbid. Mortal. Weekly Rep.* **25**, 385–386.

Anonymous authors (1979a). *Pathol. Biol.* **27**, 509–588.

Anonymous authors (1979b). *Lancet* **II**, 565–566.

Anonymous authors (1979c). *Ann. Intern. Med.* **90**, 809–811.

Acar, J.F., Cayeux, P., Goldstein, F.W. and Bouanchaud, D.H. (1974). 14th ICAAC, San Francisco, Abstract NO 339.

Appelbaum, P., Seraff, N., Bowen, A., Bhamjee, A., Hallett, A.F. and Cooper, R.C. (1977). *Lancet* **II**, 995–997.

Bastin, R., Frottier, J., Kernbaum, S. and Dournon, E. (1977). "XIVè Congrès International de Thérapeutique", pp. 325–340. Expansion Scient. Paris.

Beam, T. (1979). *Lancet* **II**, 227–228.

Brion, M., Mouton, Y. and Fourrier, A. (1979). *Méd. Hyg.* **37**, 401–406.

Brunel, D., Despaux, E., Astruc, J. and Rodière, M. (1980). *Nouv. Presse Méd.* **9**, 188.

Buogo, A. (1977). *Chemotherapy* **23**, 73–80.

Buré, A.M., Witchitz, J. and Hornstein, M. (1975). *Méd. Mal. Infect.* **5**, 156–163.

Christol, D., Boussougant, Y., Buré, A.M., Witchitz, J., Zribi, A. and Dupuis, M. (1971). *Lyon Méd.* **225**, 99–108.

Cybulska, J., Jeljaszervicz, J., Lund, E. and Munksgaard, A. (1970). *Chemotherapy* **15**, 304–316.

Dabernat, H., Bauriaud, R., Delmas, C., Lefèvre, J.C., Lemozy, J. and Lareng, M.B. (1978). *Méd. Mal. Infect.* **8**, 244–249.

Dixon, J. (1974). *Lancet* **II**, 474.

Dixon, J. and Lipinski, A. (1974). *J. Infect. Dis.* **130**, 351–356.

Dublanchet, A. and Durieux, R. (1979). *Nouv. Presse Méd.* **8**, 872.

Elwell, L.P., De Graaff, J., Seibert, D. and Falkow, S. (1975). *Infect. Immun.* **12**, 404–410.

Fleurette, J. (1977). *Encycl. Méd. Chir. Mal. Infect.* 8007 – A.10.

Frottier, J. (1977). *Ann. Méd. Interne* **128**, 521–526.

Garrod, L.P., Lambert, H.P. and O'Grady, F. (1973). "Antibiotic and Chemotherapy", 4th edn, Churchill Livingstone, Edinburgh and London.

Goldstein, F.W., Boisivon, A., Leclerc, P. and Acar, J.F. (1977). *Pathol. Biol.* 25, 323–332.

Goldstein, F.W., Dang Van, A., Bouanchaud, D.H. and Acar, J.F. (1978). *Pathol. Biol.* 26, 173–180.

Gunn, B.A. (1974). *Lancet* II, 845.

Hansman, D. (1975). *Med. J. Aust.* 2, 740–742.

Hansman, D. (1977). 10th International Congress Chemotherapy, Zurich, Abstract N⁰ 405.

Hansman, D., Glasgow, H., Sturt, J., Devitt, L. and Douglas, R. (1971). *New Engl. J. Med.* 284, 175–177.

Harves, V. and Mitchell, R. (1976). *Brit. Med. J.* 2, 996.

Hawley, B. and Gump, D. (1973). *Am. J. Dis. Child.* 126, 261–264.

Howard, A., Hince, C. and Williams, J. (1978). *Brit. Med. J.* 1, 1657–1660.

Jacobs, M., Koornhof, H., Robins-Browna, R., Stevenson, C., Vermaak, Z., Freiman, I., Bennie Miller, G. Witcomb, M.A., Isaacson, M., Ward, J.I. and Austrian, R. (1978). *New Engl. J. Med.* 299, 735–740.

Kagan, B. (1974). "Antimicrobial Therapy", 2nd edn., Saunders, Philadelphia.

Kammer, R., Preston, D., Turner, J. and Hawley, L. (1975). *Antimicrob. Agents Chemother.* 8, 91–94.

Kattan, S. (1976). *Lancet* I, 814.

Katz, S.L. (1975). *Pediatrics* 55, 6–8.

Kernbaum, S. (1979). *Méd. Hyg.* 37, 415–416.

Kucers, A. and McBennett, N. (1975). "The Use of Antibiotics". Heinemann, London.

Lambert-Zechovsky, N. and Bingen, E. (1979). *Nouv. Presse Méd.* 8, 2199.

Laverdière, M., Peterson, P., Verhoef, J., Williams, D.N. and Sabath, L.D. (1978). *J. Infect. Dis.* 137, 245–249.

Lerner, P., Gopalakrishna, K., Wolinsky, E., McHenry, M., Tan, J. and Rosenthal, M. (1977). *Medicine* 56, 457–473.

Medeiros, A.A. and O'Brien, T.F. (1975). *Lancet* I, 716–718.

Miyamura, S., Ochiai, H. and Nitahara, Y. (1977). *Microbiol. Immunol.* 21, 69–76.

Munford, R.S., Vasconcelos, Z., Philips, J., Gelli, D.S., Gorman, G.W., Risi, J.B. and Feldman, R.A. (1974). *J. Infect. Dis.* 129, 644–649.

Naragi, S., Kirkpatrick, G. and Kabins, S. (1974). *J. Pediatr.* 85, 671–673.

Neu, H.C. (1978). *In* "Seminars in Infectious Disease", Vol. 1. (L. Weinstein and B.N. Fields, eds), pp. 97–121, Straton Intercontinental Medical Book Corporation, New York.

Noble, W. and Naidoo, J. (1978). *Br. J. Dermatol.* 98, 481–489.

Paredes, A., Taber, L., Yow, M., Clark, D. and Nathan, W. (1976). *Pediatrics* 58, 378–381.

Parillo, J., Borst, G. and Mazur, M. (1979). *New Eng. J. Med.* 300, 296–300.

Peyrefitte, F., Galland, A., Mathuret, C., Goldstein, F.W. and Bouvet, A. (1979). *Nouv. Presse Méd.* 8, 872.

Pulliam, L. and Hadley, K. (1979). *New Engl. J. Med.* 300, 1442.

Rossier, A., Chabrolle, J.P., Salomon, J.L., Bergeret, M., Raymond, J. and Acar, J.F. (1977). *Nouv. Presse Méd.* 6, 3432.

Saliou, P., Ouedraogo, L., Muslin, D. and Rey, M. (1977). *Méd. Trop.* 37, 189–193.

Sorin, M. and Mozziconacci, P. (1977). Journées Parisiennes de Pédiatrie, pp. 173–180.

Sparling, P.F. and Lee, T.J. (1978). *In* "Seminars in Infectious Disease", Vol. 1. (L. Weinstein and B.N. Fields, eds), pp. 34–67. Straton Intercontinental Medical Book Corporation, New York.

Sprunt, K., Redman, W. and Leidy, G. (1968). *Pediatrics* **42**, 957–968.

Stewart, S.M. (1974). *Lancet* I, 1163–1164.

Suksuwan, M. (1975). *J. Med. Ass. Thailand* **58**, 283–286.

Tempest, B., Carney, J. and Aberle, B. (1974). *J. Infect. Dis.* **130**, 67–69.

Tometh, M.O., Stan, S.E., McGowan, J.E. Jr., Terry, P.M. and Nahmias, A.J. (1974). *J. Am. Med. Assoc.* **229**, 295.

Weinstein, L. (1975). *In* "The Pharmacological Basis of Therapeutics", 5th edn, (L. Goodman and A. Gilman, eds). McMillan, New York.

Discussion

Professor Fillastre: As a nephrologist, I wish to add a comment. For staphylococcal infections you still recommend methicillin. We now have a list of 150 case reports of immunoallergic interstitial nephropathy secondary to the use of methicillin, with serious lesions combined with haemorrhagic cystitis and also with changes in blood count. As a nephrologist I do not use any more methicillin. I should like to have your opinion since you suggest there are other therapeutic options.

Another important point is that you spoke of the possible potentiation of a toxic effect by combining cephalosporins and aminoglycosides. I wish to say that we published a great deal on this point a few years ago and I now feel that we were wrong. There are now many publications which suggest the lack of such potentiation. We have recently re-examined the problem, focusing essentially on modifications of subcellular structures, such as mitochondria and lysosomes. We have even studied intrarenal concentrations of aminoglycosides when animals have been pretreated with various cephalosporins. We now find no potentiation of the toxic effect of an aminoglycoside by cephalosporins. I think this is an important point.

The last comment I wish to make is that when nephrologists are dealing with a great number of patients undergoing haemodialysis or peritoneal dialysis, we are confronted with the problem of staphylococcal infections. As you pointed out, we should consider vancomycin in these particular patients, since drug accumulation may be considerable, and it is sometimes the most appropriate treatment for these infections which may be serious.

Professor Frottier: Thank you for your comments. I feel that it is important in a symposium like this to report your experiments on the absence of toxicity of a combination of aminoglycosides and cephalosporins. As for the first question, my account was extremely rapid and schematic, but I did not say methicillin but rather the methicillin group. In my department we do not use methicillin any more but mainly oxacillin.

Professor Chabanon: We have therapeutic problems when treating genital infections by group B streptococci in pregnant women, since when we carry out post-therapeutic monitoring we note that group B streptococci are particularly persistent in the vagina. We would like to have your opinion on this matter.

Professor Frottier: I feel that in a situation of this type we can sometimes combine systemic treatment with ampicillin at high dosages with a local treatment, depending on the antibiotic sensitivity of the organism. I personally have no direct experience in this field.

Professor Kunin: I am perplexed that Professor Frottier has found no nephrotoxicity with the cephalosporins and aminoglycosides. It is insufficient to say simply "cephalosporins" and "aminoglycosides", since patients have to be given a specific member of these two classes of antibiotics. Cephaloridine, a specific cephalosporin, is clearly nephrotoxic — and it is also clearly nephrotoxic when it is used with an aminoglycoside. Therefore Professor Frottier's statement should be modified to say that certain specific cephalosporins being used do not cause nephrotoxicity.

Secondly, if a patient is on dialysis, why not use methicillin? That patient has no kidneys to be destroyed. Methicillin is a perfectly good drug to use in these circumstances quite appropriately.

Finally, much of the information of methicillin nephrotoxicity is correct. Many of us have stopped using this drug because of the case reports of nephrotoxicity. But all the penicillins and cephalosporins may occasionally produce a lesion resembling that described with methicillin. It appears that methicillin is more commonly associated with this than other agents. I agree with Professor Frottier's recommendations, but certainly not in patients with end-stage renal failure who will not suffer from methicillin toxicity.

Professor Williams: May I add to Professor Kunin's comments that man behaves quite differently from the rat. I think that Professor Fillastre was referring specifically to the rat. Quite a lot of studies have shown that the rat kidney does not seem to suffer from the combination of cephaloridine and aminoglycoside, but the clinical evidence is that man suffers quite substantially from such a combination.

Professor Kunin: I also treat rabbits with that combination, and they also suffer.

The Evolution of Resistance Among the Common Bacterial Pathogens

J.F. ACAR, F.W. GOLDSTEIN and A. BUU-HOI

Hôpital St. Joseph, Hôpital Broussais et
U.E.R. Cordeliers, Université P. et M. Curie, Paris

Introduction

The Common Bacterial Pathogens

It is only very recently that the development of resistance to anti-biotics among common bacterial pathogens has assumed a significance that is not just bacteriological but clinical. Apart from *Staphylococcus aureus, E. coli*, shigellae and salmonellae, all responsible for digestive tract infections, the other frequent human bacterial pathogens (group A streptococci, pneumococci, *Haemophilus*, gonococci and meningococci) have for a long time retained their normal sensitivity to antibiotics. Cases of rare strains resistant to one or two antibiotics are well isolated in terms of both time and place. Hence Finland (1972) wrote that no strain of a Group A streptococcus had been found resistant to sulphonamides since the strains were observed in 1945.

Since 1973, many publications have demonstrated that the acquisition of resistance to one or several antibiotics has affected almost all microbial species. The factors which govern the epidemiology and cyclical evolution of the phenomenon are unknown.

It is customary to categorise under the term "common bacterial pathogens" the species responsible for the spontaneous infections encountered in general practice. From respiratory infections there are the group A streptococci, the pneumococci and *Haemophilus*; from cutaneous infections, *Staphylococcus aureus*; from infections of the genito-urinary tract there are *E. coli* and the gonococci; and from gastro-intestinal infections, shigellae and salmonellae. This collection of microbial species represents the principal grounds for the use of antibiotics, and it is justified to observe their behaviour in response to these agents.

Difficulties in the Study of Common Bacterial Pathogens

It is on this point that published reports are very fragmentary. There are several reasons for this:

1) Their information is founded on sampling procedures which, more often than not, are biased. Thus the more common and uncomplicated the infection, the less accurate is the diagnosis and the less likely is a bacteriological examination to be carried out. The samples are usually collected either at the time of an epidemic, when repeated isolation of the same organism is apparent, or in the hospital environment where the patient's social status or the severity of the infection dictates the importance of sampling.

2) The detection of a new resistance marker in these species is difficult. Antibiotic sensitivity testing of common pathogens is still often neglected, and when it is performed, it is based on a small number of antibiotics considered to be the most frequently used. It is therefore necessary to make use of special techniques. On the other hand, to this difficulty in detecting a new resistance marker must be added that of examining the large number of strains necessary to achieve the objectives of detection of resistance and accumulation of information. Unless a widespread programme of research is mounted, it is only when a resistance marker reaches around 10% of strains isolated that it becomes readily detectable.

3) The proliferation and persistence of one or more resistance determinants in these microbial species are hard to follow because one encounters all the difficulties associated with the problem of sampling. Furthermore, the comparison of data from one year to another assumes that the hospital admits similar types of patients. In fact, the type of hospital patients undergoes an "evolution" as a result of alterations in the prescribing habits of hospital doctors as well as community doctors.

Having set out all these reservations, the aim of this paper is to report results collected between 1973 and 1979 on common bacterial pathogens, isolated from clinical cases by our hospital laboratory.

Materials and Methods

Microbial Species

Group A streptococci, pneumococci, *Haemophilus influenzae* and *H. parainfluenzae, Staphylococcus aureus*, the coliform organisms responsible for urinary tract infections, and gonococci were all studied. No organism responsible for digestive tract infections was included in this study, owing to the small number of isolates and the limitations of our clinical and epidemiological information on these cases. The organisms were stored at $-70°$C.

Antibiotic Sensitivity Testing

Sensitivity tests were carried out by the International Collaborative Study method (ICS), using a constant range of antibiotics (Ericsson and Sherris, 1971).

Beta-Lactamase Production

The production of beta-lactamase was systematically investigated by an iodometric or acidimetric method in gonococci and in *Haemophilus* strains (Gots, 1945; O'Callaghan *et al.*, 1972; Jorgensen *et al.*, 1977).

Recognition and Determination of Resistance

Resistance was examined by the measurement of m.i c. values (agar dilution method) and by evaluation of the deviation between these m.i.c. values (or the corresponding inhibition zone diameters) and the histogram of values for normally sensitive organisms.

In some cases, specimens of organisms recognised to be resistant were studied retrospectively for their sensitivity to antibiotics, their bacteriological characteristics, and the genetic and biochemical bases for their resistance. The resistance characteristics thus observed were expressed as a "resistance profile". In this way, the groups were identified for which the relationship between serotypes or biotypes and resistance could eventually be studied.

Collection and Processing of the Data

The methods used had earlier been described by T. O'Brien *et al.* (1975). With the reservations already listed above, the validity of the sampling was considered acceptable for the Group A streptococci, pneumococci, *Haemophilus* and gonococci isolated from patients in the community or from patients in hospital with acute infections.

For *Staphylococcus aureus* and the coliform bacteria, we used the "isolation index" described by O'Brien *et al.* (1975). By grouping the strains within each species by their "resistance profile", an "index" was established for each profile, denoting the ratio between the number of strains isolated beyond the 7th day of hospitalisation and the number of strains isolated during the first week. The profiles for which the index was less than unity were deemed as belonging to organisms probably acquired outside the hospital. It was by reference to the profiles for which the index was less than unity that the distinction between staphylococci and coliform organisms of the "community" and of the "hospital" was made.

Results

Pneumococci

The number and the percentage of resistant strains are shown in Table 1 as well as the evolution of their "resistance profile" between

TABLE 1

Number and Percentage of Resistant Pneumococci and Evolution of their Resistance Profile between 1970 and 1979

Year	1970	1971	1972	1973	1974	1975	1976	1977	1978	1979
N⁰ of isolates	70	95	138	140	111	149	164	185	189	246
Resistant strains										
Total number	10	20	47	29	39	54	65	65	88	82
%	14.3	21	34	20.7	35.1	36.2	39.6	35.1	46.5	33.3
Resistance profile (a)										
(total number)										
Tc	10	20	46	24	34	46	53	51	68	52
Tc Cm			1	5	5	8	10	11	8	14
Tc Em							2		6	13
Tc Cm Em								3	4	2
Tc Cm Em Pc									2	1

(a) Tc = tetracyclines; Cm = chloramphenicol; Em = erythromycin; Pc = penicillin G

1970 and 1979. Some very rare strains with slight resistance to penicillin G have been detected since 1978. Among the other resistance features, resistance to tetracyclines revealed a modest decline in 1979. It is noted that any other resistance is always linked to tetracycline resistance. Table 2 shows the 7 most frequent serotypes, accounting for 60% or more of the strains isolated in the year, as well as other serotypes in which at least 30% of the strains are resistant to one or more antibiotics. The most prevalent serotypes are not necessarily the most resistant organisms. For example, serotype 23 is often isolated but is rarely resistant. On the other hand, serotypes

TABLE 2

Relationship between Serotypes and Antibiotypes among Pneumococci (1976–1979)

Serotype	1976		1977		1978		1979	
Nº	C (a)	R (b)	C	R	C	R	C	R
19	*	+	*	+	*	+	*	+
6	*	+	*	+	*	+	*	+
23	*	–	*	–	*	+	*	–
7	*	+	*	+	*	–		+
18	*	+		–		–		–
1	*	+		–		–		–
4	*	+		–		–		–
15		+	*	+	*	–	*	+
3		–	*	–	*	–	*	–
14		–	*	–	*	+	*	–
11		–		–		–	*	+

(a) C : (*) Classified among the 7 most frequent serotypes detected in the year.
(b) R : Rate of resistance in the serotype.
Number of resistant strains superior to 30% (+), inferior to 30% (–).

such as 6 and 19 are both frequent and resistant. This information would tend to the conclusion that the acquisition of resistance by pneumococci has diminished neither their virulence nor pathogenicity.

Haemophilus

The distribution of *Haemophilus* isolates and of their resistance profile is shown in Table 3 and, as above, indicates a slight decline in resistant strains in 1979 and clear predominance of tetracycline resistance. The resistance profiles are very varied. The existence of resistance to kanamycin and to streptomycin is puzzling since both antibiotics are as infrequently prescribed in community medicine as in hospital medicine. Resistance to ampicillin, observed since 1975, can accompany all other resistance markers (Goldstein *et al.*, 1977).

Group A Streptococci

Close to 50% of strains are resistant to tetracyclines. Resistance to erythromycin and to chloramphenicol has been observed in a small number of strains (Table 4).

TABLE 3

Number and Percentage of Resistant *Haemophilus* Strains and Evolution of their Resistance Profile between 1974 and 1979

Year	1974	1975	1976	1977	1978	1979
Nº of isolates	151	263	328	361	398	515
Resistant strains						
Total number	4	9	48	50	59	44
%	2.6	3.4	14.6	13.8	14.8	8.6
Resistance profile (a) (total number)						
Tc	4	7	35	21	23	11
Tc Km		1	2	5	3	
Tc Km Am		1	6	13	8	7
Tc Cm			2	2	5	
Cm			2	1	3	1
Tc Am Cm			1	1	2	
Tc Am				2	4	3
Am				2	2	8
Sm				3	4	2
Km					2	12
Km Sm					1	
Tc Km Am Cm					1	
Tc Km Am Cm Sm					1	

(a) Tc = tetracyclines, Km = kanamycin, Am = ampicillin, Cm = chloramphenicol, Sm = streptomycin.

TABLE 4

Number and Percentage of Resistant *Streptococcus* A Strains and Evolution of their Resistance Profile between 1976 and 1979

Year	1976	1977	1978	1979
Nº of isolates	95	102	111	67
Resistant strains				
Total number	44	44	56	27
%	46.3	43.1	50.4	40.3
Resistance profile (a) (total number)				
Tc	44	42	52	26
Tc Em		2	3	1
Tc Cm			1	

(a) Tc = tetracyclines; Em = erythromycin; Cm = chloramphenicol.

Gonococci

Forty to fifty strains are isolated annually in our hospital laboratory. This represents too limited a sample in order to detect or follow the appearance of resistant strains. In our series, only streptomycin resistance affected up to around 10% of strains examined during the past 4 years. An extensive investigation in a specialist practice has shown that out of 420 strains, penicillin resistance was due in 4 cases to the production of beta-lactamase (Thabaut *et al.*, 1980).

Staphylococcus aureus

The resistance profiles of at least 90% of the strains having no connection with hospital infections seem remarkably consistent (Table 5). They are characterised principally by the production of penicillinase and by their resistance to tetracyclines. Strains resistant to more than 5 antibiotics occur and these represent 3 to 5% of the total.

TABLE 5

Number and Percentage of Resistant *Staphylococcus aureus* and Evolution of their Resistance Profile between 1973 and 1979

Year	1973	1974	1975	1976
Nº of isolates	607	613	545	939
Resistant strains				
Total number	506	545	454	797
%	83.4	89.0	83.3	85.0
Resistance profile (a)				
(total number)				
Pc	324	409	345	550
Tc	42	18	17	18
Pc Tc	77	86	83	131
Pc Tc Em	15			14
miscellaneous (b)	48	32	19	84
(c)	(25)	(16)	(14)	(34)

(a) Pc = penicillin G; Tc = tetracyclines; Em = erythromycin.
(b) other multiresistance profiles.
(c) resistance to 5 or more antibiotics.

Coliform Organisms

The situation is very similar for the coliform organisms. We have compared (Table 6) the results from our laboratory with those obtained from routine community practice (Chabbert, pers. comm.). The most frequent resistance profiles are similar in the two series; 80% of strains are either sensitive or resistant to tetracyclines, sulphonamides and streptomycin, whilst 7% are multiresistant to 5 or more antibiotics.

TABLE 6

Comparison of the Resistance Profile of *E. coli* strains isolated at St Joseph Hospital
and from the Community

Resistance profile (a)	% Strains	
	Out patients (St. Joseph Hospital) 1973–1976 (2559 strains)	Community (b) 1974 (728 strains)
Sensible	56.8%	57.0%
Tc	8.1%	4.7%
Su	3.2%	1.2%
Tc Su	7.2%	2.2%
Su Sm	2.3%	2.7%
Tc Su Sm	5.2%	7.4%
miscellaneous (c)	17.2%	24.8%
(d)	(7.2%)	(6.9%)

(a) Tc = tetracyclines; Su = sulphamides; Sm = streptomycin.
(b) Y. Chabbert, pers. comm.
(c) other multiresistance profiles.
(d) resistance to 5 or more antibiotics.

Discussion

Common pathogenic bacterial species are not exempt from resistance and transfer factors and, for this reason, require surveillance. Throughout the results given here and those of other authors, there is the indication that a resistance marker appears on a particular date and in a particular place, defining in this way a stage in the history of the bacterial species concerned. This marker may be single or associated with other pre-existing or new markers. The time course of acquisition of these different biochemical, genetic and epidemiological characters can be monitored.

In medical microbiology what matters is overall penetration of the resistance marker within the species, that is to say the number of strains affected by the resistance. From that moment on, the genetic characterization of the marker will have real predictive value, with transferable plasmids seeming more suited to spreading throughout a species than other possible genetic support mechanisms. It must, however, be emphasised that resistance plasmids have been demonstrated in *Haemophilus* and in group A streptococci, but not in the pneumococci (Dang Van *et al.*, 1975; Goldstein *et al.*, 1977; Buu-Hoï and Horodniceanu, 1980) while tetracycline resistance has spread throughout these species in apparently similar fashion.

The frequency of resistance in common pathogenic species appears to become stable, after an initial period of spread. The level eventually reached may vary greatly, thus it occurred between 7 and 45% in the data described here. Occasionally, certain episodes of resistance remain very localised and occur with irregular annual frequency, an example being resistance to erythromycin among pneumococci and group A streptococci (Goldstein *et al.*, 1978).

Among the many factors which govern the development of resistance characters within a species, the infective capacity of the host strain and its virulence properties will, respectively, be instrumental in the immediate spread and the later limitation of the characters. The epidemics of multiresistant pneumococci or of group A streptococci resistant to erythromycin were without doubt responsive to these factors in giving rise to very substantial annual fluctuations, which were interpreted after the event in terms of a disappearance or a resurgence of the resistance (Goldstein *et al.*, 1978). On this last point, it seems that these resistance characters did not disappear but became stabilised in different species at very variable frequencies, depending on their location (and conditions of hygiene therein) and other selective pressures. In France, the relative stability of resistance to tetracycline in the pneumococci seems to be connected with the fact that for 10 years this resistance has become associated with the most common serotypes (Goldstein *et al.*, 1978). The spread of resistance from strain to strain or from species to species remains a most interesting phenomenon but one most difficult to demonstrate. It is likely that the character specifically governing the transfer of certain plasmids is an important factor. On the other hand, chloramphenicol resistance, although not plasmid-mediated in this species, has straight away pervaded 15 different pneumococcal serotypes.

The progressive monitoring of resistance and of sensitivity profiles in common pathogens is justified. Three sources of information may be available: the well characterised epidemics; studies focusing on one particular species, based on observations within a community or a region; the periodic records drawn up by public health laboratories and hospital laboratories, with appropriate sampling corrections. The ecological interest in such studies is obvious.

From the clinical standpoint, significant events of recent years (e.g. the lethal epidemic of multiresistant pneumococci, therapeutic failures in gonococcal infections and in meningitis due to penicillinase-producing *Haemophilus* strains) lead to the statement of certain objectives:

1) the early resolution of epidemics caused by organisms which are not generally resistant;
2) the modification of attitudes to therapy by taking notice of

bacteriological and statistical data. This point involves recognition of the percentage of resistant strains, which should influence the initial choice of therapy in routine medical practice;
3) the initiation of studies enabling precise recognition of those infections for which the identification of the causative organism and of its sensitivity to antibiotics are indispensable.

In practice, few resistance characters in common pathogens attain a frequency such that it justifies both the exclusion of the customary antibiotic and the need for antibiotic sensitivity testing. Thus in pneumococcal respiratory infections, for which initial treatment with tetracyclines is proscribed, the pneumococcal strains remain, with rare exceptions, sensitive to other antibiotics.

Nevertheless, in every type of infection from 3 to 10% of patients risk treatment failure if use is not made of laboratory testing. For example, 8% of infections by coliform organisms present a therapeutic problem owing to a multiresistant strain. In this case the percentage has no significance and it becomes a question of knowing how to recognise this special group of patients as distinct from the group affected by sensitive strains. We have been able to show that patients presenting with short-term recurrent urinary tract infections belong to the latter group, as opposed to those with infections recurring at intervals of about 6 months (unpub. results).

Conclusion

In summary, we believe that it is essential to identify and monitor resistance in pathogenic bacteria, to recognise the patients infected by such resistant organisms and to draw together the information on a country-wide scale in order to be able to make comparisons and to try to improve our predictive capabilities in this subject.

References

Buu-Hoï, A. and Horodniceanu, T. (1980). *J. Bacteriol.* **143**, 313–320.

Dang Van, A., Bieth, G. and Bouanchaud, D.H. (1975). *C.R. Hebd. Séances Acad. Sci. Sér. D* **280**, 1321–1323.

Ericsson, H.M. and Sherris, J.C. (1971). *Acta Pathol. Microbiol. Scand.* Section A. Suppl. Nᵒ 217, 9–90.

Finland, M. (1972). *Ann. Intern. Med.* **76**, 1009–1036.

Goldstein, F.W., Boisivon, A., Leclerc, P. and Acar, J.F. (1977). *Pathol. Biol.* **25**, 323–332.

Goldstein, F.W., Dang Van, A., Bouanchaud, D.H. and Acar, J.F. (1978). *Pathol. Biol.* **26**, 173–180.

Gots, J.S. (1945). *Science* **102**, 309.

Jorgensen, J.H., Lee, J.C. and Alexander, G.A. (1977). *Antimicrob. Agents Chemother.* **11**, 1087–1088.

O'Brien, T.F., Kent, R.L. and Medeiros, A.A. (1975). *J. Infect. Dis.* **131**, 88–96.

O'Callaghan, C.H., Morris, A., Kirby, S.M. and Shingler, A.H. (1972). *Antimicrob. Agents Chemother.* **1**, 283–288.

Thabaut, A., Durosoir, J.-L., Saliou, P., Dolivo, M., Lecam, J.-Y., Weinmann, J.-M. and Martin-Bouyer, G. (1980). *Ann. Microbiol.* (Inst. Pasteur) **131 A**, 91.

Discussion

Professor Sabath: Professor Acar's survey was comprehensive. I would like to hear his comments on some data from elsewhere about a changing sensitivity pattern in *Staphylococcus aureus*. Specifically, in Denmark in the late 1960s, as many as about 40% of bacteraemic strains were methicillin resistant. I know that the proportion has been decreasing in Denmark since then, and I recently saw figures showing that in 1978 only 0.9% of *Staphylococcus aureus* isolates sent to the Statens Seruminstitut, in Copenhagen, were methicillin resistant. Can Professor Acar comment on this dramatic change in methicillin resistance in Denmark?

Professor Acar: I cannot comment on that change, other than by mentioning a similar observation in France. In outpatients, methicillin resistant strains represent between 1.2 and 1.8%. From the data we collected and from those presented by Professor Duval, there has, during the last three years, been a decrease in resistance to both methicillin and oxacillin in infections in hospital patients, from 35 or 36% to 20%. The last survey carried out in my hospital, taking all strains together, showed that 18 to 20% were resistant.

Professor Richmond: Professor Acar's work over the years in monitoring these situations is very much to be admired. What is lacking is other people doing the same monitoring in other parts of the world, or even of Europe. In Germany, a number of the people in the German Society of Microbiology have begun to set up such a survey. It emerges that certain strains have reached truly epidemic proportions. They are found all over Europe, and even all over the world. Others, however, can be localised in one hospital. The situation is changing all the time. There may be a fairly clear idea of the situation one month, but it is neither known how it will develop nor how it has already developed. There is a strong case for some international surveillance of these things. Even in the United States, which is after all a big country, I wonder whether there is not a place for a much more comprehensive review of what is going on. For example, I do not think that the CDC (Centre for Disease Control) habitually puts antibiotic discs on strains, does it?

Professor Kunin: With regard to Professor Richmond's and Professor Acar's presentations, and also some of our other discussions relating to how to select an antibiotic in an individual without having the susceptibility tests, may I suggest that the patient should be asked what antibiotic he has had recently. That would be a critical part of the historical basis for making a decision about which antibiotic to use. If the patient has had ampicillin or tetracycline within the past few months, I would assume that, at least in the urinary tract, the probability of resistance would be greater than in the population not taking the drugs in that period of time. Part of the susceptibility testing should be to ask the patient what antibiotics he has taken over the last months.

Professor Richmond: I think that Professor Acar would also agree that in certain places where certain antibiotics are used extensively, this becomes part of the history that must be taken into account. In the Paris newspaper *Le Monde*, there was an article about gentamicin resistance in staphylococcal infections in France at a time when such resistant strains were not common outside France. I think that this was a reflection of the history of gentamicin use in France.

Professor Vilde: I have two questions about resistance of pneumococci to penicillin. I am somewhat surprised at the importance of the phenomenon from a bacteriological point of view and I agree with you that a follow-up is necessary. But don't you think that there is a discrepancy between the bacteriological side and the clinical side, which shows that penicillin is in fact capable of solving the problems at least in France? So we might really be in a sort of inflationary situation when we use too many antibiotics. My second point is: do you have any explanation for the fact that this phenomenon has been noticed only recently, whereas the phenomenon of antibiotic resistance has been observed from the earliest antibiotics?

Professor Acar: I think that the situation is totally different from one country to another. The South African epidemic was due to the epidemic spread of pneumococci within poor communities where penicillin was used at low doses and you cannot compare this with the use of penicillin in France. You cannot compare either the probabilities of pneumococcal diagnosis because a lot of pneumococcal infections are not diagnosed, so you cannot simply base yourself on a given population. There is no good answer. These strains can be dealt with by high levels of penicillin but they must be tested in the laboratory; so one must first find the proper test to detect their penicillin resistance level.

Now, the reasons why a phenomenon is not noticed before a certain time is another point. I believe personally that the phenomenon may have existed beforehand, but later spread and became significant at a certain date. I think that Dr. Tomasz had previously found a penicillin resistant pneumococcal strain, and that Dr. Sabath had also recorded one, but these were isolated events, apart from the first epidemic in Papua which was in fact due to the same penicillin resistant strain. Perhaps this type of strain more readily leads to an epidemic, simply because penicillin has been used.

Professor Chabbert: Since the topic of this meeting is the future of antibiotic therapy, I would like to raise a question which seems to be of importance. Do you think that resistance cannot be avoided? Somebody said: "all you have to do is to introduce a new antibiotic and then resistance will appear somewhere". This seems to be supported by the fact that common pathogens can acquire plasmids which then spread through the species, but there are a number of other phenomena. So should we really have to live with the idea that resistance will inexorably increase, or should we adopt for the future the idea that resistance appears and stabilizes at ecological levels which might be governed by plasmid stabilization or other mechanisms? I think this is important for the clinician, who usually rushes to use the latest antibiotic, also for the lawyers, because if they think resistance is inevitable, they are urged to try and stop the introduction of new products. I would like to know what you think about this.

Professor Acar: I would rather agree with your second idea, that resistance does appear and stabilizes at an ecological level. The important point is the original appearance of the phenomenon, because you cannot reverse such a biological effect. As soon as one strain is capable of mutating or acquiring a plasmid the character can spread. So, it is really the emergence of the phenomenon which is important ecologically, and the stabilization level may prove to be important or totally unimportant clinically.

The Needs for New Antibiotics for Infection in Man

J.D. WILLIAMS

The London Hospital Medical College, London, U.K.

Introduction

The number of antibiotic substances which are presently available for treatment in man is already very large. The usage of antibiotics is such that already in most Western hospitals 20–30% of patients receive antibiotics (Scheckler and Bennett, 1970; McGowan and Finland, 1974); in England 60% of children have already received antibiotic therapy by the time they are one year old (Percival, pers. comm.).

For the ten years after the Second World War new antibiotics appeared at a rapid rate and were just as rapidly absorbed into clinical practice. During the next decade the number of new registrations of antibiotics fell (Kurylowicz, 1976), but since the mid 1960's there has been a further rapid increase in the number and variety of new antibiotic substances available. The recent large increases stem from the change in emphasis of research from the almost random search for active substances to the deliberate manipulation of established antibiotics to produce the present bewildering array of semi-synthetic compounds. Table 1 gives a classification of some of the compounds which are at this time in common clinical use or are in a stage where the widespread use is imminent. Table 2 shows how one single group of antibiotics, the cephalosporins, are being developed for future use (Williams and Williams, 1980; O'Callaghan, 1979). It is against this background that the future needs of antibiotics in man should be considered. In order to delineate present and future needs one has to consider the existing problems. This paper attempts to outline these difficulties in antibiotic usage and state some present needs.

TABLE 1

A Simple Classification of Antibiotic Substances used in Man

Group 1: Active against Gram-positive bacteria and Gram-negative cocci	Group 2: Active mainly against Gram-negative bacilli	Group 3: Broad spectrum antibiotics	Group 4: Used for specific infections
Standard penicillins	(2a) For systemic use:	Sulphonamides	(4a) Against aerobic organisms:
Benzylpenicillin	Ampicillin	Sulphadimidine	Lincomycin (clindamycin)
Phenoxymethylpenicillin	Ampicillin esters	Sulphadiazine	Metronidazole
Other oral penicillins	Amoxycillin	Sulphafurazole	
Antistaphylococcal penicillins	Ureidopenicillins	etc.	(4b) For tuberculosis:
Methicillin	Azlocillin	Cotrimoxazole	Streptomycin
Cloxacillin	Mezlocillin	Tetroxoprim	PAS
Flucloxacillin	Carbenicillin, Ticarcillin	Cephalosporins	Isoniazid
Erythromycin and other	Carbenicillin esters	Cephaloridine	Rifampicin
macrolides	Carfecillin	Cephalothin	Ethionamide
Lincomycin	Mecillinam	Cephradine	Pyrazinamide
Clindamycin	Pivmecillinam	Cephalexin	Ethambutol
Rifampicin	Aminoglycosides	Cefazolin	Cycloserine
Vancomycin	Streptomycin	Cefamandole	
	Neomycin	Cefuroxime	(4c) Antifungal agents:
	Kanamycin	Cefoxitin	Polyenes
	Gentamicin	Tetracyclines	Nystatin
	Tobramycin	Oxytetracycline	Amphotericin B
	Amikacin	Chlortetracycline	Candicidin
	Sisomicin	Minocycline	5–Fluorocytosine
	Dibekacin	Doxycycline	Clotrimazole
	Polypeptides	Chloramphenicol	Miconazole
	Polymyxin B		Econazole
	Colistin		Griseofulvin
	Bacitracin		
			(4d) Antiviral agents:
	(2b) For urinary tract infections:		Methisazone
	Nitrofurantoin		Idoxuridine
	Nalidixic acid		Amantadine
	Cinoxacin		Arabinosides
	Mandelamine		Acyclicguanides
	Hexamine		Phosphono compounds

TABLE 2

Developments in Cephalosporin-like Antibiotics which will Probably have Clinical Uses in
the Future. Classified Primarily on a Chemical Basis with a Group of Agents Active
Against *Pseudomonas*

Group 1	
3–Acetoxymethyl cephalosporins with variable metabolism to less active compounds and susceptible to beta-lactamases of Gram-negatives.	Cephalothin Cephapirin Cephacetrile
Group 2	
Ester replaced in position 3 giving metabolic stability but susceptible to hydrolysis by beta-lactamases of Gram-negatives.	Cephaloridine Cefazolin
Group 3	
Simple chemical grouping at position 3, orally absorbed, partial stability to beta-lactamases.	Cephalexin Cephradine Cefaclor
Group 4	
Cephalosporins resistant to the beta-lactamases of most Gram-negatives. a) metabolically unstable, b) metabolically stable.	 Cefotaxime Cefuroxime Cefamandole
Group 5	
7–methoxy compounds, metabolically stable and stable to most Gram-negative beta-lactamases. a) 1–sulpha compounds, b) 1–oxa-cephems.	 Cefoxitin LY 127935 (6059–S)
Group 6	
Unclassified – some show anti-pseudomonal activity related possibly to improved cell envelope penetration.	Cefsulodin (CGP 7174/E) Cefoperazone (T–1551) Ro 13–9904 (Roche) GR 20263 (Glaxo)

Current Problems in Antibiotic Use

Antibiotic Resistance

The present problems of antibiotic therapy are not confined to the
emergence and spread of antibiotic-resistant bacteria. Nevertheless it
is the emergence of these organisms which has fuelled the search for
new effective compounds. Each year a new group of organisms
achieves prominence as a cause of some major new antibiotic resistance phenomenon. Foremost among these have been Gram-negative
rods which are able to acquire multi-resistance plasmids and so affect
rapid changes in antibiotic susceptibility and force changes in
established treatment regimens. In the community chloramphenicol-
resistant enteric bacteria such as *Salmonella typhi* and *Shigella sonnei*

have caused major epidemics in several parts of the world (Anderson and Smith, 1972; W.H.O. 1978) and, because of the inactivity of the most useful therapeutic agent available for treatment, have produced a high mortality in some of these outbreaks; a mortality equal to that of pre-antibiotic days. Furthermore the situation can be worsened where laboratory facilities are not sufficiently well established to recognise the occurrence of resistance changes. In hospital practice gentamicin resistance among Gram-negative rods responsible for nosocomial infections creates increasing difficulty. Table 3 lists the

TABLE 3

Gentamicin Resistant Gram-negative Bacilli Isolated in The London Hospital During a Six Month Period

Bacterial strains	No. of isolates	Site of isolation	No. of isolates
Providencia spp.	35	Urine	119
P. aeruginosa	32	Wound swabs	26
Pseudomonas spp.	8	Sputum	18
Acinetobacter spp.	27	Ear swabs	13
Enterobacter spp.	25	Pleural fluid	5
Alcaligenes spp.	14	Dialysis fluid	4
K. aerogenes	13	Environment	4
Klebsiella spp.	8	Cerebrospinal fluid	1
Proteus (indole-positive)	11		
E. coli	7		
Flavobacterium spp.	7		
Others	9		

From Drasar *et al.*, 1976, with permission.

range of gentamicin resistant Gram-negative rods isolated from The London Hospital during a six month period (Drasar *et al.*, 1976).

The list of organisms contains many common and well known pathogens but additionally there are less well known and less pathogenic species which do not cause problems outside hospital. This is of course a reflection of the more and more vulnerable hospital populations whose defences against infection have been weakened by natural disease progress or the unwanted effects of other pharmaceutical preparations.

The spread of resistance from the enterobacteria to other bacterial groups has been a remarkable feature of the 1970's (Williams, 1978). The acquisition of penicillinase by *Haemophilus influenzae* (Williams *et al.*, 1974) and *Neisseria gonorrhoea* (Percival, 1976) provide striking examples where a change in resistance has been acquired by plasmid transfer and where a marked change in therapeutic regimens has been forced upon us. Even pathogens which have remained antibiotic sensitive for many years can produce a surprise such as the development of penicillin resistance in *Streptococcus pneumoniae* (Jacobs *et al.*, 1978) — a change once again associated with a high mortality among the affected children.

Difficulties in Combating Antibiotic Resistance with New Drugs

It is one of the hopes of those producing new antibiotic substances that these substances will be active against bacteria which have become resistant to existing agents. Unfortunately it has not been possible to find one agent which is uniformly active against many groups of Gram-negative rods, for example. These organisms seem to be able to evade most current antibiotics and as each successive new anti-Gram-negative agent is examined the antibacterial spectrum is found to have gaps against the whole potential range of hospital Gram-negative pathogens. In evaluating the activity of amikacin against gentamicin resistant organisms we find that although active against resistant *Providencia, Proteus* and *Klebsiella* spp., it was not active against *Acinetobacter* and *Alcaligenes* spp. amongst others (Drasar *et al.*, 1976). Similarly in evaluating cefotaxime against cephalosporin resistant Gram-negative rods it was active against *Citrobacter, Serratia* and *Alcaligenes* but *Pseudomonas* and *Acinetobacter* species were relatively resistant (Drasar *et al.*, 1978). The changes which occur in antibiotic resistance in Gram-negative rods are so common and the mechanisms of resistance so variable that it may be an impossible task to find an antibiotic which will be uniformly active against this group of organisms.

Limitations in the Pharmacology of Antibiotics

It is not possible to do more than indicate that the pharmacological properties of antibiotics are far from ideal. Many of the most effective agents are not absorbed orally and have to be given intra-muscularly or by intravenous infusion which carries additional risks for the patient. Even simple questions such as whether it is better to give intravenous antibiotics by slow infusion or by bolus injection remain unanswered. The pharmacokinetic properties differ (Evans *et al.*, 1978) but the therapeutic differences are unknown. Many antibiotics have half-lives less than 1 h and need frequent application. What is the significance of protein-binding? Are dose-related kinetics relevant to antibiotic therapy? Which methods of measuring antibiotics levels in interstitial fluid are most relevant to chemotherapy? How do we get antibiotics into deep compartments such as the eye and CSF? There are many questions in the pharmacology of antibiotics to be answered. In addition there is the expanding list of toxic effects (Dukes, 1965) and the host of anti-biotic interactions — between themselves and with other drugs (Bundtzen and Kunin, 1979) — which are outside the scope of this article.

Infections which Present Problems in Chemotherapy

Some organisms are capable of producing death rapidly — these include beta-haemolytic streptococci, *N. meningitidis, S. pneumoniae, B. anthracis* and *C. perfringens.* While these remain highly susceptible to penicillin the problems are of diagnosis and rapid treatment rather than new antibiotic substances. The emergence of resistance to penicillin in pneumococci highlights, however, the limitations of chemotherapy in this and other acute infections where resistance is present. In uncomplicated pneumonia about half the children in-fected with this organism died while those with meningitis all died (Jacobs *et al.,* 1978). The latter infection points at a further limitation on therapy — the need to achieve adequate levels at the site of infection. The mortality of pneumococcal meningitis, even when the organism is highly sensitive to benzylpenicillin, is reported in different series to be between 10–50%. Here are organisms which on laboratory criteria are highly susceptible to penicillin and yet the *in vivo* failure rate is high. Streptococcal disease, especially when Group B streptococci are involved, presents similar problems. Group B streptococci are only marginally more resistant to penicillin G than are Group A streptococci and yet there is a high failure of high dose penicillin therapy in neonates with Group B streptococcal infections (Parker, 1979). It is possible that infections are detected too late for chemotherapy to be effective but it is also possible that current *in vitro* tests do not accurately predict the ability of the antibiotic to kill the microorganism in its natural habitat. Equally indicative of the limitations of penicillins and other active antibiotics are the difficulties encountered in eradicating meningococci from the throats of chronic carriers (Hoeprich, 1972).

The lack of *in vivo* activity of antibiotics is also shown in patients with deficiency of host defence mechanisms. The outcome of therapy of infection in these patients is more closely related to the polymorph count in peripheral blood than to the susceptibility of organism to the antibiotic being given. Antibiotics appear to be most effective when they are aided by the normal bactericidal mechanisms of the host. The hospital population is gradually becoming more and more limited in its natural defence mechanisms.

Special Requirements for the Community

Apart from the absence of suitable agents for treatment of viral infection, the present effectiveness of antibiotics in the community looks superficially to be in a satisfactory state. There are oral penicillins and cephalosporins for coccal and Gram-negative rod infections; suitable and effective agents exist which are active against bacterial respiratory pathogens and for those affecting the meninges; the incidence of resistance in mycobacteria remains low; provided an accurate diagnosis can be made of the causative agent, community-acquired gastro-intestinal infections with bacteria or parasites should respond to specific therapy. Community problems do exist however, some of which arise from antibiotic resistance, but also in infections of less acute type where antibiotics for one reason or another are inadequate. Two examples can be seen with chlamydial infections and with *Bordetella pertussis.*

Chlamydial urethritis is now the most common sexually-transmitted disease (STD) in the UK (Oriel *et al.*, 1976). Treatment with long courses of tetracycline is the most effective therapy but the failure rate and relapse rate are higher than in treatment of gonorrhoea. Follow-up attendance at STD clinics is difficult because clients expect to have all diagnosis and treatment carried out at one visit — as happens with gonorrhoea. Consequently the control of this infection in the community presents problems in finding more effective agents and in achieving patient compliance.

Bordetella infections are still common. The prolonged symptoms resulting from these infections are related to epithelial damage rather than to persistence of the microorganisms in the trachea. It is possible that early elimination of the organism may limit the damage caused but antibiotic trials have not shown any consistent beneficial effect. Currently studies with erythromycin are under way in the UK but these also appear to have no marked effect (Lambert, 1979).

Resistant bacteria may spread from hospital into the community. Sometimes this has obvious repercussions as shown by the isolation of penicillin resistant pneumococci mainly in those children discharged from hospitals where the organisms are prevalent, and in their siblings. The role of resistant Gram-negative rods such as gentamicin resistant klebsiellae is less obvious as these organisms have little intrinsic pathogenicity. The effects are seen mainly in highly susceptible hosts. However, there are two fairly common sequelae. Urinary tract infections in patients discharged from hospital may be associated with antibiotic resistant bacteria and surgical emergencies arising in the community, such as appendicitis, diverticulitis, cholecystitis, may be associated with antibiotic resistant Gram-negative rods. One can no longer be sure that urinary infections and surgical infections are due to organisms susceptible to a wide variety of antibiotics and monitoring of resistant bacteria in the community is necessary (W.H.O. Technical Report, 1978).

The Problems of the Clinician

The practising doctor has many problems to consider other than those of infection; keeping abreast of advances in his special field of cardiology, nephrology, neurosurgery, or whatever his particular speciality is, occupies enough of his time to preclude any detailed appraisal of the many new antibiotics which appear. In the management of such infection as he sees it, he has to balance the effect of antibiotics against the value of other forms of treatment such as the surgical drainage of abscesses, the use of immunisation against *Pseudomonas* superinfection, the value of transfused white cells and the use of immuno-modulators. Antibiotic therapy, especially in hospital, is becoming more complex and even those clinicians who regard themselves as practically full-time antibiotic workers find difficulty in keeping pace with the speed of new introductions. It is very difficult to define the precise position of a new agent in therapy of infection before some new compound arrives which might possibly be an improvement. The number of people able to make a detailed and time-consuming assessment of the role of a new agent is small. At the same time the number of doctors who take up rapidly the use of a new agent is large. In many instances this is not unhelpful to the patient because many infections are trivial and would respond to many different forms of treatment or would even be self-resolving. Practitioners become familiar with antibiotics and re-assured of their effectiveness in the management of trivial infection and consequently often feel confident of dealing with severe and complicated infection without additional advice. As more severe infections arise in more complicated patients with an increasing array of possible therapeutic agents it should become clear that more expert advice will be needed. Others will consider that control is needed over antibiotic use in order to deal with the present difficulties. However, education and advice will be more helpful to patients and clinicians than over-simplified and rigid restrictions on antibiotic use.

References

Anderson, E.S. and Smith, H.R. (1972). *Brit. Med. J.* **3**, 329–330.
Bundtzen, R.W. and Kunin, C.M. (1979). *In* "Antibiotic Interactions", (J.D. Williams, ed.), pp. 35–51. Academic Press, London.

Drasar, F.A., Farrell, W., Howard, A.J., Hince, C., Leung, T. and Williams, J.D. (1978). *J. Antimicrob. Chemother.* **4**, 445–450.
Drasar, F.A., Farrell, W., Maskell, J. and Williams, J.D. (1976). *Brit. Med. J.* **2**, 1284–1287.
Dukes, M.N.G. (1965). *In* "Side Effects of Drugs", Vol. VIII, (L. Meyler and A. Herxheimer, eds), pp. 551–693 (and subsequent annual supplements). Excerpta Medica, Amsterdam.
Evans, M.A.L., Wilson, P., Leung, T. and Williams, J.D. (1978). *J. Antimicrob. Chemother.* **4**, 255–261.
Hoeprich, P.D. (1972). "Infectious Diseases", p. 209. Harper and Row, New York.
Jacobs, M.R., Koornhof, H.J., Robins-Browne, R.M., Stevenson, C.M., Vermaak, Z.A., Freiman, I., Miller, G.B., Witcomb, M.A., Isaäcson, M., Ward, J.I. and Austrian, R. (1978). *N. Engl. J. Med.* **299**, 735–740.
Kurylowicz, W. (1976). "Antibiotics: A Critical Review", p. 10. Polish Medical Publishers, Warsaw.
Lambert, H.P. (1979). *J. Antimicrob. Chemother.* **5**, 329–330.
McGowan, J.E.Jr. and Finland, M. (1974). *J. Infect. Dis.* **129**, 431–438.
O'Callaghan, C.H. (1979). *J. Antimicrob. Chemother.* **5**, 635–672.
Oriel, J.D., Reeve, P., Wright, J.T. and Owen, J. (1976). *Br. J. Vener. Dis.* **52**, 46–50.
Parker, M.T. (1979). *J. Antimicrob. Chemother.* Suppl. A. **5**, 27–37.
Percival, A. (1976). *Lancet* **II**, 1379–1381.
Scheckler, W.E. and Bennett, J.V. (1970). *J. Am. Med. Assoc.* **213**, 264–267.
WHO Technical Report (1978) – Series 624: Surveillance and control of health hazards due to antibiotic resistant enterobacteria.
Williams, J.D. (1978). *J. Antimicrob. Chemother.* **4**, 6–7.
Williams, R.J. and Williams, J.D. (1980). *In* "Antibiotic and Chemotherapy – Current Topics", (R.N. Gruneberg, ed.), pp. 63–112. MTP Press, Lancaster.
Williams, J.D., Kattan, S. and Cavanagh, P. (1974). *Lancet* **II**, 103.

Discussion

Professor Richmond: Professor Williams said that he thought that the use of tetracycline in the community was decreasing. That may be so, but I had occasion recently to look at the DHSS statistics for the number of prescriptions written by general practitioners in Britain in 1979. There were about 9½ million tetracycline prescriptions for 55 million people, so it is still very considerable.

Professor Williams: It is amazing how long it takes for any piece of scientific information to percolate into the general body of practitioners. Professor Lambert estimated this as a quarter of a century. Tetracycline resistance in pneumococci and beta-haemolytic streptococci has now been reported for 15, perhaps 20 years, so perhaps the use of tetracycline against these organisms may fall before too long. The recognition that tetracycline affects the teeth of small children has also been known for about 20 years, yet I feel sure that there were many prescriptions for children under eight years old amongst that 9½ million in 1979.

Dr. Waldvogel: Does Professor Williams have any idea how many doses of antibiotic must be taken for an individual to become a carrier for a resistant strain? For instance gentamicin resistant klebsiellae are excreted for about 10 weeks by some patients. Does he know how many doses of gentamicin — or other antibiotics — these people had received?

Professor Williams: It varied from no doses to many — there is no need to take the antibiotic provided that the organism is able to establish itself in the patient.

Professor Trouet: Did I understand correctly that Professor Williams believes that, because of the number of drugs available in the field of the β–lactams and the cephalosporins, it would be wise to stop synthesising new derivatives, and to analyse what we already have available with regard to their clinical properties?

Professor Williams: I would not want to stop people synthesising new agents because it is possible that something extremely important will be found. However, I would like to see controlled release of the new agents into the general population of prescribers. This is a problem for the drug regulatory authorities, which, I am sure, Professor Kunin will discuss later.

Evaluation of Antibiotic Usage: A Comprehensive Look at Alternative Approaches

C.M. KUNIN

*Department of Medicine, The Ohio State
University School of Medicine, Columbus,
Ohio, U.S.A.*

Introduction

Medical practice in the seventies is caught in the bind between advances in technology and the demand for accountability. Drug usage, particularly of antibiotics, is a highly visible segment of medical progress. Antibiotics differ from other drugs in that they not only exert a therapeutic effect, but also alter the ecology of the microflora of the body and the environment. This conjures the image of fallout from antibiotic usage akin to that from a leaking nuclear reactor. There is legitimate concern about development of antibiotic resistance transmitted by plasmids under the selective pressure of excessive use of anbitiotics by physicians, veterinarians and in animal feed.

The economic consequence of antibiotic usage can be even more clearly defined. According to the U.S. Industrial Outlook published by the U.S. Department of Commerce, 1.55 billion dollars worth of anti-infectives will be shipped this year. This accounts for 17.7% of the total cost of all ethical drug products. It does not include costs of mark-up or administration of the agents which could readily double the expenditure to three billion dollars this year. How much of this expenditure is really needed to keep our population healthy? It is estimated by most investigators that about one-half of the time, antibiotics are used in hospitalised adults for an inappropriate indication, or a less expensive, equally effective agent might have been used, or the dose or duration of therapy was excessive. In addition, about 70% of antibiotics used in hospitals consist of the expensive cephalosporins and aminoglycosides. Several groups have demonstrated that costs can be reduced by half when cephalosporin use is limited to specific indications without depriving patients of effective, but less expensive treatment. We need to develop mechanisms that would enable most other hospitals to achieve the same goal.

A new antimicrobial era has emerged during the past decade, the era of the "drugs of fear" (Kunin *et al.*, 1973). By this, I mean fear on the part of the physician of failing to provide his or her patient with the very best drug for a presumed infection. Although many lives have been saved by these drugs, the underlying conditions that precipitate infection with "difficult hospital bacteria" have not been resolved. In many cases, the drugs have been used unnecessarily or have simply delayed death. Widespread use of these agents insures their own phased obsolescence as new resistant organisms emerge, and increases the costs of medical care. We would not need very many new antibiotics if we were to more wisely use those which we already have. Unfortunately, money is being spent on development and promotion of agents we really should not need.

It is essential to view the issues concerning use of antibiotics within the framework of the constraints of medical practice and social forces exerted on the physician. In my view, singling out the physician or the pharmaceutical industry for blame or adding new constraints to medical practice will not resolve the problem. Instead, we must examine the multiplicity of factors that lead to inappropriate usage of drugs and develop a strategy that recognises the complexity of the problem.

Evaluation of Appropriate Usage

Let us examine some methods to define the problem and evaluate appropriate usage. Most of the studies reported in the literature employ different criteria for appropriateness of usage. This makes it difficult to compare data gathered in different institutions. Broad categories of surveillance methods are presented in Table 1, together with a brief account of the advantages and disadvantages of each.

The simplest and least expensive method is to obtain gross utilisation data from hospital pharmacies. This method can often identify a special problem such as overusage of chloramphenicol or a newly introduced agent. Attention can then be focused upon individual services, particularly on patterns of usage in a major problem area such as surgical prophylaxis. Drug orders can also be audited in relation to specific indications, such as use·of antibiotics for upper

TABLE 1

Methods of Surveillance of Antimicrobial Agent Usage in Hospitals. Reprinted from
Kunin (1978) with permission.

Gross utilisation data based on pharmacy records
Inexpensive; provides secular trends on usage of individual agents and costs; may be used for
interhospital comparisons when adjusted for patient hospital days; may identify unusual
practices which may lead to more detailed studies.

Utilisation by services
Inexpensive if pharmacy record system is on unit dose system or can identify shipment to
specific wards; will provide data on problems of use by different groups of physicians and
may lead to detailed studies of potential problem areas; will refine gross utilisation for more
appropriate interhospital comparisons.

Survey of routine orders for prophylaxis in surgery
Requires chart review of all cases for specific operations; provides data on actual practices
of individual surgeons; permits comparison of practices in different hospitals; identifies
unusual practices and can be used for feedback to the surgical service.

Survey of orders for specific infectious diseases
Based on discharge diagnosis such as pneumonia, bronchitis, urinary tract infection; provides
data on actual practices of individual physicians; permits comparison of practice according
to specialty groups and can be used for feedback in education programs.

Case review by independent experts
Requires establishment of strict criteria to avoid subjective or varying standards; requires
establishment of feedback loops to practicing physicians; may identify specific problems of
individual physicians.

Guidelines audit
Hospital staffs establish standards of practice and guidelines based on national criteria; audit
is used to evaluate compliance with self-imposed standards; enables peer pressure to provide
checks and balances; mutes external judgmental evaluations; must be altered as new
knowledge of new agents is introduced.
    Audits may be used for interhospital comparisons.

---

respiratory infections. Case reviews can be conducted using broad
criteria established by specialists in the field.

An advisory committee on infectious diseases to the Veterans
Administration established specific guidelines and audits for antibiotic usage to aid individual hospital staffs, in conducting their own
programmes of surveillance (Kunin and Efron, 1977). The guidelines
were prepared for 18 common problem areas including prophylaxis
in surgery, evaluation of high-cost or potentially toxic agents,
criteria for obtaining blood and other cultures, and services that
should be available in a competent clinical microbiology laboratory
to perform antibiotic susceptibility testing. It is important to
emphasise that these are guidelines, not commandments written in
stone. They can potentially be used to establish policy for individual
hospitals after they have been thoroughly reviewed and debated by
the staff. Some, such as the guidelines on surgical prophylaxis, may
have to be modified to meet special, local problems. Others, such as

indications for bacteriological culture, can be applied without much adaptation. The essential point, however, is that once these guidelines are adopted, the physicians and surgeons should be expected to adhere to them and respond to questions that will arise when actual practices are audited.

Several groups have experimented with methods to evaluate appropriate use of antimicrobial agents in ambulatory practice. This is somewhat more difficult to assess than in hospitals because of the widely dispersed nature of office practice. Nevertheless, useful data is being gathered by the Kaiser–Permanente group in California and by others. Ray *et al.* (1976, 1977) have reported that Medicaid data can be used as part of a surveillance method of individual practitioners. As third party payment for drugs becomes more extensive, excellent data should be generated by using this approach. The major advantage is the ability to detect a small group of aberrant physicians who account for most of the inappropriate usage.

Causes of Inappropriate Usage

Let us now examine the constraints of medical practice which lead to inappropriate usage. In order to solve the problem of inappropriate usage, we must understand the constraints under which the physician works and the pressures that are exerted on him to prescribe drugs. An overall scheme of the elements that motivate the patient to seek help and comply with the physician, and the forces that lead the physician to prescribe drugs is outlined in Figure 1 (Kunin, 1978).

Some of the major factors which appear to influence physicians to use antibiotics to resolve some of the constraints of practice are as follows:

1) Motivation of the physician to help his patient regardless of the uncertainties of diagnosis and management.
2) Adequacy of the physician's knowledge of diagnosis and management of patients with infectious disease.
3) Belief that, if a drug might do some good, and probably is not likely to do harm, then why not try it, even though it is not clear that it is needed at all.
4) Belief that if a small amount of drug will be effective, higher and more prolonged usage might be better.
5) Inappropriate use of resources or poor support and high costs of the clinical microbiology laboratory.
6) Use of multiple antimicrobial agents or "broad spectrum agents" to "cover" unusual organisms.
7) Pressure from the patient to be treated with an antimicrobial agent.

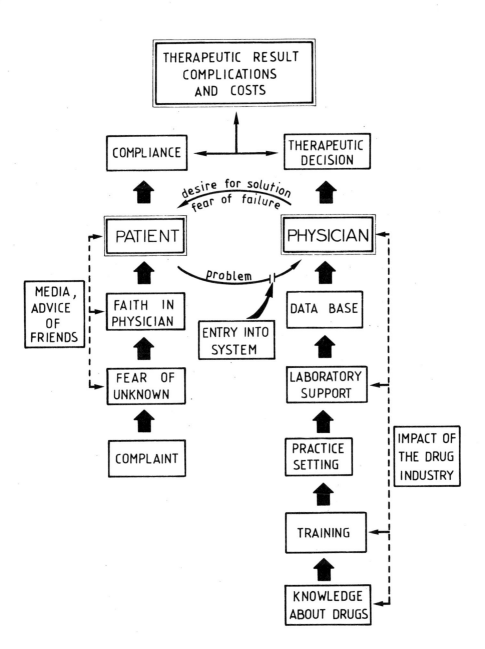

FIG. 1 Outline of the elements and complex interrelationships which influence the patient and physician to use drugs. Reprinted from Kunin (1978) with permission.

8) Cost and availability of x-rays and diagnostic tests in relation to ready solution offered by drugs.
9) Malpractice considerations.
10) Solution to 1–9 provided by pharmaceutical manufacturers.

Proposals for Improvement of Antibiotic Usage

The efficacy of each of the proposed methods to control the misuse of antibiotics (shown in Table 2) depends upon whether they meet the needs of the practicing physician.

The first method is education. Neu and Howrey (1975) demonstrated that there were major deficiencies in the physician's knowledge of antibiotic use, and they emphasised the need for further postgraduate education in this field. However, even though continued medical education is expanding in this country, there is no concrete evidence that it improves actual practice. One study evaluating the effect of education was conducted by Jones *et al.* (1977). Hospital staff did not show improvement in antibiotic usage following an intensive educational programme. Gilbert and Jackson (1976) reported success in improving usage by targeting their campaign for one drug, gentamicin. Achong *et al.* (1977) reported remarkable success which in large part was attributable to improved usage of antibiotics in surgical prophylaxis.

My own belief is that education should emphasise familiarity with how to make a diagnosis of a bacterial infection that might require antimicrobial therapy. Only after this is mastered should we provide information about use of antimicrobial agents. Heavy emphasis should be placed on simple measures such as use and interpretation of the Gram-stain, in aspirates of abscesses and examination of specimens of sputum. The technique of transtracheal aspiration, for example, has revolutionised our understanding of pneumonia. Simple office procedures for urine and throat cultures and greater use of blood cultures in febrile patients with leucocytosis will enable the physician to be more confident in his diagnostic judgement and better define when antimicrobial agents are needed. Antimicrobial agents should not be used as a substitute for careful diagnostic measures. Imagine how much more frequently these procedures would be used if their cost were paid to the physicians by third party payers. It is the third party payers who have made endoscopy so lucrative. Why not infectious disease as well? This responsibility cannot be defaulted to the clinical diagnostic laboratory.

Another method, control of contact between pharmaceutical representatives and staff physicians, is only sporadically enforced in a few institutions. The representative is usually visualised as a helpful

TABLE 2

Methods Used to Control Use of Antimicrobial Agents in Hospitals. Reprinted from Kunin (1978) with permission.

Education programmes on use of antimicrobial agents:
1. Staff conferences
2. Lectures by outside authorities
3. Audio-visual programmes
4. Clinical pharmacist consultants
5. Hospital-Pharmacy Committee "newsletters"
6. Independent sources of information ("Medical Letter", AMA Drug Evaluations)

Control of contract between pharmaceutical representatives and staff physicians:
1. Registration in the pharmacy
2. Visits to staff physicians by appointment only
3. Policy concerning entry of salesmen to patient care areas
4. Restricted time and place of displays
5. Policy on free samples
6. Policy on sponsoring speakers

Hospital formulary:
1. Restriction of formulary to minimum number of agents needed for most effective therapy
2. Elimination of duplicative agents
3. Substitution rules for least expensive, most effective agent among a given class of agents
4. Generic terminology required for all orders and labels

Diagnostic microbiology laboratory sensitivity tests:
1. Appropriate selection of sensitivity tests for organism and site
2. Use of generic class disks
3. Restriction of reports on "specialised" agents unless specifically requested or indicated
4. Print own report forms with generic terminology

Automatic "stop" orders for specific high-cost agents

Written justification for high-cost agents:
In cases where alternative, equally effective, less expensive or toxic agents may be used, e.g. oral cephalosporins, new parenteral aminoglycosides and cephalosporins, lincosamides, chloramphenicol.

Required consultation:
This is to be done after first three doses of specific high-cost agents are ordered, e.g. aminoglycosides, parenteral cephalosporins, carbenicillin–ticarcillin, lincosamides.

Controlled agents:
Release of specific agents which may alter ecology of hospital flora requires approval by infectious disease consultants, e.g., amikacin, carbenicillin–ticarcillin.

Guidelines and audits of antimicrobial usage:
These permit the hospital staff to set standards of usage based on local needs and judgements, guided by independent criteria. Audit is based on compliance with these standards, but requires a well-structured, authoritative feedback loop.

colleague who provides quick information, favours, and is properly obsequious. His entry is aided by advertising gimmicks and gifts, provision of funds for education, guest speakers, and funds for research or fellowship training. It is extremely difficult, even for the academic physician, to restrict these people since the information they bring is often valuable and the companies they represent do develop many excellent antimicrobial agents. However, I believe that contact with drug representatives should be limited and restricted only to provision of new information in a physician–hospital controlled setting. Some have proposed that "counter–detailing" by clinical pharmacists may help (Hendeles, 1976), but this remains to be proven.

The hospital formulary committee can be extremely useful in examining the claims and need for new agents. It is in this area that the clinical pharmacist may be of greatest help by advising the committee on the relative benefits of adding or deleting agents from the formulary. In many ways, the diagnostic laboratory plays a key role in selection of antimicrobial agents by physicians. Therefore, it is exceedingly important that the laboratories be open discussion areas for clinicians and antibiotic susceptibility test results be reported by generic name and class and be tailored to the best agents according to the organism and site of infection.

Another way to control antibiotic usage is to employ automatic "stop" orders for specific high-cost agents. In a recent paper (Shapiro *et al.*, 1979), it was shown that antibiotic use correlates more with length of patient stay than the need for the agent. Almost 80% of usage and costs were beyond the effective peri-operative period. Consequently savings can be accomplished simply by using proper timing of prophylaxis.

Written justification for use of antibiotics on the prescription is an effective method to decrease inappropriate usage. This forces the physician to explain his actions and the requirement to write even a brief justification tends to blunt unnecessary prescribing. McGowan and Finland (1974) have demonstrated that removal of this requirement has been followed by increased usage of these agents.

Recommended Procedure for Preparing and Conducting an Antimicrobial Audit

My own interest has been directed at attempting to develop practical procedures for conducting antibiotic audits. Outlined in Table 3 is a process which may be helpful to those who wish to conduct these audits. Prophylactic use of antibiotics in surgery is emphasised since it is the most expensive and potentially most correctable problem area.

TABLE 3

Preparing and Conducting an Antimicrobial Audit

Reasons for audit
The primary reason for audit is to improve medical care and lower costs. Therefore:
1) Do not use audits to find fault or police the staff.
2) Do not use audits simply to satisfy the authorities.
3) Do not allow audits to produce conflicts among physicians or between the hospital administration and staff.

Basis of audit
Audits must be based on thorough knowledge by the staff of the literature in the field and understanding of the principles of antimicrobial therapy. Therefore:
1) Prepare a selected bibliography of the important papers dealing with the topic.
2) Photocopy the title and abstract of each paper. Submit audits and guidelines obtained from the literature at meetings. Distribute the material to the medical staff in an attractive binder.
3) Photocopy each article in entirety for reference only. Place in attractive binder. To be used only when questions arise.
4) Audits are a function of the medical staff. The function of the administration is to provide support to the staff.
5) Designate a physician or surgeon leader in the discipline for which the audit is being prepared. Pharmacists, infection control nurses and medical records librarians are supporting staff.
6) The leader and staff should review the literature. Then review suggested guidelines or audits from the literature. Select those which are most simple to use and best represent the current "state of the art" on appropriate usage.
7) Ask the leader to present the most appropriate guidelines and audits to his/her peers for adoption. Vigorous discussion is encouraged. A guest "expert" can help in these deliberations. A copy of the adopted audit should be sent to each member of the staff for his/her information.
8) The medical staff is expected on "good faith" to adopt these standards for their practice.

Outline of the guideline
Prepare an outline of the guideline-audit to be considered by the hospital staff.
For example for surgical prophylaxis:
1) List procedures for which routine antimicrobial prophylaxis is indicated or established.
2) Indicate drugs route and dosage which are considered appropriate for each procedure.
3) Be sure timing is agreed as "perioperative", that is, the first dose is given 1–2 hours before the procedure, during the procedure and stopped 24 hours after the procedure is completed.

Benefits of audit
Audits should be demonstrated to effect a change.
   It is exceedingly difficult to demonstrate in any one hospital that audits improve medical care by decreasing resistance to antibiotics or decreasing complications of antimicrobial therapy. It is more realistic to expect that total usage and costs of antimicrobial agents will be reduced. Therefore, employ usage and cost data to demonstrate the efficacy of your programme.
1) General: Collect data on overall expenditures for antibiotics in your hospital for the three years prior to introduction of the antibiotic audit. This should be broken down for each year into:
   a) total expenditure for antimicrobial agents,
   b) proportion of expenditure for antimicrobial drugs compared to all drug costs, and
   c) costs and gram usage expended by each service (e.g. surgery, medicine and specialty services).
These data will only be meaningful if the hospital census and number and type of

TABLE 3 (contd.)

surgical procedures are stable. If these are changing, you will need to adjust costs by relating them to patient days or number of operative procedures per year.

Compare rates of usage and costs as described above to similar rates obtained in the year after guidelines and audits have been accepted by the staff.

2) Specific: Collect data on costs and usage for the procedures for which the audits are designed for a three-year period prior to adoption of the audit-guidelines. Then compare these with costs and usage for the year after the guidelines are adopted. (See method described below)

Mini-Audits for Rapid Assessment of Critical Areas of Antimicrobial Usage

It is recommended that audits be as simple as possible. This will enable you to obtain useful information with minimum effort. Prophylaxis in surgery is potentially the most productive audit since most of the excessive use of antibiotics in hospitals can be traced to usually excessive duration of prophylaxis. In addition, there is now a substantial literature based on studies by surgeons, indicating that short-term peri-operative prophylaxis is as effective as more prolonged use and results in fewer complications and lower cost. A recommended procedure for conducting a mini-audit on prophylaxis in surgery is outlined in Table 4.

TABLE 4

Mini-Audit for Prophylaxis in Surgery

Definition of prophylaxis

For operational use in chart review, one must be able to distinguish the patient who receives antibiotics for prophylaxis from those who are receiving antibiotics for treatment of presumed infection.

The patient should be considered to be receiving prophylaxis if the chart indicates the following:

1. Antibiotics are begun: within 2 days of, *or* the day of, *or* the day after the operative procedure, and
2. There is no record in the chart within a week prior to the operation of: fever, leucocytosis, pneumonia, urinary tract infection, wound or other infection.
3. Prophylaxis is considered to be terminated when: the last dose is given, *or* the antimicrobial drug is continued but the chart indicates that the patient developed fever or leucocytosis or pneumonia, urinary tract, wound or other infection.

Audit of timing, route and duration of prophylaxis

The following criteria are to be considered:

1. Antimicrobial agent should be begun 1—2 hours prior to the procedure.
2. The last dose should be given no more than 24 hours after the procedure.
3. The total number should not exceed six doses.
4. The drug should be given by injection.
5. Prophylaxis is used for the appropriate procedure.

These can be used for your entire audit without necessarily going into further detail.

TABLE 4 (contd.)

Procedures currently considered acceptable for prophylaxis
1. Cardiovascular (valve and open heart, coronary artery bypass)
2. Orthopedic (prosthetic joint)
3. Intestinal (colonic)
4. Biliary (patient more than 70, acute cholecystitis, obstructive jaundice or common bile duct stones)
5. Gynaecologic (vaginal hysterectomy, caeserian sections)
6. Urologic (bacteriuric patients prior to urologic procedures)

Analysis of data on surgical prophylaxis
1. Perform audit on 100 consecutive surgical procedures each year in your hospital. These should be in addition to certain routine "scopies" and dilatation and curettage that tend to fill operating room schedules. List all of these separately, e.g. cystoscopy, bronchoscopy, gastroscopies, colonoscopies, D and C (dilatation and curettage), etc., but do not include in the calculations described below.
2. Divide surgical procedures by the following classes:
   a. No preceding evidence of infection   Number   %
   b. Preceding evidence of infection (fever, leucocytosis, peritonitis, active pyelonephritis, pneumonia, abscess, etc.)   Number   %
3. Analyse only those with *no* preceding evidence of infection
4. List each by major and subcategory

For example:	Performed	Received prophylaxis	
Cardiovascular	Number	Number	%
Valve replacement			
Coronary artery			
Coarctation			

5. For each procedure analyse by a separate column:

	Number	%
a. Received prophylaxis		
b. Prophylaxis appropriate for this indication		
c. Began 2–4 hours prior to the procedure		*
d. Completed 24 hours after procedure		*
e. No more than six doses given		*

   *Calculate as per cent of those receiving prophylaxis appropriate for this condition.
6. Calculation of excessive usage
   a. For each procedure, add up total grams and days for each drug actually used for "prophylaxis" regardless of whether or not it was appropriate.
      e.g. Patient A received 40 g of cephalothin for 10 days.
      Patient B received 8 g of methicillin for 2 days.
   b. For each procedure, add up total grams of each drug and days recommended in the guideline–audit which could have been used instead. If prophylaxis was not indicated, list as zero days and cost. You may use Veterans Administration guidelines for Peer Review or other sources in the literature to assess recommended drugs and doses.
   c. Add the totals for a and b and subtract b from a. This will give excessive grams and days. You can then multiply grams by unit cost to your pharmacy to obtain an estimate of "wasted" expenditure. You can also extrapolate these data for the year, based on the number of procedures performed each year. This is the most important economic justification of the audit programme.
      e.g. If you conducted your audit over a one-month period, then you can multiply excess costs by 12 months to obtain yearly "wasted" expenditures.

Conclusions

Overuse of antibiotics is not simply an economic problem, even though it is easily measured by these standards; nor is it just poor practice because of the heavy price paid for ecological changes with new, resistant microbial strains. Most importantly, it reveals how effectively we as health care workers use scientific technology to help our patients. The solution to the problem rests on our willingness to use this technology wisely. We cannot do this alone, nor can we accomplish our goals by taking over the job of the practicing physician. We must work with the people on the firing line, understand their problems and constraints and help them to do the job for which they have been trained.

Audits are only one among several means of attempting to solve the problem of excessive use of antimicrobial agents. They are not an end in themselves, but simply provide a data base to know how well or poorly we are accomplishing our goals in rational chemotherapy. Audits combined with other methods to improve usage, hopefully, will improve medical care by reducing the ecologic and financial costs of excess use of those valuable drugs.

References

Achong, M.R., Theal, H.K., Wood, J., Goldberg, R. and Thompson, D.A. (1977). *Lancet* II, 1118–1121.

Gilbert, D.N. and Jackson, J. (1976). *Clin. Res.* 24, 112A.

Hendeles, L. (1976). *Am. J. Hosp. Pharm.* 33, 918–924.

Jones, S.R., Bratton, T. and McRee, E. (1977). *Am. J. Med. Sci.* 273, 79–85.

Kunin, C.M. (1978). *Ann. Intern. Med.* 89, 802–805.

Kunin, C.M. and Efron, H.Y. (1977). *J. Am. Med. Assoc.* 237, 1001–1008; *ibid.*, 1134–1137; *ibid.*, 1241–1245; *ibid.*, 1366–1369; *ibid.*, 1481–1484; *ibid.*, 1605–1608; *ibid.*, 1723–1725; *ibid.*, 1859–1860; *ibid.*, 1967–1970.

Kunin, C.M., Tupasi, T. and Craig, W.A. (1973). *Ann. Intern. Med.* 79, 555–560.

McGowan, J.E., Jr. and Finland, M. (1974). *J. Infect. Dis.* 130, 165–168.

Neu, H.C. and Howrey, S.P. (1975). *N. Engl. J. Med.* 293, 1291–1295.

Ray, W.A., Federspiel, D.F. and Schaffner, W. (1976). *Ann. Intern. Med.* 84, 266–270.

Ray, W.A., Federspiel, D.F. and Schaffner, W. (1977). *J. Am. Med. Assoc.* 237, 2069–2074.

Shapiro, M., Townsend, T.R., Rosner, B. and Kass, E.H. (1979). *N. Engl. J. Med.* 301, 351–355.

Discussion

Professor Sande: Both Professor Kunin and I, when training house officers in a university institution, tend to take care of very complex patients. Many of them are leukaemics, neutropenics, impaired hosts or they develop bacteraemia in the hospital, frequently with resistance to drugs. In our house officers, we tend to develop a reflex pattern of therapy. Initially they "cover the waterfront" with broad spectrum drugs but such therapy is altered within 48 hours, when the cultures have been reported. Therapy can then be tailored to an individual agent with a narrow spectrum and minimal toxicity. Unfortunately this approach to the complex infection in the impaired host is often carried over to the simple straightforward pneumococcal pneumonia. It is thus critical for those of us in the business of training physicians to clearly distinguish between these two patient populations since antibiotic therapy must clearly differ between the two.

Professor Kunin: Professor Sande and I agree not to leave out clinical medicine. For example if a woman, aged 72 years, comes in with pneumonia, and she does not have either leukaemia or lymphoma we should select the drugs corresponding to the diagnosis of pneumonia as Professor Sande does. Not everybody has leukaemia who is taken care of in a university hospital. Somebody may have a catheter in place, or someone may have a heart murmur in which case he will certainly not be treated with the same drugs as would be used to treat a leukaemic. A patient with a heart murmur and fever would not be treated with broad coverage. There is much more to this whole question than "sepsis of unknown origin", which I think is deceptive. Infectious disease is really not very complicated. The principle is to put a needle into a spot, or to look at some pus. The mistake that is made is to consider infectious disease as sepsis, and that it must be treated broadly.

Professor Trouet: One way in which to control the use of drugs is used in Belgium, where the Social Security will no longer pay for oral cephalosporins.

Professor Kunin: That is excellent — it sounds like a major advance in Belgium.

Antimicrobial Drugs in Veterinary Medicine

Y. RUCKEBUSCH

*Station de Pharmacologie, Institut National de la
Recherche Agronomique, Toulouse, France*

Introduction

Antimicrobials represent approximately one third of all the chemicals used in veterinary medicine. Moreover, the chemicals used for both plants and animals constitute nearly one third of the market value in 1978 of the output of the pharmaceutical industries in France (19.10^9 francs). The use of antimicrobials by practitioners involves mainly therapy in bovine species, 75%, compared with 25% for the treatment of infections in horses, pigs and domestic animals. The "in-feed use" concerns mainly calves, pigs and poultry.

Veterinary Aspects of Clinically Used Drugs

The concept of true selective toxicity applies, for example, to drugs which act by inhibiting cell wall synthesis in bacteria and not in host cells. Penicillins are inhibitors of the transpeptidases involved in peptidoglycan biosynthesis, and their activities are destroyed by opening of the lactam ring. Cell wall biosynthesis is also inhibited by cephalosporins, bacitracin, ristocetin and vancomycin. Other agents exhibit relative toxicity, e.g. polymyxins, by an alteration of cell membrane permeability.

Inhibition of protein biosynthesis (i.e. inhibition of translation and transcription of genetic material) involves each type of subunit of the 70S bacterial ribosomes, which are different from the 80S mammalian ribosomes. Inhibition is effected by low binding (30%) and high binding (80%) tetracyclines, by aminoglycosides (streptomycin, kanamycin, gentamicin and neomycin), by macrolides (erythromycin, spiramycin, and tylosin) and, to a lesser extent, by lincomycins.

Inhibitors of DNA synthesis form a heterogeneous group, with dihydrofolate reductase inhibitors like pyrimethamine and trimethoprim, also sulphonamides etc.

Other antimicrobial agents are used for their antiprotozoal and antifungal activities, e.g. nitrofurans (nitrofurazone, furazolidone, nitrofurantoin) and imidazoles (metronidazole, dimetridazole, miconazole). Quinoxalines are used as feed premix.

The deficiencies in the use of these drugs in veterinary medicine are: too low dosage, the usual absence of sensitivity tests, the large variation in drug distribution between species and some adverse reactions and side effects (Table 1).

TABLE 1

Adverse Reactions and Side-Effects of Some Antibiotics in Dogs

Sulphonamides	a) Renal damage due to formation of crystals in urine. b) Nausea and vomiting.
Penicillin	a) Hypersensitivity to penicillin in animals. b) Procaine toxicity from large doses of procaine penicillin.
Streptomycin	a) Neuromuscular blockade and respiratory failure (cats, neonates). b) Hearing loss.
Gentamicin	a) Nephrotoxicity in both dog and cat. b) Unsafe if dose is more than 5 mg/kg used for long periods.
Tetracyclines	a) Vomiting and diarrhoea. b) Discoloration of teeth and bones. c) Pyrexia and hair-loss.
Broad-spectrum agents	a) Gastrointestinal upsets. b) Anorexia and lethargy. c) Hepatotoxicity (nalidixic acid).

Drug Concentration and Susceptibility

The difference between antibiotics in terms of whether they kill bacteria i.e. are bactericidal (penicillins and cephalosporins, aminoglycosides, polymyxins) or prevent bacterial growth i.e. are bacteriostatic (chloramphenicol, tetracyclines, macrolides and sulphonamides) is dictated by the fact that both activities depend on the concentration of the drug relative to the sensitivity of the organism. Low dosages are frequent in veterinary practice thus permitting only a bacteriostatic rather than a bactericidal effect. A high tissue concentration resulting from impairment of hepato— renal function is also infrequent in young animals. Since it is essential for the antibacterials to reach the infected area, advantage is taken of the varied distribution of antibacterials in the body: penicillins accumulate at high concentrations in the bladder, streptomycin in the kidney, erythromycin in the mammary gland and spiramycin in pulmonary tissue (Videau, 1978); there are enteric acting sulphonamides and there is enterohepatic cycling of tetracyclines. Another possibility is to achieve the level of antibacterial drug by local injections, e.g. by the intramammary (Le Louedec, 1978), intra-uterine (Oxender, 1976), intra-articular and, recently, the intra-tracheal route in calves (Hjerpe and Routen, 1976).

The emergence of drug resistance in bacteria is an enormous ecological change which mirrors the use of antibiotics in animals and in humans, and there is no essential difference between the resistant strains of bacteria resulting from the use of antibiotics in the treatment of clinical diseases and from their use as feed additives; the presence of an antibiotic provides the selection pressure resulting in the removal of the sensitive strains. Resistance patterns developed in scouring calves corresponding to the widespread use of some antibiotics are given in Table 2. In herds where low levels of antibiotics

TABLE 2

Antibiotic Sensitivity of *E. coli* from Healthy and Scouring Calves

Drugs	% of sensitive strains of *E. coli*	
	Healthy calves (n = 46)	Scouring calves (n = 181)
Ampicillin	43.5	14.4
Streptomycin	34.8	5.0
Kanamycin	60.9	42.5
Chloramphenicol	60.9	30.4
Tetracycline	37.0	17.1
Minocycline	69.6	44.2
Sulphonamides	32.6	6.1
Trimethoprim + sulphonamides	63.0	70.6
Gentamicin	100	100
Colistin	100	100

From Dubourguier *et al.* (1979).

are fed for growth purposes, members of the same antibiotic group are avoided for therapeutic purposes. The resistance possessed by most of the *E. coli* inhabiting the pig alimentary tract is transferable. Transfer *in vivo* also occurs in the rumen of sheep, provided that the animals have been deprived of food for 24–48 hours; without the starvation period, the inoculation of 10^{10} cells of the same organisms resulted in almost undetectable transfer (Smith, 1976). Finally, although a natural, continuous process of R–factor exchange between animals and humans has not been clearly established, it is necessary to reduce the size of the human and animal reservoir of R–factors by careful use of antibiotics. Resistance is rare and never found on R–factors for nalidixic acid, furan derivatives and polymyxins, all widely used in both man and animals; flavomycin, a feed additive for livestock and poultry, is specifically effective against bacteria with R–factors.

The purpose of sensitivity tests is to determine if the organism under consideration is likely to be susceptible to the action of an antimicrobial agent at the drug levels that can be achieved physiologically. However, resistance or susceptibility is not an all–or–none phenomenon but is dependent upon drug concentration. An organism that is susceptible to benzylpenicillin at 0.1 μg/ml would be considered sensitive because such a level of benzylpenicillin can be easily achieved physiologically. One susceptible to only 10 μg/ml or more would be considered resistant because it is difficult to maintain such a concentration in the tissues.

The need for sensitivity testing is limited in large animal practice, because the results frequently come too late to be useful. According to the volume of distribution and thus the cell penetration of an antimicrobial agent, previous clinical experience also suggests the exact antibiotic to be used and allows a confident prediction of success of the therapy. However, taking samples may be important to confirm the initial choice of therapy. For example, diarrhoea in postweaned pigs may be due to coliform gastroenteritis or salmonellosis. Neomycin sulphate could be used for initial therapy of the outbreak but samples are taken for culture to differentiate between salmonellosis and coliform gastroenteritis. In small animal practice, sensitivity testing is intended to give a rational basis for the choice of an antimicrobial drug.

Drug Distribution and Residues

Factors governing distribution involve a multicompartmental system with all body compartments being in contact directly or indirectly with the blood. The rate of exchange between the blood and the compartments is governed by the concentration of the drug and blood flow through the tissues. The extent of protein binding of the drug in blood and in the tissues, pH differences in the compartments, the lipid solubility and pKa of the drug strongly influence the efficacy of therapy. For example, the percentage of protein bound oxytetracycline in bovine serum is about 36%, that of minocycline and doxycycline reaches 80% and 90%, respectively. The extent of their penetration into milk (Ziv and Sulman, 1974b) as well as their transplacental passage correlated with the degree of protein binding of ampicillin (20% bound) and cloxacillin (90% bound).

When the volume of distribution exceeds or even approximates total body water, antimicrobials can enter cells. Such large diffusion which includes brain, cerebro-spinal fluid, eye, placenta and foetus, applies to sulphonamides, chloramphenicol, tetracyclines and macrolides (Siddique and Simunek, 1977). Weak acids like penicillins or weak organic bases like aminoglycosides have a low volume of distribution and thus remain in the extracellular compartment.

The blood–milk barrier represents a major consideration for therapy and residues since milk is traditionally the staple diet in infants. Besides the intramammary antibiotics which are dyemarked, systemically administered antibiotics may appear in the milk: the highest ratio between drug concentrations in milk and in serum is found for macrolides (erythromycin, spiramycin, tylosin) and for lipophilic tetracyclines (minocycline, doxycycline). However, the withdrawal period depends more on the sensitivity of the method of analysis and on the country's regulations than on a pharmacokinetic basis. For example, the 10–15 days required for benzathine–penicillin, dihydrostreptomycin and oxacillin, and 5–7 days for chloramphenicol, tetracyclines and sulphonamides do not reflect the amount persisting in the milk of a lactating cow following mastitis.

Antibiotics are transported across the placenta to varying degrees (Kauffman *et al.*, 1973). From cord plasma obtained at birth, it has been shown that for low binding substances the amount crossing the placenta will be maximal. The stage of gestation is another factor involved in the foeto–maternal blood ratio of sulphadimidine which increases from 0.5 to 0.9 in pregnant goats (Siddique and Simunek, 1977). The placental transfer of chloramphenicol occurs in cattle as in the human, with no untoward effect despite the well-described "gray syndrome". Tetracyclines, due to their affinity for skeletal structures, are incorporated irreversibly into the matrix of the foetal osseous tissue.

Residues in edible tissues are usually those of antibiotics used for therapeutic purposes by the rearer without having allowed an appropriate interval to elapse between the last treatment and slaughter. The withholding time is strongly influenced by assay sensitivities and by differences in drug persistence in diseased as opposed to healthy animals. In cattle, taking the kidney cortex as a reference and considering muscle, the withdrawal times vary from 2–3 days to 3 weeks for penicillins and aminoglycosides, respectively, and these values could be threefold increased in nephrotic animals (Nouws and Ziv, 1978). In pigs, the withdrawal period set at 10 days for sulphamethazine and tylosin could be shifted by placing animals on bedding in pens formerly occupied by medicated pigs. The tendency to root out and consume part of the bedding accounted for sulphamethazine concentrations developing in excess of 0.1 ppm (Samuelson *et al.*, 1979).

Useful and Useless Combinations

A major breakthrough in sulphonamide therapy has come about with the discovery of trimethoprim, an antimetabolite of folic acid and which has antimicrobial properties of its own. It prevents conversion of folic acid into folinic acid by inhibiting the enzyme dihydrofolate reductase. The mechanism of antimicrobial action differs from that of sulphonamides, which compete with PABA in folic acid synthesis. The double attack by the combination sulphonamide + trimethoprim synergically produces "thymine—less death" of the organism. However, the biological half-life of trimethoprim is shorter than that of the sulphonamides in the human and even in domestic animals, thus emphasizing the need to search for sulphonamides other than sulphadiazine of sulphamethoxypyridazine to maintain the optimal blood ratio.

Adverse reactions and side effects may result from useless combinations of antibiotics. The true hazard of some combinations is unknown beyond the classical antagonism between the group penicillins, aminoglycosides and the group sulphonamides, tetracyclines, macrolides, chloramphenicol. The following interactions are well documented: poorly absorbable tetracyclines—calcium complex in milk-fed calves; muscle weakness by aminoglycosides potentiated by anaesthetics, barbiturates, sodium citrate; altered antibody production by chloramphenicol and erythromycin; decreased antibacterial action of aminoglycosides, erythromycin and chloramphenicol in acidosis (Craig and White, 1976). The combination of antibiotics with other compounds (e.g. corticosteroids) is difficult to justify on grounds other than convenience. The danger of these products is that it is too easy to administer the combination to every case on the grounds of vague feeling that it must be doing some good, without thinking about the specific indications for each component (Davis and Faulkner, 1976).

Antibacterial Chemotherapy in Cattle

Enteric infections (associated with *E. coli* and *Salmonella* spp. in calves), respiratory diseases in feedlot heifers (associated with mycoplasma in 82% of cases, *Pasteurella haemolytica* in 52% or *P. multocida* in 26% and *Corynebacterium pyogenes* in 12%), mastitis and metritis (associated with *Streptococcus* spp., *Staphylococcus* spp., *E. coli* and other coliform organisms) are the major diseases encountered in cattle.

Undifferentiated Pneumonia, Diarrhoea and Coccidiosis

Routes of administration, dosage rates and cost of antibacterials were defined by Hjerpe and Routen (1976) for a 13,000-head capacity feed-lot in California, thus giving the relative importance and values of the drugs used in calf pneumonia as well as others available to the owner.

Among sulphonamides, the most used and the least expensive in large animal practice is sulphadimidine (sulphamethazine) given orally as tablets once daily. Therapy should be initiated with parenteral administration of 150 mg/kg of the sodium salt in ruminants, since rumen stasis may markedly influence the absorption, and since peak blood levels may not occur for periods up to 15 hours following oral administration. The blood level is maintained by the use of oral sulphadimidine (Blood *et al.*, 1976), 68% of an oral dose being absorbed (Koritz *et al.*, 1978b). Comparative studies showed that daily oral dosing of sulphadimethoxine at 27.5 mg/kg serves to sustain the plasma concentration achieved by an initial intravenous dose of 55 mg/kg given as a loading dose (Boxenbaum *et al.*, 1977). Sulphonamides are excreted through the ruminal wall and salivary glands, and they are acetylated (Atef *et al.*, 1979). Sulphathiazole is more extensively acetylated (16.2%) than sulphadiazine (7.1%) or sulphamerazine (8.4%) and is thus more rapidly excreted. Since no synergic effect is seen for cotrimazine against organisms which are sensitive to only sulphadiazine or trimethoprim alone, the discrepancy between the biological half-lives of the sulphonamide (5 h) and trimethoprim (0.5 h) seems to be detrimental in ruminants (Hungerford, 1979).

Among antibiotics, the serum concentrations obtained after oral and parenteral routes of administration in calves are related to weaning. Ampicillin which is acid stable is well absorbed following oral administration: milk either suckled or taken from a pail bypasses the rumen and enters the abomasum directly from the oesophagus by contraction of the reticular groove forming a closed conduit to the reticulo–abomasal orifice. When given orally to 2–6 weeks old calves, ampicillin (400 mg) dissolved in milk is detected in the plasma within 57 min. Atropine administration slowed the appearance of the drug in the plasma but did not decrease the efficiency of absorption (Thompson and Black, 1978), which was similar to that seen after parenteral administration. For chloramphenicol to reach a tissue level of 5 μg/ml in bovines, a dose of at least 50 mg/kg must be administered intramuscularly and at two sites (Nouws and Ziv, 1979). Oral administration before weaning at a dose of 50 mg/kg permitted a level of only 5 μg/ml for 2–3 hours to be reached, even in the newborn. At 12 weeks, the plasma chloramphenicol level rarely reached 1 μg/ml, thus suggesting that rumen function may interfere even in relatively young animals (De Backer et al., 1978). Oxytetracycline has been subjected to a great deal of sophisticated formulation technology to obtain stable solutions for injections. Polyvinylpyrrolidone enabled more concentrated solutions, e.g. 100 mg/ml, to be prepared, and now long-acting injectable solutions of 200 mg/ml, superior in terms of viscosity, freezing point and syringeability to some of the more dilute formulations are available. A single intramuscular injection of 20 mg/kg maintains a therapeutic blood level of 0.5 μg/ml over a 3–4 day period. Deep intramuscular injections in the rump or thigh (minimum needle length of 3 cm) are well tolerated and all edible tissues are negative for the drug within 28 days.

A comparative study of resistance of E. coli in scouring calves infected first by rotavirus shows the inefficacy of oxytetracycline, sulphonamides and streptomycin, the relative inefficacy of ampicillin and chloramphenicol, while gentamicin, colistin and quinolines are always active (see Table 2). The variety of oral antibiotic and sulphonamide preparations available for the treatment of calf diarrhoea is testimony to the lack of complete understanding of the therapy of this condition (Moon et al., 1978). Amoxycillin (7 mg/kg), an ampicillin derivative (Kirby et al., 1974), neomycin sulphate, the combination erythromycin–colistin (Jobard et al., 1975), and combinations of trimethoprim with sulphonamides are claimed to be of value in nearly 75% of the cases.

Coccidiosis occurs commonly in calves of more than 2 months of age. A count of 5,000 oocysts/g of faeces, considered as significant, occurs for a short period of 3–6 days after the peak of clinical signs. Coccidiosis is a self limiting disease, with increased host susceptibility after dexamethasone and cold stress. Sulphonamides, e.g. sulphadimidine and sulphathiazole, are effective at a dosage of 1 g/75 kg of body weight. Other drugs used for chemosuppression are nivaquine, mepacrine hydrochloride, metronidazole and dimetridazole which, like other imidazole derivatives, were recently found to be of interest in the treatment of anaerobic bacterial infections. The signs of coccidiosis in lambs range also from loose diarrhoeal faeces to severe dysentery. Monensin suppressed the development of *Eimeria* infection until a week after the drug was discontinued (Bergstrom and Maki, 1976). Aureomycin (10 mg/kg of feed) is equally active but the two drugs fed together have a detrimental effect, since the mean daily gain was 0.23 kg instead of 0.33 kg (Samizadeh-Yazd *et al.*, 1979).

Bovine Metritis and Mastitis

Bovine metritis varies from a very acute postpartum septic metritis to an endometritis barely detectable clinically. In order to treat an overcoming suspected uterine infection, general therapy may be used; in this case, intramuscular doses of antibiotics must be repeated in order to maintain a sufficient serum concentration (Table 3).

TABLE 3

Intramuscular Complementary Doses of Antibiotics Necessary to Maintain a Required Serum Concentration in Cattle

Antibiotic	Initial dose (mg/kg)	Required serum concentration (μg/kg)	Maintenance dose (every 12 hours) (mg/kg)
Benzylpenicillin	10	0.05	4.2
		1.00	93.2
Ampicillin	10	0.05	7.6
		1.00	75.4
Dihydrostreptomycin	20	5.00	55.0
Oxytetracycline	20	1.00	48.6
Erythromycin	10	0.05	2.1
		1.00	42.4
Lincomycin	10	0.10	1.8
		1.00	17.8
Spiramycin	10	2.5	0.6
		5.0	1.2
Chloramphenicol sodium succinate	50	2.5	59.1
		5.0	118.2

Usually a dilute iodine solution (250 ml of 2% Lugol) or large doses of broad spectrum antibiotics (e.g. 2–4 g of oxytetracycline, 1 g of streptomycin or around 5 g of benzylpenicillin) are given by intra-uterine infusion (Arbeiter *et al.*, 1979). Rapid absorption occurs from the uterine lumen or possibly by escape into the peritoneal cavity at the time of proestrus and oestrus (Ayliffe and Noates, 1978). Ancillary therapy is to mobilise the uterine defence mechanisms by oestrogens followed within 2 weeks by infusion of an antibiotic preparation.

Increased conception rates is another aspect of intra-uterine antibacterial treatment. The most common bacteria isolated are *Streptococcus* spp. which account for about 50%, others being *E. coli, Klebsiella, Staphylococcus* and *Corynebacterium*. The conception rate of 20 cows was 54% compared with 23% in controls after an antibiotic infusion or an irritating solution which causes premature luteolysis (Oxender, 1976). Nitrofuran derivatives or sulphonamides and gentamicin are indicated when *Pseudomonas* is involved (Ensley and Hennessy, 1979). Evidence of latent infection was that the first service conception rate of cows infused with sulphonamides 24 h after insemination was 73% compared with 43% for untreated controls in clinical trials (Oxender, 1976).

Retained foetal membranes is a common sequel to induction of parturition using corticosteroids. Injection of diethylstilboestrol (60 mg) and of calcium borogluconate (100 ml of a 24% solution) at the time of injection of corticosteroids reduces the incidence of retained foetal membranes: 24% as against 62% with dexamethasone alone. It is also a common practice to treat all cows retaining membranes with an injection of benzylpenicillin or one of the other widely used antibiotics, whether or not there appears to be an increase in metritis following induction.

Antibiotics are administered via the intramammary route in the treatment of chronic or mild mastitis, and parenterally in acute clinical cases of mastitis (Cecyre *et al.*, 1979). For parenteral use, high availability to the infection site is desirable. A drug which is weakly basic or otherwise highly ionized in serum and sufficiently lipid soluble is indicated, e.g. a macrolide like erythromycin (Ziv and Sulman, 1974a). However the bioavailability of erythromycin (pKa = 8.8) is influenced by "ion trapping" in the rumen, especially when the animal is fed on concentrates, i.e. at a pH close to 5.5. The mean tissue concentration in the udder, which is about 8 times that of the plasma, decreases during mastitis due to pH changes (pH 7.5). Changes occur also during urinary acidosis (pH 7.5) (Fig. 1). By contrast, the milk pH changes during mastitis may enhance the tissue concentration of substances like sulphonamides, penicillins which are usually poorly distributed to the udder (McDiarmid, 1978).

For local use during lactation, penicillin, especially in peanut oil base containing 3% aluminium monostearate (Roguinsky, 1972), could give a success rate close to 100% in the case of infection with *Streptococcus agalactiae*, at a dose of 100,000 I.U. at 48 h intervals. Cloxacillin which is not degraded by the staphylococcal penicillinases

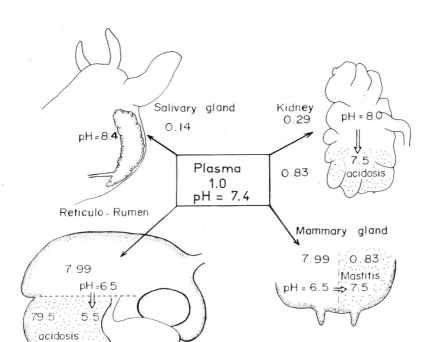

FIG. 1   Concentration in μg/ml of erythromycin in various tissues of lactating cow, about 10 h after an intramuscular injection of 12.5 mg/kg.

is widely used (200 mg daily for 3 days) alone or combined with ampicillin (75 mg) against *Staphylococcus aureus* (Le Louedec, 1978). Novobiocin (25 mg daily for 3 days) is able to cure clinically 96% of cases affected by *S. aureus* as against 16% for penicillin--streptomycin. Other antibiotics like rifamycin SV (Ruffo *et al.*, 1973), kanamycin–spiramycin (Deschanel *et al.*, 1976), ampicillin (Pepin and Boudene, 1977), tylosin (Launay *et al.*, 1977) or nitrofurans like nifuroquine (100 mg at 12 h intervals) are claimed to cure 70 to 80% of cases affected by *S. aureus* and mycobacteria.

Antibiotics for infusion in dry cow therapy must be non-irritant to the udder. Benzathine--cloxacillin eliminates 84% of *S. aureus* and 94% of *S. agalactiae* infections. Penicillin with novobiocin or with neomycin are other major active ingredients. In a clinical trial on the bacteriological efficacy of benzathine–cloxacillin (500 mg) versus erythromycin (600 mg) in dry cow therapy, Clegg *et al.* (1975) obtained a successful treatment of *S. aureus* in 72.9 and 75.4% of the infected quarters, respectively. Erythromycin efficacy (88.6% and 100%) also compares favourably with that of cloxacillin (84.4%

and 86%) against *Corynebacterium bovis* and *Streptococcus uberis*, respectively.

Antibacterial Drugs in Swine

A closer veterinary involvement in the pig industry is warranted for any restriction in the use of certain antibiotics in feed at subtherapeutic levels and for more emphasis on the use of therapeutic levels of antibiotics for disease control.

Major Bacterial Infections

Clostridial infections are sporadic, except for gas gangrene in wound infections or at the site of iron injection in piglets: penicillins are the drugs of choice, as for erysipelas. *E. coli* is very common in intensive piggeries. Products commonly used parenterally are oxytetracycline (4–10 mg/kg daily), neomycin sulphate (10–20 mg/kg) cotrimazine (10–20 mg/kg) and ampicillin (2–6 mg/kg). In the case of ampicillin, recent pharmacokinetic studies advise the use of higher doses (Galtier and Alvinerie, 1979) possibly with enhancement of its bioavailability by probenecid (Fig. 2). The plasma clearance (Cp) of ampicillin is decreased after forced feeding of probenecid (40 mg/kg) and its biliary excretion rate is increased by sodium dehydrocholate (DHC) at 20 mg/kg. Since the elimination half-life of oxytetracycline is about 4.5 h in pigs, in contrast to 15 h in horses (Mercer *et al.*, 1978), again higher daily doses must be used. Sulphonamides, especially sulphadimethoxine, a long acting sulphonamide as compared with sulphamerazine or sulphadiazine, are of interest in both treatment and control of *Haemophilus, Bordetella bronchiseptica* and *Listeria* infections. The longer action of sulphadimethoxine is attributed to a higher degree of binding of the drug to plasma proteins and its reabsorption by non-ionic diffusion from renal tubular fluid. It has been shown also that tissue concentrations were 3 to 8 times higher in suckling pigs than in growing pigs which eliminate the drug more efficiently (Righter *et al.*, 1979).

In-Water and In-Feed Disease Control

Mycoplasmal infections with polyserositis, arthritis and sudden onset of lameness are often associated with pneumonia. They are poorly controlled by an injection of tylosin or spectinomycin or oxytetracycline unless followed up by the use at therapeutic level of 100 g per tonne of feed of tylosin and lincomycin or spectinomycin for 10 days. A concentration of 40 g per tonne of feed is then given

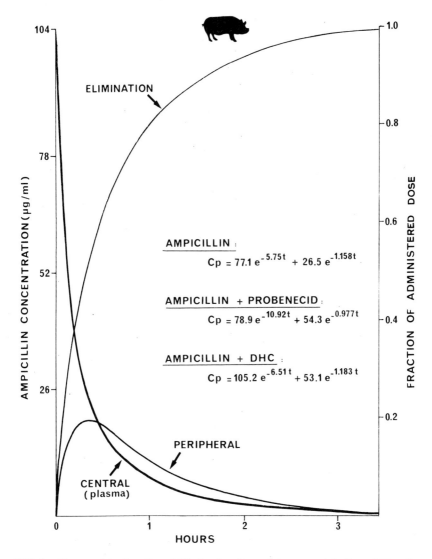

FIG. 2 Pharmacokinetics of ampicillin in pigs after an intravenous injection of 20 mg/kg, with comparative plasma clearance (Cp) equations when the antibiotic is administered alone or together with probenecid (40 mg/kg) or dehydrocholate (DHC) (20 mg/kg). Reprinted from Galtier and Charpenteau (1979); Galtier and Alvinerie (1979) with permission.

continuously. Sulphadimidine or sulphaquinoxine (200 g/tonne) is used after a parenteral loading dosage of sulphadimidine (100 mg/kg daily for 3 days intraperitoneally) for pasteurellosis, which may or may not be secondary to mycoplasmal pneumonia. When severe respiratory distress and laboured breathing occur, long-acting penicillins are required.

Salmonellosis may be a secondary infection following swine dysentary due to *Treponema hyodysenteriae* and is controlled by appropriate drug injection or by medication via drinking water, followed by carbadox (50 g per tonne of feed), dimetridazole (100 g per tonne of feed), etc. fed continuously and withdrawn 70 days prior to slaughter.

The injection of long-acting penicillins which are very effective for the control of streptococcal and staphylococcal infections, mastitis, agalactic syndrome, etc. is followed up by sulphadimidine (500 g/ tonne) or chloramphenicol (200 g/tonne) for 7 days. However, both chloramphenicol and corticosteroids are avoided for sows prior to farrowing since they pass through the milk to the piglets and cause immunosuppression.

Antibacterial Chemotherapy in Horses

The penicillin group of antibiotics, the first of the true antibiotics to be introduced into medicine, remains by far the most potent and effective in horses. The use of antibacterials which has been extensively reviewed in this species also includes sulphonamides (English and Roberts, 1979; Tobin 1978).

Peculiarities of Penicillin Therapy

Penicillins are active against Gram-positive organisms at the minimum effective concentrations of 0.1 unit/ml for streptococci and 2.5 unit/ ml for staphylococci. The use of broad spectrum penicillins active against Gram-negative bacteria, including *E. coli, Shigella, Proteus*, e.g. ampicillin in aqueous solution, is thus indicated in enteritis and septicaemia. The excretion of penicillin by the kidney is five times faster than inulin (Knudsen, 1960), hence a half-life of about 30 to 40 minutes, so that the drug is useless except for urinary tract infections (Table 4). Prolonged plasma levels are obtained by the administration of insoluble preparations such as procaine or benzathine penicillin. The minimum effective concentration of 0.1 unit/ml for 24 h requires 2 million units of procaine–penicillin for a 500 kg horse. However, the horse is about 20 times more sensitive than the human to plasma levels of procaine (about 30 million units are sufficient for procaine toxicity) and embarrassing procaine "positive" urine may be recorded in racehorses up to two weeks after a usual therapeutic dose (Tobin and Blake, 1977). Because of its very low toxicity, the dosage of penicillin is not limited and high doses may be used to pass cellular membranes, e.g. into joint cavities, pleural cavities, and cerebrospinal fluid. Five million units of procaine–

TABLE 4

Mean Plasma Concentration and Half-Life of Antimicrobial Drugs in the Horse

Drug and usual active concentration (μg/ml)	Protein binding	Dosage mg/kg bodyweight	Half-life (hours)	Mean plasma concentration (μg/ml)	References
Sodium benzyl penicillin (0.01 to 5)	45%	15 30	0.9	0.15 at 12 h	Doll and Dimock (1946)
Sodium ampicillin (0.03 to 4)	10%	40	1.5		Durr (1976)
Gentamicin (0.1 to 1)		4.4 (i.m.)		1.4 at 9 h	Beech *et al.* (1977)
Chloramphenicol (1 to 5)		20 (i.m.)	0.9	2.5 at 8 h	Sisodia *et al.* (1975)
Oxytetracycline (2)	50%	4.4 (i.v. & i.m.) 4.4 (i.v. & i.m.)	15.7 & 10.5 24.0 & 48.0	0.5 at 36 h	Teske *et al.* (1973) Eidt *et al.* (1976)
Trimethoprim (0.5 to 2)		5.5	3.4	1 at 12 h	Alexander and Collett (1974)
Sulphadimidine (10 to 50)		60 (i.v.)	9.8	20 at 24 h	Tschudi (1972)
Sulphamonomethoxine (10 to 50)	40%	60 (i.v.)	5.5	10 at 12 h	Stewart and Paris (1962)

penicillin are sometimes used as a loading charge for a 500 kg horse followed up by lower doses twice daily.

Among other drugs listed in Table 4, gentamicin is used for uterine lavage, and chloramphenicol has a very short life in the horse. By contrast, oxytetracycline is slowly eliminated after enterophepatic cycling: its half-life is 4 times that seen in cattle and it is currently used by some practitioners.

Sulphonamide Loading and Maintenance Dosages

New interest has been attracted by sulphonamides like sulphadiazine or sulphamethoxypyridazine which are potentiated by trimethoprim (TMP). The combination should aim to provide a plasma concentration of 2.5 and 50 μg/ml respectively, i.e. a ratio of 1:20. Due to the larger volume of distribution of TMP, the commercial combination ratio is 4:20. However, TMP and sulphonamides are not handled similarly by the horse body and the optimum 1:20 ratio is not reached for a long time. Other sulphonamides may be used. Pharmacokinetic studies suggest an intravenous loading charge of

26.5 mg/kg for sulphamidine, 53.2 mg/kg for sulphadimethoxine, 250 mg/kg for sulphaphenazole and only 9.7 mg/kg for sulphamerazine. The corresponding half-life (hours) and volume of distribution (l/kg) values suggest the following daily maintenance dosage rate starting 12 h after the loading dose: 9.8 h and 0.37 l/kg i.e. 21.6 mg/kg for sulphamidine; 11.3 h and 0.37 l/kg i.e. 41 mg/kg for sulphadimethoxine; 8.8 h and 0.33 l/kg i.e. 210 mg/kg for sulphaphenazole; 11.9 h and 0.47 l/kg i.e. 7.3 mg/kg for sulphamerazine.

In practice, for acute infection, the penicillin–ampicillin group is of considerable use, with an antibacterial action persisting for a period after plasma levels of the drug decline. Sulphonamides are of interest for bacteriostatic cover (e.g. cover for virus infections). The rule is that the desired effect must be obtained within 12 hours after a loading dose. If not, a change of drug should be made. Combinations should be treated with caution. For example, the synergy which occurs with a combination such as procaine–penicillin and dihydrostreptomycin (a cell wall inhibitor and a cell membrane inhibitor) will be only of value if the daily dose is divided, owing to

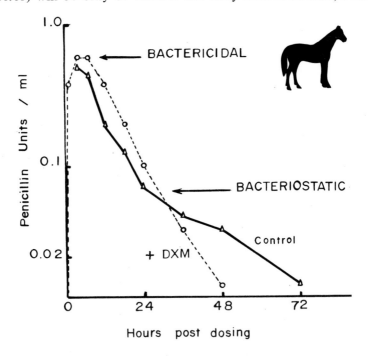

FIG. 3   Mean plasma concentration in U/ml of penicillin in horses, after intramuscular administration of a mixture of procaine penicillin G (4000 IU/kg) and dihydrostreptomycin (4000 IU/kg) alone (– △ –) or associated to dexamethasone (DMX) (– – ○ – –). Reprinted from Tobin (1978) with permission.

the rapid excretion of dihydrostreptomycin. It is also necessary to avoid enhancement of elimination by association with corticoids (Fig. 3).

Canine Antibacterial Chemotherapy

The clinician in small animal practice also bases his choice of treatment on his clinical experience and on the order of frequency of causal organisms (Table 5). As claimed by Hird (1979), the diagnosis must be firstly that the patient is suffering from a bacterial infection.

TABLE 5

Suggested Antibiotics to Treat Canine Bacterial Infections

Site of infection	Causal organisms	First choice antibiotic	Second choice antibiotic
Skin and appendages	a. *S. pyogenes*	Penicillin	Erythromycin
	b. Staphylococcus with β–haemolytic streptococcus	Neomycin (topically)	Cloxacillin
	c. Mixed infections	Lincomycin	Amoxycillin Cotrimazine
Urinary tract	a. Mixed infections with coliforms	Cotrimazine	Nitrofurantoin Gentamicin
	b. Pure coliform infection	Amoxycillin (possibly)	
External ear	*S. pyogenes*, the predominant organism, with β–haemolytic streptococcus and *Pseudomonas*	Neomycin (topically)	Framycetin Nystatin Cloxacillin Erythromycin Tetracycline
Oral cavity	Mixed infections with *Bacteroides* spp. Flagellates may also be pathogenic	Penicillin	Tetracycline
Eye	*S. pyogenes*	Neomycin	Framycetin Chloramphenicol

Antibiotic Selection

Gram-positive organisms, especially *Staphylococcus aureus*, are usually the significant pathogens in dermatitis and osteomyelitis. An extremely soluble antibiotic like lincomycin penetrates well into bone and will be effective if started early, while the bone still retains its blood supply. Antibiotics like erythromycin and ampicillin are able to attain high cerebrospinal fluid levels when the meninges are inflamed, but only trivial levels otherwise. Brain levels of chloramphenicol appear to remain adequate for as long as 12 hours, even though the blood level will have diminished to a minimal value in this period (Waston and McDonald, 1976). Since there is little protein in the cerebrospinal fluid, sulphonamides will mostly be free and able to exert their antimicrobial action, thus making cotrimazine suitable.

Broad-spectrum agents, such as neomycin or chloramphenicol without addition of a corticosteroid, are the first line of approach for the eye. Subconjunctival injection has the advantage of introducing the antibiotic at the site but chloramphenicol is capable of crossing the blood—humour barrier, when given systemically.

Penicillins, streptomycin, erythromycin, gentamicin, nitrofurantoin and soluble sulphonamides attain satisfactory high urinary concentrations. Because of this high concentration, even narrow-spectrum antibiotics, such as penicillin G, may be present in concentrations sufficiently high to kill even insensitive bacterial species such as *E. coli* (Ling and Gilmore, 1977). Moreover, amoxycillin achieves much higher blood levels than the same dose of ampicillin in the dog and should thus be regarded as a drug of choice. TMP is concentrated in the canine prostate when given in combinations with sulphamethoxazole or with sulphadiazine and may be of value in urinary tract infections associated with chronic prostatitis (Robb *et al.*, 1971).

Advantages claimed for combinations are: a broader spectrum of antimicrobial activity, synergic actions and lower toxicity of each component drug. The disadvantage of a fixed-dose combination is that the antibiotics may have totally different pharmacokinetic characteristics. The indications for antibiotic combination therapy are overwhelming infection and mixed infections, e.g. contamination of surface wounds. Useful synergy can be reliably obtained from some penicillin and cephalosporin mixtures and from penicillin with streptomycin, etc.

Some antibiotics, such as penicillins, are remarkably free of adverse reactions in veterinary usage. The reasons for lack of success are failure to start treatment early enough (since antibiotics work best during the logarithmic phase of bacterial growth) or to select the correct antibiotic. Another cause is lack of penetration into the site of infection, due not only to natural barriers (e.g. blood—humour and blood—brain barriers) or to pathological processes (e.g. fibrosis around an abscess, pH of pus) but also to underdosing.

Antibiotic Dosage

Antibiotic treatment commonly results in an overdosage in cats and an underdosage in dogs. Overdosage is less serious than underdosage which results in selection of resistant organisms without improvement in the condition under treatment. Weighing of patients and knowledge of bioavailability of the drugs used are therefore necessary, since blood concentrations of drugs given subcutaneously may never reach therapeutic levels, because clearance from the body is proceeding as rapidly as the drug is being released from the injection site. Tylosin, which belongs to the macrolide group is highly distributed (1.7 l/kg) but is cleared at 22 mg/kg/min (Weisel *et al.*, 1977). Obviously the recommended dose of 6–11 mg/kg which produces a serum level of 1 μg/ml for only 30 min is insufficient to treat infections by *Pasteurella* spp. and some *Staphylococcus* (m.i.c. values around 0.4 μg/ml). By contrast, rapid achievement and maintenance of therapeutic levels for oxytetracycline (i.e. a serum concentration from 1.25 to 5.00 μg/ml) are easily obtained by a priming dose (10 mg/kg intravenously) followed by maintenance doses (7.5 mg/kg) at 12 h intervals (Baggot *et al.*, 1978).

The importance of clinical trials and pharmacokinetic studies for antibiotic dosage has been shown for amoxycillin, cotrimazine and gentamicin. Two formulations were used for clinical testing of amoxycillin in 351 dogs and 264 cats: oral capsules (4 to 11 mg/kg) given twice daily and an aqueous suspension by injection at doses ranging from 2 to 7 mg/kg. Overall percentage success was 80.1% (Francis *et al.*, 1978), with 80.9% for oral capsules and 73.8% for injectable suspension. These results emphasize that it may be worthwhile to consider oral administration three or four times daily rather than relying upon a single daily injection to achieve reliable tissue concentrations (Bogan, 1977). Similar observations have been made for ampicillin (Bywater, 1978).

Since TMP, a weakly basic drug (pKa 7.3), is extensively metabolised in the dog (unlike in man), variations in urinary pH will alter the optimum ratio of TMP and sulphadiazine, a weak acid (pKa 6.8). In spite of these drawbacks clinical trials show that cotrimazine is effective in the treatment of urinary tract infections (Weaver and Philinger, 1977) and that adequate tissue levels of cotrimazine are maintained for up to 24 h following oral administration (Craig and White, 1976).

The serum concentration of gentamicin drops below the therapeutic level within 12 h of administration, and the injection of 4 mg/kg of bodyweight twice daily seems necessary to maintain adequate levels in tissues for treatment of a variety of canine bacterial diseases including cystitis, nephritis, tonsillitis, pneumonia, tracheobronchitis, and skin and soft-tissue wounds. In practice, when a single subcutaneous injection of 20 mg/kg of bodyweight is substituted for the first three injections of the multiple-dose regimen, the drug concentrations in many tissues tested are higher than with the multiple dosage regimen (Spreat and Van Horse, 1979), thus suggesting the benefits of a single elevated dose.

The Future in Veterinary Medicine

The great screening effort for antibacterials has passed its peak although there is still the need for antibiotics for growth promotion in animal husbandry (Visek, 1979) and for better chemotherapy against infections caused by some Gram-negative bacteria such as some coliforms, by protozoa and by viruses. Although some antibiotics are available without veterinary prescription, problems of an ethical nature arise in the use of antibacterial drugs in therapeutics and in feed, the risk being to human health. There is a need for more sophistication in feed additives, including the use of non-therapeutic antibacterial drugs for the purpose of growth, and their use at therapeutic concentrations only at times of stress and for a limited period of time. Similarly, in the treatment of infections, one must beware of the feeling that if one antimicrobial drug is good, two or three should cure almost everybody of everything. Accordingly, the true challenge should be the penetration of drugs to the sites of infection for greater efficiency, and the use of an adequate total dose at proper intervals. The selection of the right drug for the right species in the right amounts would be a gargantuan task involving specific veterinary drugs. Moreover, diseases must be controlled according to the appropriate parameters: clinical, with analysis of hyperthermia, pain, anorexia in small animal practice; and economic ones, taking into account death loss, relapse rate, average daily gain and treatment time for response in large animals.

Penetration of Drugs to the Sites of Infection

The final proof of a drug's value is whether or not it controls the disease. Better knowledge of pharmacokinetics using models such as embedded "tissue cages", and clinical trials taking advantage of the closure of the reticular groove to by-pass the rumen are a prerequisite to improve the dosage regimen. Another approach may be to introduce more directly the antibacterials where they must act, for example in the lung, by intratracheal route in feedlot pneumonia (Hjerpe, 1979), or in the cells, by the use of liposomes as carriers for membrane penetration. The preparation of drugs with a large volume of distribution is another promising way. Assessment of the hepato— renal function prior to treatment may be of interest since diminished renal clearance results in an increased retention in the body, as with the use of probenecid to compete with cephalosporins in calves (Ziv *et al.*, 1978) and with ampicillin in pigs (Galtier and Alvinerie, 1979). The percentage of protein-bound antibacterials may be decreased as a result of hepato–renal disorders.

Adequate Dosage and Choice of Specific Antibacterials

When the results of pharmacokinetic studies in farm animals become available, it is probable that they will suggest changes in the dose levels and intervals for several antimicrobial drugs. The behaviour of a drug may differ from one species to another slightly, e.g. spiramycin (Videau, 1978), or to a large extent e.g. oxytetracycline (Baggot *et al.*, 1978), or sulphamethoxypyridazine (Stewart and Paris, 1962). The following example will illustrate the corresponding outcome: the average minimum inhibitory concentration (m.i.c.) for oxytetracycline against organisms considered to be sensitive varies from 0.13 μg/ml (*Sphaerophorus necrophorus*) to 1 μg/ml (*Listeria monocytogenes* and *Corynebacterium pyogenes*) and 2.54 μg/ml (*E. coli*). If we have to sustain a concentration at five times the m.i.c. for each of the three classes, i.e. from 0.65 to 12.7 μg/ml, the calculated maintenance dose to treat *E. coli* infections is, according to Teske *et al.* (1973) for 6 h and 12 h intervals, 14.5 and 37.3 mg/kg in cattle, and 15.5 and 38.6 mg/kg in the horse. The corresponding daily dose is well tolerated in cattle but harmful for horses.

The availability of drugs with a broad spectrum of activity (ampicillin, oxytetracycline) has lessened the need for drug combinations even for antibiotic prophylaxis. There is no more evidence in animals than in man that prophylactic antibiotic therapy reduces the incidence of postoperative infection whether given systemically or instilled into the wound. Antibiotics given to sterilise the gut prior to and after intestinal surgery are probably less effective than mechanical cleansing of the bowel by purgation and/or enema, which reduces the population of all organisms. By contrast, antibiotic prophylaxis is indicated in viral diseases if there is a distinct likelihood of bacterial secondary infection; e.g. tetracyclines may be used to prevent the development of *Bordetella bronchiseptica* pneumonia in dogs suffering from distemper; sulphonamides may be used to prevent infections in cattle with respiratory diseases. Knowledge of pharmacokinetics may predict from drug levels in blood or urine the time required for residues in edible tissue to decline to a sufficiently low level to allow their use for meat (Koritz *et al.*, 1978a).

An open question for the appropriate choice of antibacterials is the immunosuppressive effect of some antibiotics (chloramphenicol, erythromycin), as well as the concurrent usage of corticosteroids. This is especially true in calves where dexamethasone always suppresses anorexia, and in horses where excitatory effects are observed. Conclusive evidence that corticosteroids are detrimental or that they are beneficial to animal recovery is still lacking. Their routine use in infectious diseases should thus be discouraged and reserved to counteract specific effects. Canine blastomycosis becomes a fulminating infection and bovine coccidiosis diarrhoea progresses to dysentery with an oocyst production 10 times the previous level if they are used in these conditions.

For example, specific antibacterials are needed in the future for the treatment of herbivores, where excretion rates are often 3 to 4 times faster than in carnivores. Specificity is also the way to avoid idiosynchratic toxicity such as that of chloramphenicol in cats, which is due to their lack of glucuronyl transferase which detoxifies the drug. Chloramphenicol, which inhibits the liver microsomal enzymes involved in barbiturate inactivation, increases the duration of anaesthesia by barbiturates by 120% in dogs and by 260% in cats. The decrease in body temperature during penthiobarbital anaesthesia lasted about 3 hours in cats after an oral dose of chloramphenicol at 22 mg/kg of body weight compared with only 55 minutes in controls or after a subcutaneous injection of chloramphenicol which is not bioavailable from this route of administration (Ruckebusch and Richez, 1980). Peripheral respiratory paralysis due to neuromuscular blockade is a potential side effect of some antimicrobial drugs in pigs. At a dose of 30 mg/kg, both neomycin and streptomycin decreased by 44% the muscle twitch strength in pigs; a decrease by 20% was also recorded for tetracycline (40 mg/kg). The intravenous administration of calcium chloride (10 mg/kg) antagonized this neuromuscular blocking effect (Mathew *et al.*, 1978). Conversely, the use of aminoglycosides should be avoided at the time of calving because of an interaction with calcium metabolism. Displacement of drug bound to protein through interaction with a substance with a greater affinity for binding may occur with the expected side effects. Consequently, the effect required could thus be obtained through a lower dosage of the active drug, e.g. by supplementary injection of an antibiotic instead of thiopental to prolong anaesthesia (Fig. 4).

A survey of adverse reactions, such as those of antibiotics in cattle over a 3-year period in Canada, showed also the importance of specific reactions. Anaphylaxis was characterised by dyspnoea, swelling of the eyelids and perineum, and staggering. The overall mortality was 2%, a percentage also recorded by Stowe (1975) concerning the adverse effects of oxytetracycline and penicillins in

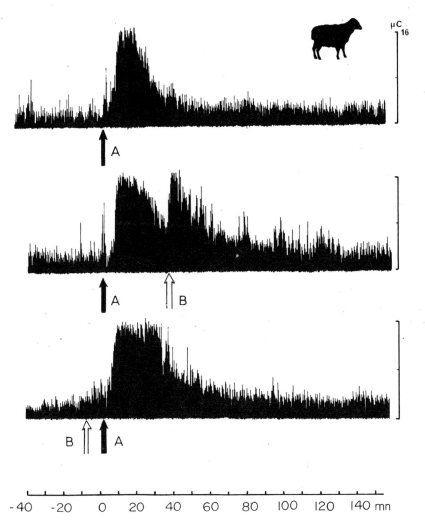

FIG. 4 Effect of injection of a highly protein bound antibiotic or non steroidal anti-flammatory drug on anaesthetised sheep by thiopental (pentobarbital). A: Injection of thiopental (25 mg/kg); B: Injection of doxycycline (10 mg/kg) or phenylbutazone (5 mg/kg). Electroencephalogram is recorded every 20 seconds. (From Ruckebusch and Richez, 1980.)

the state of Iowa. Analysis of the disposition in swine of sulphathiazole following intravenous administration of 72 mg/kg of body-weight revealed the presence of "fast" and of "slow" acetylators (Bourne *et al.*, 1978). Reports so far on polymorphic acetylation of drugs have been in humans and concern the metabolism of sulphadimidine, isoniazid, monoacetylhydrazine, hydralazine and the sulphone dapsone. The alleles controlling the acetylation of sulphadimidine are inherited in a simple Mendelian fashion, the "slow" acetylators being homozygous while the "fast" acetylators are either homozygous or heterozygous. The genes are probably controlling the production of acetyltransferase, the liver enzyme involved in the transfer of acetyl groups from acetyl CoA to the sulphonamide. After daily intravenous administration of oxytetracycline for 3 days, a positive dose–effect correlation was observed between 11 and 33 mg/kg, not for alleviation of clinical signs but for hepato–renal lesions, the lesions being similar to nephrosis produced by exogenous toxins (Griffin *et al.*, 1979). Sudden absorption of toxins from the uterus is probably the origin of adverse reactions to the injection both of stilboestrol, which increased blood flow, and antibiotics, in acute metritis.

Within the last 3 years, *Salmonella* strains, which represent one quarter of all the organisms found in bovine species in France (see Table 1), belonged to 31 serotypes; two species, *S. typhimurium* and *S. dublin*, accounted for 96% of all the strains. The number of resistant strains increased from 39% in 1976 to 96% in 1978. Such multiresistant strains, mainly those of *S. typhimurium*, would be a danger to man if strict observance of sanitary regulations during slaughtering of (sick) animals was not followed.

Conclusions

The era of modern chemotherapy was ushered in following the announcement half a century ago that Prontosil protected mice from experimental streptococcal infection. At the same time, it was found that a *Penicillium* mould and staphylococcal colonies produced a state of antibiosis. Nowadays, fungal and viral infections are antagonised by drugs capable of increasing the natural defence mechanism, e.g. by induction of interferon.

Since the use of antimicrobial drugs has become as sophisticated as that of cardiovascular drugs, it seems important to have a better understanding of their pharmacological properties in domestic animals. The LD50 of a true antibiotic like pure penicillin G administered intravenously is 3,500,000 units/kg of bodyweight for mice, but only 500,000 units/kg for an anaesthetised cat. A fatal 10 million-fold increase in the number of faecal coliforms is observed in guinea-pigs and also probably in pigs after the administration of penicillin. The future of veterinary antimicrobial chemotherapy is more likely to involve the search for the best way to provide a pause in microbial activity through specific drugs administered at an adequate dosage at proper intervals.

Two groups of antibiotics are in general use: "feed antibiotics", a safe and inexpensive way for intensive livestock husbandry, and "therapeutic antibiotics" with problems of residues due to injudicious use of an inadequate dosage. It may be unwise to follow the philosophy of the Swann report, influenced by the outbreak of *S. typhimurium* 20 years ago, without a better understanding of microbial ecology and the contribution of R–factor-bearing resistant strains to morbidity. The currently held doctrine is directed towards the uneconomic prescription of "therapeutic antibiotics"; it must be remembered that the sharper the weapon, the more completely can it be blunted.

References

Alexander, F. and Collett, R.A. (1974). *Br. J. Pharmacol.* **52**, 142.

Arbeiter, K., Awad-Maselmeh, M., Kopschitz, M.M., Lorin, D. and Willinger, H. (1979). *Tierärztl. Umsch.* **34**, 673–678.

Atef, M., Salem, A.A., Alsamarrae, S.A. and Zafer, S.A. (1979). *Res. Vet. Sci.* **27**, 9–14.

Ayliffe, T.R. and Noates, D.E. (1978). *J. Vet. Pharmacol. Therap.* **1**, 267–271.

Baggot, J.D., Powers, T.E., Powers, J.D., Kowalski, J.J. and Derr, K.M. (1978). *Res. Vet. Sci.* **24**, 77–81.

Beech, J., Kohn, C., Leitch, M., Weinstein, A.J. and Gallacher, M. (1977). *Am. J. Vet. Res.* **38**, 1085–1087.

Bergstrom, R.C. and Maki, L.R. (1976). *Am. J. Vet. Res.* **37**, 79–81.

Blood, D.C., Henderson, J.A. and Radostits, O.M. (1976). "Veterinary Medicine" (5th edn), pp. 75–97. Bailliere and Tindall Publish., London.

Bogan, J.A. (1977). *Vet. Rec.* **101**, 473–477.

Bourne, D.W., Dittert, L.W., Koritz, G.D. and Bevill, R.F. (1978). *J. Pharmacokinet. Biopharm.* **6**, 123–134.

Boxenbaum, M.G., Fellig, J., Hanson, L.J., Snyder, W.E. and Kaplan, S.A. (1977). *Res. Vet. Sci.* **23**, 24–28.

Bywater, R.J. (1978). *Vet. Rec.* **102**, 44–46.

Cecyre, A., Larouche, Y. and Malo, R. (1979). *Med. Vet. Quebec* **3**, 11–13.

Clegg, F.G., Halliday, G.J. and Hardie, H. (1975). *Br. Vet. J.* **131**, 639–642.

Craig, G.R. and White, G. (1976). *Vet. Rec.* **98**, 82–86.

Davis, L.E. and Faulkner, L.C. (1976). *In* "Proceedings of the Colorado State University Symposium (Sept. 1975)", C.S.U. Press, Fort Collins.

De Backer, P., Debackere, M. and De Corte-Baeten, K. (1978). *J. Vet. Pharmacol. Therap.* **1**, 135–140.

Deschanel, J.P., Desmoulins, M., Oudar, J. and Richard, Y. (1976). *Bull. Soc. Sci. Vet. Lyon* **78**, 97–100.

Doll, E.R. and Dimock, W.W. (1946). *J. Am. Vet. Med. Ass.* **108**, 209–214.

Dubourguier, M.C., Contrepois, M. and Gouet, P. (1979). *In* "Gastroentérites Néonatales du Veau" (Réunion Soc. Franc. Buiatrie, Vichy, Oct. 1979), pp. 161–171.

Durr, A. (1976). *Res. Vet. Sci.* **20**, 24–29.

Eidt, E., Anhalt, G. and Forehner, H. (1976). *Dtsch. Tierärztl. Wochenschr.* **83**, 489–492.

English, P.B. and Roberts, M.C. (1979). *J. Equine Med. Surg.* **3**, 259–268.

Ensley, L.E. and Hennesy, P.W. (1979). *Vet. Med. Small Anim. Clin.* **74**, 864–870.

Francis, M.E., Marshall, A.B. and Turner, W.T. (1978). *Vet. Rec.* **102**, 377–380.

Galtier, P. and Alvinerie, M. (1979). *J. Vet. Pharmacol. Ther.* **2**, 181–186.

Galtier, P. and Charpenteau, J.L. (1979). *J. Vet. Pharmacol. Ther.* **2**, 173–180.

Griffin, D.D., Amstutz, H.E., Morter, R.L., Hendrix, K.S. and Grandall, R.A. (1979). *Bov. Practitioner* **14**, 29–35.

Hird, J.F.R. (1979). *In* "Pharmacological Basis of Small Animal Medicine" (A.T. Yoxall and J.R.F. Hird, eds), pp. 63–84. Blackwell Sci. Publ., Oxford.

Hjerpe, C.A. (1979). *Bov. Practitioner* **14**, 18–26.

Hjerpe, C.A. and Routen, T.A. (1976). *Bov. Practitioner* **11**, 97–140.

Hungerford, T.C. (1979). Proceeding No. 39 (August 1978), University of Sydney, NSW Australia.

Jobard, A., Scheid, J.P., Grandadam, J.A., Boisson, J.M. and Benet, A. (1975). *Bull Soc. Vet. Prat.* **59**, 487–492.

Kauffman, R.E., Boulos, B.M. and Zarnoff, D.L. (1973). *Am. J. Obstet. Gynecol.* **117**, 66–72.

Kirby, W.M.M., Gordon, R.C. and Regamey, C. (1974). *J. Infect. Dis.* **129**, 154–155.

Knudsen, E. (1960). *Acta. Vet. Scand.* **1**, 188–200.

Koritz, G.D., Bevill, R.F., Bourne, D.W.A. and Dittert, L.W. (1978a). *Am. J. Vet. Res.* **39**, 481–484.

Koritz, G.D., Bourne, D.W.A., Dittert, L.W. and Bevill, R.F. (1978b). *J. Vet. Pharmacol. Therap.* **1**, 155–161.

Launay, M., Dintrans, J. and Gauthier, P. (1977). *Bull. Soc. Vet. Prat.* **61**, 27–37.

Le Louedec, C. (1978). *Ann. Rech. Vet.* **9**, 63–88.

Ling, G.V. and Gilmore, C.J. (1977). *J. Am. Vet. Med. Assoc.* **171**, 358–365.

Mathew, B.P., Teske, R.H., Robinson, J.A. and Adams, H.R. (1978). *J. Vet. Pharmacol. Therap.* **1**, 171–175.

McDiarmid, S.C. (1978). *New Zealand Vet. J.* **26**, 290–295.

Mercer, H.D., Teske, R.H., Lond, P.E. and Showalter, D.H. (1978). *J. Vet. Pharmacol. Therap.* **1**, 119–128.

Moon, H.N., McClurkin, A.W., Isaacson, R.E., Pohlenz, J., Skartuedt, S.M., Gillette, K.G. and Baetz, A.L. (1978). *J. Am. Vet. Med. Ass.* **174**, 577–583.

Nouws, J.F.M. and Ziv, G. (1978). *J. Vet. Pharmacol. Therap.* **1**, 47–56.

Nouws, J.F.M. and Ziv, G. (1979). *Vet. Quart.* **1**, 47–58.

Oxender, W.D. (1976). *J. Am. Vet. Med. Ass.* **168**, 217–219.

Pepin, G. and Boudene, C. (1977). *Rec. Med. Vet.* **153**, 565–571.

Righter, H.F., Showalter, D.H. and Teske, R.H. (1979). *Am. J. Vet. Res.* **40**, 713–715.

Robb, C.A., Carroll, P.T., Tippett, L.O. and Langston, J.B. (1971). *Invest. Urol.* **8**, 679–685.

Roguinsky, M. (1972). *Bull. Soc. Sci. Vet. Med. Comp. Lyon* **74**, 195–206.

Ruckebusch, Y. and Richez, P. (1980). *Ann. Anesth. Analg. Rean.* (to be published).

Ruffo, G., Nani, S. and Aliprandi, L. (1973). *Rec. Med. Vet.* **149**, 751–764.

Samizadeh-Yazd, A., Rhodes, C.N., Pope, A.L. and Todd, A.C. (1979). *Am. J. Vet. Res.* **40**, 1107–1109.

Samuelson, G., Whipple, D.M., Showaller, B.S., Jacobson, W.C. and Health, E. (1979). *J. Am. Vet. Med. Ass.* **175**, 449–452.

Siddique, A.B. and Simunek, J. (1977). *Acta Vet. Brno* **46**, 95–100.

Sisodia, C.S., Kramer, L.L., Gupta, V.S., Lerner, D.J. and Taksas, L. (1975). *Can. J. Comp. Med.* **39**, 216–223.

Smith, M.G. (1976). *Nature* (London) **261**, 348.

Spreat, S.R. and Van Horse, L.M. (1979). *Vet. Med. Small Anim. Clin.* **74**, 337–341.

Stewart, G.A. and Paris, R. (1962). *Aust. Vet. J.* **38**, 535–541.

Stowe, C.M. (1975). *J. Am. Vet. Med. Ass.* **166**, 980–981.

Teske, R.H., Rollins, L.D., Condon, R.J. and Carter, G.G. (1973). *J. Am. Vet. Med. Ass.* **162**, 119–120.

Thompson, S.M. and Black, W.D. (1978). *Can. J. Comp. Med.* **42**, 255–259.

Tobin, T. (1978). *J. Equine Med. Surg.* **2**, 475–479.

Tobin, T. and Blake, J.W. (1977). *J. Equine Med. Surg.* **1**, 188–194.

Tschudi, P. (1972). *Pferd Zbl. Vet. Med. A.* **19**, 851–861.

Videau, D. (1978). *Cah. Med. Vet.* **47**, 155–164.

Visek, W.J. (1979). *J. Anim. Sci.* **46**, 1447–1469.

Waston, A.D.J. and McDonald, P.J. (1976). *Am. J. Vet. Res.* **37**, 557–566.

Weaver, A.D. and Philinger, R. (1977). *Vet. Rec.* **101**, 77.

Weisel, K., Powers, J.D., Powers, T.E. and Baggot, J.D. (1977). *Am. J. Vet. Res.* **38**, 273–275.

Ziv, G. and Sulman, F.G. (1974a). *Am. J. Vet. Res.* **35**, 1197–1201.

Ziv, G. and Sulman, F.G. (1974b). *Res. Vet. Sci.* **17**, 68–74.

Ziv, G., Nouws, J.F.M., Groothuis, D.S. and Van Miert, A.S. (1978). *Refuah Vet.* **35**, 147–152.

Antibiotics as Feed Additives for Livestock

R. BRAUDE

c/o Commonwealth Agricultural Bureaux,
Reading, United Kingdom

Introduction

I welcome the opportunity to participate in this Symposium and assess the present situation concerning the use of antibiotics as feed additives in order to improve the performance of livestock. I am avoiding the well established term "growth promoters" because, as I will explain later, it is misleading on at least two accounts: other criteria than growth may be more important, and in future "growth" may not be involved at all.

I find myself in some difficulty because it can be genuinely argued that there is really nothing new to report in this field. In 1976 two symposia were held in the U.S.A., one in Texas organised by the American Society of Animal Science on the theme "Antibiotics in Animal Feeds: Human and Animal Safety Issues" (Solomons, 1978) the other at Iowa State University on "Nutrition and Drug Inter-relations" (Hathcock and Coon, 1978), incidentally two of many Symposia on this subject held in many places throughout the world. One can truly say that early in 1980 there is very little that one can add that could constructively advance the arguments in the controversy that existed then and continues to exist. What I intend to do today is to up-date some of the established facts and stimulate discussion on an issue which, I strongly believe, should no longer be controversial.

Use of Antibiotics as Feed Additives: A Controversial Issue

Time has moved very rapidly — it is now thirty years since the discovery that antibiotics can have a subsidiary function to their main use as therapeutic drugs, namely as a supplement to animal feed, capable of boosting food production for the growing population of the world. Just as the discovery of antibiotics was a milestone in the field of medicine and social sciences and contributed tremendously to improvement of health of people in the world, so did their application as feed additives contribute tremendously to our food resources, and is destined to continue to do so in the future. The picture is marred by a controversy which, unfortunately, is partly based on lack of adequate knowledge and partly on partisan interpretations by some authors of their own limited experimental data and extrapolation in terms of time, species and environmental (in the widest sense) circumstances. Controversy only exists when the scientific evidence is incomplete. As long as one has to deal with hypothesis there is room for different interpretations. One is quite entitled to adopt a tentative view and a temporary attitude, but one should be prepared to withdraw from, however well entrenched, positions, when the passage of time makes the hypothesis no longer tenable.

In the field of antibiotics as feed additives we are experiencing similar reactions to those in the surrounding political arena. A small group of militant activists picks on an established fact, like the one that poverty still exists, to build up their hypothesis on how to remedy the situation and save the world from disaster. A small group of individuals have launched a crusade to save the world from the imaginary "menace" connected with the use of antibiotics as feed additives for livestock, which is based on one or two facts established in the laboratory with no corroboration in the field, and all sorts of hypothetical speculations. They continue to extrapolate and exploit their limited data to create a public anxiety. However legitimate this attitude may have been in the early stages of the controversy, it seems to me futile to ignore the passage of time, and persist with such activities. I particularly deprecate the fact that politicians are brought in to adjudicate; this in turn brings into action the bureaucratic machinery and allows a few individuals to exert undue influence on subsequent developments. I have in mind the FDA in U.S.A., the various bodies in E.E.C. and in slightly different context, the Swann Committee in U.K. I have expressed my views on the latter elsewhere (Braude, 1978), and I will make only one comment here, namely that one should not take it for granted that, because in the U.K. the use of penicillin and tetracyclines as feed additives is controlled by veterinarians, there is convincing and scientifically sound evidence to support such a restriction. Fifteen years have passed since the Swann Committee's deliberations — nothing of significance emerged in U.K., but hectic battles continue to be fought in different parts of the world. FDA has been trying to "sort things out" in U.S.A., but became "politically" involved and can no longer be considered an impartial assessor. However, time has progressed rapidly and time is now ripe for a cease-fire to be called, with impartial observers appointed to guide and monitor future developments. In this field one should no longer indulge in speculations into what may or may not happen. If the evidence is adequate for present day conditions, one should not stifle both scientific and industrial progress by giving priority to misgivings for which there is no adequate proof.

If I may, I would like to digress here and comment on one other "political issue". At present the sale of antibiotics in premixes (carrier with a relatively small amount of active antibiotic) to supplement diets is directed through the channel of feedingstuffs merchants. There is a considerable pressure from the veterinarian to rope in this activity within the scope of their activities. Unless one opposes this tendency we may soon find other feed additives in the same orbit. After all, lack of vitamins creates clinical deficiency signs, excess of minerals may lead to bone abnormalities, both in some circumstances may result in residues in animal tissues. I hope that, in the future as up to now, these dietary additives will not call for a veterinary prescription, and I believe that antibiotics as feed additives fall into the same category. If some additional safeguards are needed there is not a better one than that antibiotics could be effectively withdrawn overnight should events justify it. And after all, they have been in use for 30 years and one should not expect a disaster to strike suddenly.

Benefit Assessment for Food Production

Meat production is a difficult task, and too easily taken for granted by the consumers, welfare people and legislators. Today, it is essential to take every possible measure to make this task easier. Obviously, one should encourage new developments, and provided all reasonable precautions are taken, one should welcome them. One wonders why the consumer sometimes, and public health authorities often, resent the use of antibiotics as feed additives? They do not appreciate, or perhaps sometimes are ignorant of the magnitude of the benefits these substances contribute to food production and modern methods of livestock management. Of course, one could have done without them and, of course, one could do without them in the future, but at what cost and why should one?

Here a few facts may be helpful. The population of the world has been increasing rapidly and Table 1 provides the relevant statistics for the last 10 years. I have subdivided the totals into figures for

TABLE 1

Population Changes (millions)

	1969	1978	Difference	% increase
Total	3,530	4,182	652	+18.5
Developed countries	1,070	1,146	76	+ 7.1
Developing countries	2,460	3,036	576	+23.4
France	50.3	53.3	3	+ 5.9
U.K.	55.4	56.7	1.3	+ 2.3

(From FAO, 1979)

developed and developing countries and added figures for U.K. and our host country. These are interesting figures, but obviously this is not the right place to analyse them in depth and interpret them, except to justify the conclusions which I intend to draw after presenting some other facts. In Table 2, corresponding figures are

TABLE 2

% Economically Active Population Employed in Agriculture

	1969	1978	Difference	% reduction
Total	51.5	46.2	−5.3	−10.3
Developed countries	16.8	13.6	−3.2	−19.0
Developing countries	67.3	60.7	−6.6	− 9.8
France	14.5	9.5	−5.0	−34.5
U.K.	2.9	2.2	−0.7	−24.0

(From FAO, 1979)

given for the percentage of economically active population employed in agriculture. Table 3 shows the changes in the population of cattle,

TABLE 3

Farm Animals in the World (millions)

		Total	Developed countries	Developing countries
Cattle	1969	1,097	390	707
	1978	1,213	432	781
	% increase	+10.6	+10.8	+10.4
Pigs	1969	625	269	356
	1978	732	314	418
	% increase	+17.1	+16.7	+17.4
Chickens	1969	5,315	2.468	2.847
	1978	6,468	2,886	3,582
	% increase	+21.6	+16.9	+25.8

(From FAO, 1979)

pigs and poultry during the last 10 years. Table 4 brings the data together.

TABLE 4

World Changes (%) Between 1969 and 1978

	Human	Employed in agriculture	Cattle	Pigs	Chickens
Total	+18.5	−10.3	+10.5	+17.1	+21.6
Developed countries	+ 7.1	−19.0	+10.8	+16.7	+16.9
Developing countries	+23.4	− 9.8	+10.4	+17.4	+25.8

(From FAO, 1979)

It is clear that the human population of the world has increased markedly, and much more in the developing than in the developed countries. Manpower employed in agriculture has been declining and obviously much more rapidly in the developed than in the developing countries. The number of livestock has increased, but only in the case of poultry on a sufficient scale to cater for the increase in human population. Pigs kept close, but cattle numbers failed to keep up with it. The comparison between developed and developing countries is also very constructive. However, all that I wish to conclude on this occasion is that the world is faced with an enormous problem of feeding the rapidly increasing human population. We all appreciate the fact that many and varied factors contributed to the increase in livestock population, but today I wish to state dogmatically that the use of feed additives, and I would put antibiotics in front of the list, have made a substantial impact. Obviously poultry and pigs benefited most. The achievements could not have been realised if it was not for the use of antibiotics. How great was the contribution in economic terms? It is virtually impossible to give an authoritative answer. However, I have attempted to assess the situation in several different ways, and having made certain assumptions, I have arrived at some figures, presented in Table 5, which give the value of profit estimated for a 100% usage of antibiotics and also for a more realistic 10 or 20% usage, assumed for the developing and developed countries respectively. In 1978 the benefit from usage of antibiotics as feed additives for calves, pigs and poultry was estimated at 68.1 million pounds sterling. The figures in Table 5 are only meant to indicate the magnitude of values involved − obviously very large amounts of money.

The monetary benefits stem, of course, from improved efficiency in livestock production. Here, certain facts are relevant: we still do not know what is the mode of action of antibiotics as performance

TABLE 5

Profit to Animal Producers in 1978 from the Use of Antibiotics as Performance Promoters (million £)

Usage	100%	10%	20%
Calves			
Developed countries	70		14.0
Developing countries	64	6.4	
Pigs			
Developed countries	125		25.0
Developing countries	167	16.7	
Chickens			
Developed countries	23		4.6
Developing countries	14	1.4	
Total	463	24.5	43.6

promoters. Of course, after 30 years, everyone has his favourite hypothesis. I am increasingly inclined to believe that there is more than one valid explanation, and that different mechanisms apply in different circumstances. Whether antibiotics are effective because they spare nutrients by lowering dietary requirements, or because they suppress organisms causing clinical or subclinical disease, is obviously of little importance to the livestock producer. The result is important to him. In the past the criteria were simple: improvement in growth rate (average 9–10%) and efficiency of feed utilization (average 5–6%), reduction in losses (mortality and morbidity) and making possible more intensive production. However, a new situation is developing as far as some of these criteria are concerned.

During the last 50 years great progress has been made in pig performance, as illustrated in Figure 1, in which the reduction in feed: gain ratio (F:G) is presented as an example. It was reduced from 4.5 to 2.5 with normal diets containing 12 Megajoule of digestible energy per kg. Obviously progress on such a scale cannot continue – somewhere there must be a ceiling. There must be a physiological limit to biological processes involved. It may be un-realistic to expect further improvement of more than say 20%, leading eventually to a F:G of around 2.0, or if one is inclined to wishful thinking, a F:G of 1.8 may be put as the ultimate target. One must realise, however, that the better the performance of the pig, the smaller becomes the possible improvement due to whatever measures one initiates and obviously this applies to responses to dietary antibiotics. Another aspect needs stressing; the smaller the responses the more difficult it is to measure them. For example, in Figure 1, figures are shown to illustrate that a 5% response is of such

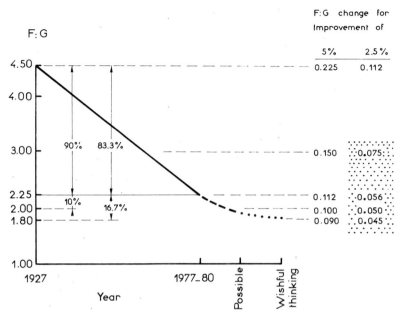

FIG. 1   Annual improvement of Feed : Gain ratio (F : G) for pigs. The extent of changes in F : G values related to improvements of 2.5 and 5% are also tabulated.

magnitude that we can measure it in a reasonable experiment, but when it comes to 2.5% improvement, (the shaded area) it becomes rather unlikely that statistically meaningful results can be obtained from a, however well-designed, experiment. Certainly the experiments of the future will have to be more sophisticated and use a larger number of animals. It may also become debatable whether the small improvements at the end of the road are of practical value in economic terms. Eventually a point may be reached where further improvement may not be possible and then the target will become how to maintain the maximum performance already attained? One other point is relevant; with the better performance and smaller responses the profitability from the use of antibiotics declines. One should not be misled by claims of higher profits which simply reflect higher cost of feed due mainly to inflation (Table 6). For instance, with F : G ratio = 3.0, there was a profit of 42 p./pig when the cost of feed was £40/ton and 126 p. when it increased to £120/ton.

One should also keep in mind the possibility that an antibiotic may be effective in some conditions and not in others, and that different antibiotics may be effective in different circumstances. I have never seen eye to eye with the claim (incidentally, made also in the Swann Report without any evidence to support it) that one

TABLE 6

Bargain in Feed Expenses for One Pig* by a 5% Gain on F : G at Different Values,
According to Feed Prices

Value of F : G	Bargain (in pennies)		
	Feed price in £/ton		
	40	80	120
4.5	60	120	180
4.0	56	112	168
3.5	49	98	147
3.0	42	84	126
2.5	35	70	105
2.0	28	56	84

* Assumption of a weight increase from 20 to 90 kg.

antibiotic can be replaced by another without necessarily affecting the response of the animal. I much prefer the attitude of freedom of choice and selection of the antibiotic which, in given circumstances, is most effective. And here the cost of the antibiotic should not be overlooked. It can differ considerably and what matters is cost effectiveness.

I have intentionally refrained from quoting up-to-date evidence to substantiate the claims that antibiotics are effective in improving performance. I have also intentionally refrained from mentioning any antibiotic by name, and there are many new names competing in the field. In fact, there are now many hundreds of reports from all over the world involving the old and the new, the general and the "feed" antibiotics (what a meaningless distinction introduced by the Swann Report) which extol the virtues of antibiotics as effective and attractive feed additives. There are of course some, relatively few in number, which dispute these claims.

As many biological responses follow a normal distribution pattern, it is unrealistic to expect perfect reproducibility of results. With feed additives, the response to which is often affected by many interacting and sometimes antagonistic factors, one must be very careful what value one should attach to experimental results. I will illustrate this point with evidence concerning copper sulphate as performance promoting additive for diets of growing pigs. Recently, I have reviewed this subject (Braude, 1976). In Figure 2 results from 205 experiments of the response in daily liveweight gain accruing from the addition of 250 mg Cu/kg diet, when compared with control animals, are diagrammatically presented. The mean response of +9.1% was statistically highly significant, and the two extreme values are also given. It can be appreciated that one more result, or

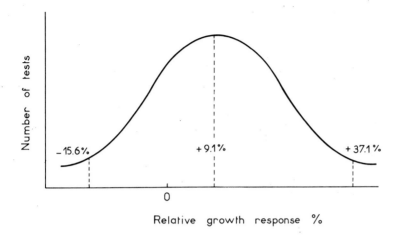

FIG. 2   Improvement of growth in pigs by addition of 250 mg copper/kg diet. Distribution curve of relative mean responses by comparison with controls for 205 separate experiments.

even several, could not alter substantially the conclusion that the addition of 250 mg Cu/kg diet has a greatly beneficial effect on growth. It follows that if an author wishes to challenge a well established response he cannot shelter behind "statistical significance" in experiments of very limited size carried out under highly specialised conditions, but must produce evidence of new factors emerging and confirm them in extensive trials.

Reasons for Ending the Controversy

The first part of this paper discussed the background for the use of antibiotics as feed additives. We have arrived at a point that the substantial economic advantages associated with it are no longer disputed. The need for prevention of clinical and subclinical disease in animals and birds is unquestionable and antibiotics in feed have proved to be very effective for this purpose. Notwithstanding this, there seems to be a lot of confusion and uneasiness in some circles about the need and the value of feed additives in animal production. One often hears a statement, which I wish to repudiate, namely, that antibiotics as feed additives are purchased because of advertising and company appeal. In fact antibiotics are used because they perform important biological and economic functions. Some believe, in their ignorance, that the improvement in animal production is brought about by obscure and dangerous drugs which jeopardise the health of the public.

After 30 years of very widespread use of antibiotics as feed additives one can dispose, I hope without fear of contradiction, of two of the arguments which were the subject of prolonged controversy:

1) The issue of allergic reactions is still raised occasionally. However, I believe that the only allergies so far encountered have resulted from the use of antibiotic in human and animal therapy. Be it as it may, should it be encountered in animal attendants, it could only prove an advantage as it would ensure proper and timely monitoring. Allergic response in hypersensitive people (e.g. to penicillin) must be recognised early and acted upon.

2) The question of residues. Tiny amounts of residues are unavoidable: obviously as long as the additive, or a portion of it, is absorbed from the digestive tract, some amounts must be found somewhere in tissue. With present day methods of detection, the amounts can be very small indeed, so small that not many years ago they would have remained undetected. It is also true that as the dietary intake increases, the residues in tissue remain at a constant low level. There just is not any evidence anywhere that these small amounts could jeopardise human health. There can be no reason to doubt that man can excrete the traces of absorbed antibiotics in the same way as the animal does. There is no tendency to accumulate antibiotics in the animal's body. There are some exceptions, none material to the arguments discussed here. For example, there is some evidence that tetracyclines have some affinity to bone material, but the bone does not release the traces of the material even after being subjected to long periods of cooking.

Accepting that small residues from therapeutic uses are unavoidable, the paramount question is what levels can be tolerated, and I mean tolerated by the body and not by the busy-body legislators. Nobody is prepared to stick his neck out and claim to know what is the answer to the first part, but there are some people who adjudicate on the second. However, already the Swann Report has rightly reassured the public by stating "We see no reason to suppose that residues present any danger", and today the whole controversy on antibiotic residues in the context of animal feed supplementation is no longer seriously entertained. One should also perhaps mention that the possibility of indirect transfer of the resistant organisms developing in the human intestines due to frequent exposure to residues in food must be considered very doubtful; there just is not any convincing data to indicate that this has occurred.

This leads to the remaining aspect of the controversy associated with the many and varied claims concerning the development of bacterial resistance in general, and the phenomenon of transferable resistance, the latter being discovered in the late fifties but obviously existing in nature before that. Some people have the impression that risks associated with resistance are very great, others that they are small. Many will claim that it has little to do with use of antibiotics as feed additives, but rather with the use, or perhaps misuse of antibiotics in human and veterinary medicine. On the other hand, there still are some who contend that the risk is associated with the continuous feeding to livestock and poultry of low levels of antibiotics. There are those who theorise that new resistant pathogens could emerge and defy known treatments. Examples are sometimes quoted of acute outbreaks, even epidemics, involving resistant pathogens, but nobody as far as I know has yet provided sound evidence that the developments were in any way connected with, and/or aggrevated by, feeding antibiotics as performance promoters to pigs or poultry.

And then you have the celebrated classic story of *Salmonella typhimurium* strain 204 initiated by Anderson in 1962 and pursued vigorously by his successor at the Central Health Laboratory at Colindale. The latest publication is as recent as November 1979 (Rowe *et al.*, 1979). The cases of resistance and cross resistance are clearly established *in vitro. In vivo* the evidence of transfer is claimed for calves and circumstantial, and rather doubtful is the evidence of transfer from calves to man. Pigs and poultry have not been involved by the Anderson school, not because of lack of endeavour in that direction but simply because of lack of evidence. Certainly, as a layman, I am increasingly puzzled that after about 20 years of thorough investigations, attempts are continuing to stir up public anxiety.

The case for combating salmonellosis in man is as strong today as ever, and all endeavours to eradicate this scourge are justified, but I am more and more convinced that it has nothing to do with feeding of small amounts of antibiotics to pigs and poultry. The fact that resistance of *Salmonella typhimurium* has been increasing is undeniable, as is the fact that acute food poisoning can be due to salmonellae, but it is also a fact that the source of infection is usually contaminated human food, and that when an outbreak of salmonellosis in man occurs, antibiotics should not be used for treatment.

Before finishing I would like to digress once again: when discussing the relationships between the host and microorganisms, and worrying on one hand about the protection from harm, and on the other hand about any man-induced changes, one should spare a thought for natural antibiotic systems which function in the body. Recently I have been particularly impressed by the lactoperoxidase system on which my colleague Dr. B. Reiter has been researching and reporting (Reiter, 1976). The enzyme lactoperoxidase which occurs in saliva, cervical mucus, milk and other secretions, forms compounds with peroxide and oxidises the thiocyanate, which is also present in body fluids and secretions, to a short-lived intermediary oxidation product which is bactericidal for pathogens such as coliforms, salmonellae, shigellae, pseudomonads and others. It appears that a natural antibiotic is involved, and all that is required is to activate the system when circumstances call for it. If confirmed, one will be able to argue that nature supplies in the milk of all species a dietary antibacterial system for the protection of the young. In this context the idea of adding antibiotics to the diets of livestock may be more acceptable to the people who argue against their use.

Conclusion

To end, I would like once again to quote Sir Derrick Dunlop: "The public which demands therapeutic progress must be prepared to take some risk" and just as I started this paper, I wish to focus attention on the time factor; antibiotics have now been used as feed additives for 30 years, and many billions of animals received diets supplemented with low levels of antibiotics. In contact with these animals were millions of people – can one really argue in 1980 that any risk whatever is involved? Fourteen years have passed since the publication of the Swann Report in U.K. Ten years ago, Dr. D.G. James at the Symposium on "Aspects of infective drug resistance" commented: "I believe that the Swann Report is providing breathing space so that we can assess, and hopefully, bury this ogre" (the claim that resistant germs in the intestines of animals are a hazard to man). I respectfully submit that not only the scientific evidence but also the time factor now unconditionally support the case for use of antibiotics as additives for diets of livestock and poultry.

References

Braude, R. (1976). *Proc. Nutr. Soc.* **35**, 377–382.
Braude, R. (1978). *J. Animal Sci.* **46**, 1425–1436.
F.A.O. Production Yearbook 1978 (published in 1979).
Hathcock, J.N. and Coon, J. (1978). "Nutrition and Drug Interrelations", Monograph of the Nutrition Foundation. Academic Press, New York.
Reiter, B. (1976). *Soc. Appl. Bacteriol. Symp. Ser.* **5**, 31–60.
Rowe, B., Threlfall, E.J., Ward, L.R. and Ashley, A.S. (1979). *Vet. Rec.* **105**, 468–469.
Solomons, I.A. (1978). *J. Animal Sci.* **46**, 1360–1369.

Discussion

Professor Chabbert: For many years, I have participated in France in discussions concerning the use of antibiotics in animals, as therapeutic agents and as feed additives. All of us know the position of the Swann Committee, but now we see that Professor Braude has a completely different one. The position in France has ever been intermediate. If one compares the different ways in using antibiotics to several flows from a common tank, a large hose-pipe represents treatment in humans, a smaller one treatment in animals and a very small one represents animal feedstuffs. This is why the Commission for animal feeding in France is always very "cool" about this problem. I regret that Professor Braude has been unable to convince the Swann Committee that they should be "cooler" about this problem. Recently, the Commission in Brussels suppressed the use of the macrolides in animal feedstuffs, something I was totally against.

Secondly, on microbiological and "plasmidological" grounds, I do not agree with the statement that plasmids are completely transferable *in vivo* in animals.

Dr. Braude: With regard to the Swann Report, I believe that if the Swann Committee was sitting now, it would not produce the Report that it adopted in 1967. If the Report is read carefully, it is clear that the Committee went out of its way to indicate that the required scientific evidence was not available, but being conscious that a decision was called for, they found it necessary to advocate that certain action should be taken, in order to remove the public anxiety created by the media. The Swann Committee sat 15 years ago; look at what has been happening since in the United States, where the FDA is still trying to convince the scientists that the Swann Report is applicable in their country. The arguments continue, but no common ground can be found. The fact that many countries have adopted the Swann Report would suggest that it has been assumed that the Report is correct. They had no evidence of their own, they have simply followed the lead of Britain, assuming that because Britain has published the Swann Report, its conclusions must be right. As I see it, in Britain 15 years have now passed, and the Swann Report has not contributed anything, neither has it done any damage. So why should anyone wish to do anything about it? The scientific evidence to support the Swann's Committee recommendations was never there, and is still not there. When the French, who are at present selling meat to Germany, use the argument that the antibiotic residues in that meat must be measured in order to comply with German request, the question that should be asked is why do the Germans insist on it? Such a demand should not be accepted by the French simply because they wish to export meat. Why should they agree to measure residues which are of a magnitude which is of no significance whatsoever? The Germans obviously wish to cut imports of meat from various countries, but the French, rather than accept the unreasonable demand for monitoring residues, should ask for evidence on which the demand was based.

Professor Davies: We cannot submit to a double standard. On the one hand, we say that we must avoid inappropriate or irrational use of antibiotics in hospitals in human beings. On the other hand, we cannot adopt the same approach of throwing antibiotics into other places and I am not referring only to animal feedstuffs. Antibiotics work, they are very good at promoting growth; nobody will deny this, nor that, at the present time, there is no evidence that there has been any health problem for humans as a result of such use, but it is surely better to use different antibiotics in animal feedstuffs from those used in human beings. I am very disturbed at the moment that, at least in the United States, the incidence of gentamicin resistance in turkeys is very high. It is hard to find turkeys that are not shedding gentamicin-resistant salmonellae. I think that this is an inappropriate and irrational use of gentamicin, and that the development of such gentamicin resistance should be avoided. Although I am willing to admit the points made by Professor Braude, the problem should be avoided by developing and using antibiotics that may not potentially cause problems in human use.

Professor Williams: Is gentamicin used as a food additive or for therapy in the turkeys in the United States? If it is the latter, for what disease are the turkeys being treated such that they develop gentamicin-resistant salmonellae?

Professor Davies: Gentamicin is used as a prophylactic, not as a food additive. In the United States turkey eggs are dipped in gentamicin solution as soon as they are laid.

Regulations and Uses of Antibiotics in Veterinary Medicine

G. MILHAUD

Ecole Nationale Vétérinaire, Maisons-Alfort,
France

Introduction

In France, the use of antibiotics as feed additives was regulated earlier than was their use as veterinary medicinal products. Indeed, in the latter field, to which the present paper will be devoted, measures were taken about 10 years ago pursuant to the law on "Repression des Fraudes" of 1st August 1905; yet it was only after the adoption by Parliament of the law on Veterinary Medicinal Products, of 29th May 1975, that an overall policy emerged. To further these rulings, the Sub-Committee for Veterinary Medicines of the Pharmacopoeia investigated the criteria on which proposals for tolerances of antibiotic residues in animal-based foodstuffs could be established.

Regulations Pursuant to the Law on "Repression des Fraudes", of 1st August 1905

First, we shall report on the measures designed to prevent the presence of antibiotic residues in milk, then we shall briefly report on the same problem in meat.

Legislation Concerning Milk

A Statutory Regulation dated 4th January 1971, amending a Statutory Regulation dated 25th March 1924, stipulates "that which cannot be considered as milk fit for human consumption ..." includes: "5. Any milk containing antibiotics or antiseptics". The text adds that such milk cannot even be considered as fit for animal consumption.

Two decrees dated 6th August 1971 were passed in application of the Regulation of 13th August 1965. One stipulates that antibiotic substances intended for intramammary administration to animals whose flesh and products are consumed by man can only be sold against veterinary prescriptions. The other stipulates that veterinary medicines containing penicillins which are to be injected into the udders of dairy cows through the teat canal must be of a specific colour (acid green BS or blue FCF). By concentrating these dyes on a resin column, milk containing more than 0.003 I.U. of penicillin/ml should be identifiable.

How have such regulations been enforced? The rule requiring a veterinary prescription for the supply of medicines containing antibiotics for intramammary administration has certainly been the more commonly infringed. In spite of some technical difficulties, the dyeing of penicillin-containing preparations has been achieved. This has undoubtedly led to a drop in the use of penicillins. Nevertheless, a decree dated 3rd March 1978 released these preparations by allowing "authorised farmers' groups" (placed under the direct control and responsibility of a veterinarian) to supply to breeders who are members of these groups slow-release products containing penicillins for dry cow therapy.

It has proved to be much slower and more difficult to withdraw from consumption all milk containing antibiotics, for prior to such withdrawal the means necessary to detect antibiotic residues in the milk have had to be developed and implemented. At the same time, the hazards of milk contamination resulting from normal veterinary therapy have had to be clearly defined.

Significant advances were achieved in June 1977, thanks to an inter-professional agreement between producers and the dairy industry which laid out a number of measures during a 30 month transition period before the strict enforcement of the provision. The major measures comprise the following. First, separate collection of normal milk and milk obtained from animals treated with antibiotics, and second, a fortnightly analysis of antibiotic residues in random samples of supposedly normal milk, followed by price cuts in cases of positive results and possible legal action through "Repression des Fraudes" in the event of repetition of the offence.

The period of transition came to an end on 1st January 1980. For the decree of 4th January 1971 to be strictly applied and for all milk containing antibiotic residues to be withdrawn from the market, veterinarians must be in a position to instruct breeders how to use medicines containing antibiotics.

Considering that up to now, few veterinary medicines have

received market authorisation with their withdrawal times given, a decree of 23rd December 1979 requires the manufacturers of veterinary medicines "to be responsible for providing within 6 months a withdrawal time for medicines likely to leave bacteriostatic, antibiotic or antifungal residues".

It is at this stage worth noting that the simple term "residue" is used and not "residue likely to present a hazard to the health of the consumer". This point will be re-examined below.

Legislation Concerning Butcher's Meat

When, owing to disease, animals are slaughtered in emergency, the decree of 15th May 1974 makes it compulsory to submit them to bacteriological tests and tests for the detection of antibiotics, if the animals are not immediately seized for other reasons. According to statistics supplied by the Ministry of Agriculture (Direction de la Qualité), 13,271 such tests were carried out in 1977. As regards other meat, more freedom is left to the veterinary inspectors. It is recommended, among other things, that "the good condition of meat is expressed in terms of absence of any antimicrobial substance of therapeutic origin; an examination for such substances must be carried out whenever the inspector knows that treatment has been administered within the 6 days prior to slaughtering".

Finally, since 1st July 1979, examinations for residues from antibiotics have been carried out on fresh butcher's meat exported to West Germany. A means of bringing the regulations of the member-states of the E.E.C. into line is under consideration in Brussels.

Legislation Resulting From the Law on Veterinary Medicinal Products, of 29th May 1975

The law on veterinary medicinal products clearly distinguishes antibiotics used as feed additives, which are not referred to in this text, from antibiotics in veterinary medicinal products in the form of either proprietary medicinal products, ready-made veterinary medicinal products, premix for medicated feeds or medicated feeds themselves.

Supplemented feeds containing additives are subject to control by the Statutory Regulation of 28th November 1973, applied and revised according to the E.E.C. directives.

No industrial veterinary medicinal products, whether or not they contain antibiotics, can be marketed without authorisation. The latter is granted only when the manufacturer guarantees analytical control of the medicine, its innocuity under normal conditions of use, its therapeutic effect, and an adequate withdrawal time, i.e. a period of time between administration of the medicine to the animal and the use of food products from this animal sufficient to "guarantee that these food products contain no residue that could be hazardous to the health of the consumer".

Notwithstanding the above-mentioned disagreement on the nature of the residues that are to be taken into consideration, the law on veterinary medicines abides by the legislation adopted in pursuance of the law on "Repression des Fraudes". In the legislation adopted in pursuance of the law on veterinary medicinal products, two important points concerning antibiotics can be mentioned.

First, the list of active ingredients which can be supplied to their members by 'authorised farmers' groups" according to the Article L 612 from the "Code de la Santé Publique" contains no antibiotics in the form of proprietary medicinal products except for dry-cow preparations which contain penicillins. However, most antibiotics can be supplied by the "groups" in the form of medicated feeds or premix for medicated feeds.

Second, according to pharmaco-toxicological evaluation, antibiotics should not be entitled to the more lenient provisions applied to occasionally used medicines. Moreover, for these medicines, attention must be given to the risks of emergence of resistant pathogenic organisms and to the harmful implications of their residues in the industrial processing of animal-based foodstuffs.

Proposals for the Sub-Committee on Veterinary Medicinal Products of the Pharmacopoeia

Since 1972, the Sub-Committee on veterinary medicinal products of the Pharmacopoeia has investigated the terms of application of the concepts of tolerance and withdrawal time in veterinary medicinal products.

The first tolerances, published in the 49th propharmacopoeia notice primarily concern antiparasitic medicines, or medicines with oestrogenic activity. As regards the few antibiotics mentioned in that paper, withdrawal times were determined such that "no residue should be detectable in foodstuffs".

Because the sensitivity of a method of analysis does not presuppose in any way the toxicity of the residue analysed, the need to calculate toxicological tolerances for antibiotics soon becomes apparent. To do so, three difficulties must be overcome. The first results from the above-mentioned legislation on "Repression des Fraudes" in so far as it applies simply to "residues" and not to "residues hazardous to the consumer". The second has to do with allergenic antibiotics, the sensitising doses of which are extremely low and hard to determine. The third results from the risk of emergence of resistant organisms in the flora of the digestive tract by antibiotic residues, and of the possible transmission of this resistance by plasmids.

On this third point three major elements must be considered in the evaluation of the risk:

1) the bacterial composition of the digestive tract flora;
2) the m.i.c. values of the antibiotic concerned against the various species;
3) the factors of dilution and reconcentration of antibiotics in the digestive tract.

The method of evaluation of the risk of emergence of resistant organisms through antibiotic residues is certainly far from perfect. Yet it enables the risk to be worked out approximately and to be compared with other risks which may result from repeated ingestion and which may be evaluated using the now classical toxicological methods.

Since hygienists set great store by the notion that antibiotic residues should be undetectable in animal-based foodstuffs, it would be interesting to compare the tolerances thus obtained with the sensitivity of the analytical methods used at present. The first comparative tests we have carried out show that in certain cases, the sensitivities of the methods are largely sufficient and that it is unnecessary to persist in trying to improve their performance. However, in other cases, seemingly sensitive methods may prove insufficient to guarantee that foodstuffs offer no hazard to the consumer.

Conclusion

In conclusion, we feel that an extensive debate is necessary to reconcile the different points of view. This debate should first be at national level, and then should be extended to all members of the E.E.C. in order to establish the means of protecting the health of the consumer without inflicting unjustified losses upon the farmer through over-prolonged withdrawal times, and without needlessly impairing E.E.C. and international trading in animal-based foodstuffs.

Part 2

Suggestions on Methods for Selection and Assessment of New Antimicrobial Agents

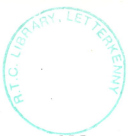

Improvement of Management of "*In Vitro*" Evaluation

Y. A. CHABBERT

Institut Pasteur, Paris, France

Introduction

As the subject of this conference is to elicit new ideas, it would be an excellent occasion to be provocative or paradoxical. However antibiotics have been satisfactorily evaluated *in vitro* for more than 30 years, so I would be extremely ambitious if I pretended to propose any really new criteria. However I do think that originality today resides not in the methods employed but in the organization of research.

In vitro studies and toxicology and pharmacology studies are part of the first phase of a product assessment. These three types of studies must be sufficiently well documented before any further study at the clinical level. *In vitro* evaluation guides clinical study, but it also delineates the framework: potent activity against a bacterial genus such as *Haemophilus* focuses attention on studies of penetration into the CSF and the effect on meningitis; moderate activity at concentrations similar to those expected in the body fluids draws attention to debatable activity at the clinical level. All these classical concepts reveal *in vitro* evaluation to be a necessary but insufficient condition.

Moreover, I believe that, in the future, we cannot be satisfied with antibiotics which are simply active since a large number of active products already exist; antibiotics of the future must be better than existing products. Tomorrow's problem in evaluating antibiotics is therefore a problem of comparison. But comparative clinical studies have limitations for various reasons: scarcity and severity of diseases, difficulty in establishing objective criteria of cure, lack of means to follow the disappearance of bacteria from the focus of infection, etc. Although clinical studies are necessary to conclude that a product is active, they are frequently insufficient in establishing the statistical superiority of a product. But when all laboratory evaluations are in favour of the product, its preferential use can be recommended. Comparative *in vitro* evaluation is therefore an essential element in establishing product hierarchy.

Comparative "In vitro" Evaluation

Relationship between "In vitro" and "In vivo" Activities

In vitro evaluation must integrate bacteriological and pharmacological data, as a whole. Here, I will be speaking almost exclusively about concentrations which are active *in vitro* but, in my mind, the most important point is not the concentrations themselves but the relationship between the levels which are active in the body fluids and tissues and concentrations which are active *in vitro*. *In vitro* evaluation is intended to make a value judgement on the product. This appraisal is not easily made since factors, sometimes contradictory, must be considered, for example: highly specific activity against one bacterial genus and "wide spectrum" activity; activity against the most sensitive strains and activity against bacteria resistant to other members of the same family or other types of antibiotics.

In the history of antibiotics, tendencies to favour one point or another have been cyclic and very variable. Any prediction of future trends is hazardous. Nevertheless I can state that successes between 1965 and 1975 primarily involved the development of semisynthetic derivatives of the large families, aminoglycosides and beta-lactams, which act on strains made resistant by enzymatic mechanisms related or not to plasmids; however these products did not provide any significant increase in activity against sensitive strains. In the last few years, we have, on the contrary, seen the emergence of products which, while remaining extremely potent against resistant bacteria, have increased activity against several bacterial genera. I would say that, for the time being, resistance to antibiotics is no longer the urgent problem and that the possibility of developing products with superior activity against an increasing number of bacterial genera must be considered.

Recent Approaches

In vitro study techniques are too well known to need long explanations: most studies are based on the determination of minimum inhibitory concentrations in agar or liquid medium and of minimum bactericidal concentrations. Many specific methods have recently been developed, dealing with:

1) survival kinetics in the presence of fixed and variable concentrations;
2) effect on the bacterial cell mass;
3) various biochemical modifications;
4) individual morphologic modifications;
5) exact duplication of *in vivo* conditions (bacterial colonies, serum, granulocytes, lymphocytes, etc.).

Not all of the new technical methods constitute evaluation criteria. The technical results obtained with a method do not become an evaluation criterion until the relationship to the real activity of the antibiotic in the clinical setting can be definitely established. For example, inhibitory concentration values were related to clinical efficiency for 30 years and there is a general consensus that an antibiotic will be active in systemic infections when local concentrations exceed *in vitro* active concentrations. The m.i.c. is therefore an evaluation criterion. As another example, a certain relationship was established between *in vivo* survival of bacteria and the formation of filaments by these bacteria when they are submitted to subinhibitory concentrations of beta-lactam antibiotics. However, the number of specific cases is insufficient to make this relationship a definitive evaluation criterion. For this reason, I will now emphasise more specifically on organisation in studying inhibitory concentrations.

In vitro evaluation of the inhibitory effect of a product against various bacterial species currently involves different approaches which can only be termed stochastic. In fact, chance is a determining factor in the choice of strains. Schematically, the initial approach is made at the industrial stage when a so-called "study of the antibacterial spectrum" is made; this study involves determining the m.i.c.'s for a series of strains representing the different bacterial genera. This bacteriological basis is insufficient as all species are not always represented and, above all, there are very few representatives of the various biochemical and genetic mechanisms of resistance. At the same time, useless redundancy occurs because many bacterial genera behave in similar fashion in the presence of an antibiotic family and could be represented by a single genus. To complete the data on this spectrum, as soon as a product shows interesting properties, it is usually supplied to several investigators who study the m.i.c.'s on a few dozen strains of each main species, selected without any rational basis among the regular collection strains of the laboratory or the clinical isolates collected over a certain period of time. The results are generally expressed as cumulative percentages, i.e., the product concentrations needed to inhibit 50, 75 or 95% of strains from each species are often calculated. The amount of information gathered in this way is of great importance particularly as these studies often involve comparisons with other antibiotics of the same or different families. This approach may however be criticized: on one hand the strains are not sampled on a statistical basis and sampling may be biased by specific recruiting of laboratory strains; a national collection will provide many "problem strains" and strains from a hospital laboratory will depend on the hospital's specialities. The activity percentages will not have any real value until multicentre studies involving a large number of investigators have been conducted. All this represents considerable waste of time and money if the product does not really have any great qualities.

New Approach

The question we are faced with is whether this approach can be improved by basing the selection of strains on a different principle and whether we can make satisfactory comparative evaluation over a very short period.

This new approach, which we could term "analytic", is based on the permanent study of the individual behaviours of the main species, when faced with antibiotics of one family. The primary goal is not the global study of a series of strains and expression of results as cumulative percentages but is rather the individual study of the resistance profile of each strain, i.e. a diagram of the respective m.i.c.'s of the products ranked in an arbitrary and variable order. If the profiles of a large number of original strains are analysed, strains which have very similar profiles (taking experimental errors into account) can be classed together and a list of strains representing the different profiles can be drawn up. An antibacterial spectrum established with representative strains would allow us to rapidly determine the worth of a product and, if the relative frequencies of the strains are also known, we could predict the frequency of activity in clinical practice.

Choice of Representative Strains

Statistical Distribution of Strains

How to choose these representative strains? If we consider the m.i.c. distribution of an antibiotic which is active against a group of bacteria belonging to either one genus or one species, we can identify two strain populations. On one hand, there is a population of so-called sensitive strains which have a roughly normal distribution; this population could be called the "Main Sensitive Population"; it may vary in size, it may not be the largest population (staphylococci penicillinase⁻) nor the most sensitive (*P. aeruginosa* sensitive to carbenicillin) but the existence of such a population results from the fact that the product was selected for its activity (without this activity the product would not have been retained and marketed). On the other hand, there are strains corresponding to various m.i.c.'s which do not belong to this population. These strains are more resistant, because they were biochemically altered in their genetic information. These changes are well known and could be listed briefly: changes in permeability, modification of active site and enzymatic inactivation. These phenotypic modifications can vary greatly, due to gene amplification, regulatory gene mutation, variability in the number of plasmid copies, etc. This sometimes results in diphasic distribution due to a single preferential mode of resistance with unequivocal expression. But, frequently, all these biochemical and genetic factors associate to give a relatively continuous distribution.

Representative Strains

"Main Sensitive Population" and the "More Resistant Strains" could be selected as follows.

Sensitive strains   Using the previous distribution, a sufficiently large sample (60 to 100) of strains with m.i.c.'s in the modal region is chosen and their distribution is studied again. We then obtain a statistically normal distribution, but with values scattered over ranges of 1 to 4, 8 or 16. Does this dispersion reflect the minor differences between the strains or the variance of the method? These strains can be tested once again using two other methods giving respectively the 99% inhibitory concentration (IC_{99}) and the 50% inhibitory concentration (IC_{50}). If the variance of strain distribution is compared with that obtained using the methods on one strain, it becomes obvious that the largest part of the variability in sensitive strains is due to the method. A single strain from the sensitive population can therefore represent this population. If the concentrations of 10 beta-lactams which inhibit 50% of the growth of the "sensitive" strains are compared to the IC_{50} of *E. coli* K 12 J 5, it can be demonstrated that the profiles are parallel; in this case, this confirms that a single strain will provide sufficient information on the comparative value of a new product. For antibiotics of this family, it can also be demonstrated that the profiles of *Escherichia, Salmonella* and *Shigella* are very similar and that it is useless to have a strain representing each of these genera.

More resistant strains   The selection of strains representing the population of strains which do not belong to the sensitive population may, *a priori*, seem impossible due to the many genetic and biochemical characteristics shown by different phenotypes. But the aim in evaluating a product must be kept in mind. Above all, we must know if the product is active against strains with different mechanisms of resistance, whatever the level of phenotypic expression. In fact, if the product is very active against the strain with the highest level of expression of a given mechanism, it will be active against all strains of the same phenotype which have weaker expression. If the level of activity on this strain is questionable (i.e. if the m.i.c.'s obtained are similar to body fluid concentrations), there is a good chance that the product will act on strains which express this mechanism less intensely. Anyway, the real statistical distribution of cases in which the product is clinically active cannot be determined until after a long period of experimental and clinical use.

Analysis of Factors of Choice

We will now examine a few practical situations to analyse the factors which should be considered in selecting the strains. As an example, I will discuss the case of the beta-lactams and the various resistance profiles (IC_{99}) obtained for selected strains producing beta-lactamases characterised by their isoelectric points (pI), as determined by electrofocusing in polyacrylamide gel and detection with nitrocefin (Glaxo).

Phenotypic profiles and mechanisms   We compared the profiles of *E. coli* K12 and three variants of this strain: one contains plasmid pIP111 which produces a TEM1 type penicillinase, the second is an amp^R mutant obtained by selection on ampicillin which produces a high level of cephalosporinase, the third was isolated on a gradient containing cefoxitin. Since this does not produce more cephalosporinase than the initial strain its resistance apparently does not involve the production of beta-lactamase. It is obvious that each of these mechanisms of resistance produces a different profile.

Plasmid coded penicillinases We compared the profiles of *E. coli* strains containing: (a) pIP111 (A^{TEM1}), a non-autonomously-transferable plasmid with relaxed replication, represented by 20 to 30 copies per chromosome; thus the enzymatic activity of the strain is very high; (b) RP1 (A^{TEM2}KT), an autonomously-transferable, stringently replicating (1 to 2 copies) plasmid of the P group with lower enzymic activity; (c) pIP71a (A) which produces an enzyme precipitating in immunotype 2 Pitton serum, with an isoelectric point of 7.7 which is similar to that of enzymes observed in *Klebsiella* (PUB5451 and SH1); and (d) pIP55 IncC (A oxaIII) representing the oxacillin-hydrolyzing enzymes. The phenotypes are not very different in spite of important differences in resistance. If the activity observed against *E. coli* K12 pIP111 is close to that observed against *E. coli* K12, which has been the case with all the recent cephalosporins, it seems useless to test for the effect on the others. By transferring these plasmids to *Salmonella, Shigella, Klebsiella* and *Proteus*, very significant differences in phenotypic expression can be obtained but, if the β—lactam is stable in the presence of an enzyme in *E. coli* K12, it will also be stable towards these species. Study of strains of genera containing these plasmid coded penicillinases is not justified.

E. coli cephalosporinases We studied the profiles of 30 strains of *E. coli* which do not contain plasmids coding for a penicillinase but which have increased production of the cephalosporinases in "sensitive" *E. coli.* From their isoelectric points, four different enzymes were found. The levels of resistance to cephalosporins appeared to be related to the specific activity of these enzymes, but the resistance profiles of these strains were parallel among themselves and with *E. coli* K12 LA002 amp^R mutant strain. This mutant can be considered as an analogue of mutant D11 in which hyper-production of cephalosporinase is due to amplification of *amp* genes. It can be reasonably assumed that increased resistance to cephalosporins in the strains studied here is due to the same mechanism and that the phenotypic effect is the same, whatever the pI of the enzyme. A product which is active against *E. coli* K12 LA002 at concentrations similar to those active against *E. coli* K12 will therefore probably be active against all *E. coli* strains.

Species-specific cephalosporinases It is known that different species of enterobacteria produce cephalosporinases which differ greatly from one to another. This property, joined to other intrinsic factors, produces specific profiles for each species, as it can be seen by comparing the phenotypic profiles of cephalothin resistant strains from the following species: *Enterobacter cloacae, Serratia marcescens, Citrobacter freundii, Proteus morgani, Proteus rettgeri* and *Proteus inconstans.* This fact therefore compels us to study representatives of each of these species.

Phenotypic profiles and enzymes   Taking *Proteus morgani* as an example, recent studies show that there exists a wide variety of enzymes with different isoelectric points but, if we compare the phenotypic profiles of the most frequent strains, no significant differences can be seen. Conversely, if we compare cephalothin resistant strains of *Klebsiella pneumoniae* which produce enzymes with pIs of 7.1 and 7.7, the profiles are quite different. It may be concluded that it is unnecessary to use all the strains producing enzymes with different pIs as representative strains; this needs to be done only if the pI and the phenotype are related. However as a different pI could appear with a new product, different activity should not be excluded and an inventory of enzymes is needed to select the representative strains producing the most frequent enzymes.

Regulation mutants   Enterobacteria belonging to the genera *Enterobacter, Citrobacter, Serratia, Proteus* (*P. morgani* and *P. rettgeri*) produce inducible cephalosporinases. Using "sensitive" strains, it is easy to obtain increasingly resistant mutants which produce a larger amount of one enzyme with the same pI. Conversely, strains highly resistant to cephalothin can be used to isolate "sensitive" variants producing less enzymes with the same pI. Even though the enzymatic and genetic study of these variants is still incomplete, the generally accepted hypothesis is that variability could be due to the existence of regulation variants. If the phenotypic profiles of "sensitive" and "resistant" variants are compared, notable differences are found. These differences reflect the absolute activity of the products and their stability towards these enzymes. In fact, increased production of an enzyme brings a more marked phenotypic modification with a very unstable product than with a more stable one. In selecting strains representing the cephalosporinase-producing species, the approach is the same as for the plasmid coded penicillinases. Since a product which remains active against a variant with a very high enzyme level will also be active against strains with lower levels of expression, the latter are not needed.

Conclusion

This rapid overview of the behaviour of enterobacteria when faced with cephalosporins demonstrates that comparative analysis of genetic and biochemical mechanisms of resistance and of phenotypic behaviour can lead to the selection of a limited number of representative strains which can rapidly reveal a product with real qualities. The example given here can easily be extended to other groups of antibiotics and other groups of bacteria. Several points should be specified: such collections can only be obtained by constantly monitoring resistant strains isolated in clinical laboratories and intensive studies of the biochemistry and genetics of these strains must be conducted. It is far from evident that relationships between research in universities and hospitals and the needs of industry were sufficient or that industry realised the interest of these studies and gave sufficient support. In addition, we cannot try to rapidly determine the particular qualities of a product while we strive to discover what its real frequency of activity will be in the clinical setting. The analytical approach is an initial approach which can show whether a product has a real advantage, it does not replace the statistical approach which later requires much time and effort. For normal commercial reasons, a considerable number of products without evident advantages when compared to existing products have been tested and marketed. As a result, the medical mind is now somewhat saturated, therefore large financial efforts are required, long delays are needed before launching a product; finally successes are questionable and product lives are decreasing. I hope that research on antibiotics in the future will be aimed at the real advantages, in terms of activity and resistance, but for this, the management of research must, more than in the past, take into account the fundamental results on the mechanisms of activity and resistance which were, or will be, acquired.

Acknowledgements

This work was undertaken with the technical assistance of E. Derlot.

Discussion

Professor Waldvogel: May I come back to what you said about m.i.c. and IC_{99}? The second technique gives standard deviations that are much smaller than the first one. So my question is the following: when you change the technique, do you change your measurement method?

Professor Chabbert: Yes, we change the measurement method, and also the number of bacteria/ml of inoculum.

Professor Waldvogel: So this is my question. When you switch from m.i.c. technique to IC_{99} technique and decrease the standard deviation, is there any decrease in the standard deviation of the measurement, or do you believe that the bacterial population you are testing is heterogeneous enough to reproduce systematically such an error? This would mean that some cells are probably in a metabolic condition which changes their sensitivity to the antibiotic being tested.

Professor Chabbert: I think that there is a primary and simple cause of inaccuracy: it is the 2 fold dilution factor. Very often, you can be more accurate and you find the inhibition of a strain can be in fact more precise by using a 1.25 dilution factor instead of 2; 1.25 is a quite good dilution factor, but 2 is more often used because it is more handy. Furthermore, if you have only 10,000 or 100,000 bacteria per spot on an agar you end up with an heterogeneous population. In toxicology, no one studies the 100% toxic dose as we do in bacteriology. In fact you often observe what is called the "tail effect" which is due to the Gaussian distribution of the bacterial population and also to some variants which might be studied apart specifically.

Professor Waldvogel: Did you study such variants?

Professor Chabbert: Not really. However, I found some different values in the IC_{50} on a number of auxotrophic E. coli K12 strains. All mutants do not have the same IC_{50}; there is a small but clear-cut difference of 3—4%.

Professor Richmond: In his presentation, Professor Chabbert divided the isolates into sensitive, resistant and more resistant. What criteria are used to decide where this division occurs? Is it anything to do with the pharmacokinetics of the molecule, or is it only an arbitrary decision?

Professor Chabbert: All the statisticians told me that it is impossible to define these populations, when they are mixed with resistant variants. In many cases, it is only a pragmatic decision in taking the most sensitive part of the curve distribution. Apparently, there is no real statistical definition — except in a few cases, for instance with penicillinase producing staphylococci.

Professor Richmond: Is there really no merit in the idea of trying to define that boundary in terms of the levels of antibiotic which might be expected to be achieved in blood or tissue?

Professor Chabbert: No. It looks to me to be a quite different problem to be studied afterwards.

Professor Williams: Professor Chabbert is suggesting that there should be a third group of people assessing the antimicrobial activity of new antibiotics. At the moment, we have industry's ideas about the activity and also the clinical laboratory's ideas. Professor Chabbert is suggesting that neither gives a true picture, and a specialised group doing different tests would give a truer picture. I would support Professor Chabbert in this proposal. The tests that he is suggesting ask the critical questions — what are the mechanisms of resistance, and does this relevant organism have it or not? These are not the only valid questions; Professor Richmond, for example, examines the hydrolysis of new compounds by bacteria which also provides rapid answers to important questions.

I offer two criticisms of the other approaches. From the industrial side, we receive long lists of susceptibility tests against organisms such as *Pasteurella pestis*, and various other organisms, some of which have not appeared in Europe since the Middle Ages. These are not very relevant to antibiotic activity today.

In the hospital laboratory there seems to be undue reliance placed upon simple disc diffusion tests which are supposed to give accurate answers for all antibiotics and all organisms. There is, in fact, no simple test which will do this.

Professor Davies: Obviously, one of the main problems with antibiotics is getting them to work in animals, especially in humans. Professor Sande will discuss animal models for evaluation.

Animal Models in the Evaluation of Antimicrobial Agents

M. A. SANDE

University of California and San Francisco General Hospital, San Francisco, California, U.S.A.

Introduction

Activity of antibiotics *in vitro* may not always be reproduced in clinical infections. Thus, new *in vitro* observations should be confirmed in *in vivo* systems prior to clinical trials. Numerous experimental models of infection have been utilised. This paper will deal with the rabbit models of endocarditis and of meningitis. Advantages and disadvantages of each will be discussed and specific areas where these models have been used to advance our understanding of the correlations between *in vitro* laboratory testing and effects *in vivo* will be described. It is hoped that, by a critical examination of these two widely used techniques, the value and pitfalls of animal models for the study of new therapeutic approaches in the future will become apparent.

Rabbit Endocarditis

The rabbit model of infectious endocarditis was developed by Freedman *et al.* in the 1960's (Garrison and Freedman, 1970). Over the last 12 years we have learned a great deal about the factors that influence the therapy of endocarditis by studying this model. The advantages of the rabbit endocarditis model are straight forward. First of all it is reproducible and simple. Secondly, the pathogenesis of the disease, the clinical, bacteriological and pathological findings are very similar to those found in man. Thirdly, there are clear-cut end-points to therapy:

1) presence of disease versus no disease,
2) the number of bacteria (colony forming units) per gram remaining in the vegetation after therapy,
3) relapse versus cure.

It has been well-known for nearly a hundred years that the endothelial surface of a normal aortic valve is nearly impossible to colonise with microorganisms. But by passing a polyethylene catheter across the aortic valve and traumatising this surface for several minutes, colonisation becomes possible. On Fig. 1 (Calderone *et al.*, 1978) one can see the results of a trauma to the aortic valve and

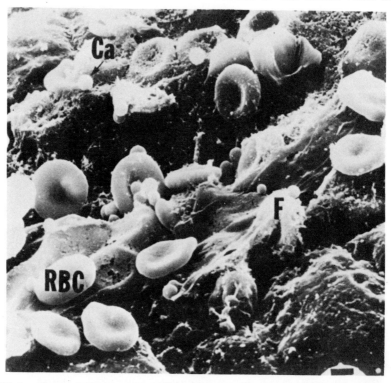

FIG. 1   Traumatised heart valve endothelium showing adherent erythrocyte (RBC) and fibrin (F). Note the erythrocyte covered by fibrin. Yeast cells (Ca) are also present on the developing vegetation. Bar = 2.0μm (Calderone *et al.*, 1978; reprinted with permission of American Society for Microbiology).

of the injection of *Candida* species: deposition of fibrin, red cells and platelets. The blastospores can be seen adhering to fibrin and platelets on the surface. Within hours to days, the surface is further covered by fibrin resulting in the mature vegetation, consisting of very large numbers of organisms tightly encased within the meshwork.

There are very few phagocytic cells in the vegetation, and thus the infection seems to exist in an area of impaired host defenses. Infection can be produced with numerous species and therapeutic studies are relatively easy to conduct. Figure 2 shows the rate of response of penicillin sensitive *Staphylococcus aureus* endocarditis

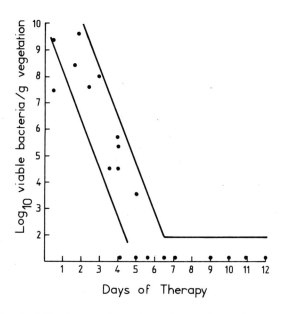

FIG. 2   Penicillin therapy of experimental staphylococcal endocarditis.

with penicillin treatment. The number of organisms remaining in the vegetation predictably decreased with treatment and after six days of treatment, all vegetations were sterile. Microscopic examination confirmed the lack of organisms after successful treatment.

The disadvantages of this model for treatment studies should also be stressed. First, a very large (and perhaps artificial) inoculum is usually necessary to produce infection in studies dealing with prophylactic antibiotic therapy. Secondly, in those studies in which the catheter was left in place, therapy is complicated by the artifact of the foreign body, making results more difficult to interpret. Thirdly, the pharmacokinetics of the drugs vary among species and are considerably more different in the rabbit than in the human. In order to be able to extrapolate results of therapy to man, comparable serum and/or tissue antibiotic concentrations must be achieved. In most instances, much larger dosages per unit weight must be used in small animals in order to reach levels that are considered therapeutic in humans. Next, statistical analysis requires large numbers of animals, and thus most studies have been conducted using a single bacterial strain. This should be remembered since antimicrobial sensitivity between strains varies considerably. Finally, regimens can only be compared, and data relevant to the effectiveness of a single regimen in a rabbit model cannot be directly extrapolated to the therapy in man. However, useful information can be derived by comparing new regimens with those known to be effective in man and principles of therapy can be carefully studied.

Thus, the major usefulness of this model has been to study the principles relating to prophylaxis and treatment of endocarditis. We have been able to critically examine traditional regimens by testing the validity of basic hypotheses, and examine innovative approaches with the goal of identifying techniques that reduce infection rate, increase cure rate, reduce duration of therapy and reduce valve damage. We have learned that the relative rate at which antimicrobial agents alone or in combination kill microorganisms in broth is, in general, predictive of the relative rate that they eradicate organisms from cardiac vegetation *in vivo*. This has been demonstrated with various strains of streptococci, staphylococci and Gram-negative bacilli.

For instance, we have known for many years that penicillin plus streptomycin exerts a more rapid bactericidal rate against *viridans* streptococci than penicillin alone, as shown by Fig. 3 (Wolfe and Johnson, 1974). The implication of this observation has been studied by several investigators in the rabbit model of endocarditis. Figure 4 (Sande and Irvin, 1974) demonstrates the results of one such study. When therapy with penicillin alone was discontinued after 3, 4, 5 and 7 days, the animals relapsed with positive blood cultures. After 8 days of therapy, all vegetations were sterile and all animals were cured. When gentamicin or streptomycin was added to the regimen, only three days were required to sterilise all of the vegetations. None of the animals relapsed after three days of therapy.

Are these observations applicable to man? Data collected by Wolfe and Johnson (1974) and others suggest that the therapy of non-enterococcal, streptococcal endocarditis with penicillin for 4 weeks and with the addition of streptomycin for the first two weeks is successful in essentially all patients with a relapse rate approaching zero (see Table 1). However, Karchmer *et al.* (1979) have recently published data relating to a series of 100 patients treated for 4 weeks with penicillin alone with only a 1% relapse rate. Wilson *et al.* (1978) have also published results of 99 patients treated for 2 weeks with a

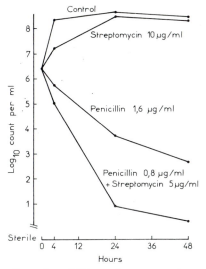

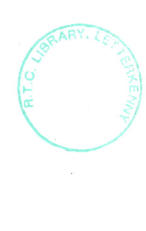

FIG. 3   Synergistic action of penicillin and streptomycin on 48 strains of *viridans* streptococci isolated from endocarditis patients between 1944 and 1947 and between 1967 and 1971 (Wolfe and Johnson, 1974; reprinted with permission of the authors and of The American College of Physicians).

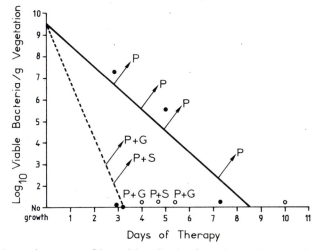

FIG. 4   Approximate rate of bacterial eradication from the cardiac vegetations of rabbits with *Streptococcus viridans* endocarditis during therapy with penicillin (P) alone (———) or penicillin plus either streptomycin (S) or gentamicin (G) (– – – –). Rates were determined by titres of viable *S. viridans* (●) per g of vegetation removed from animals sacrificed during therapy and by the presence (↗) or absence (○) of bacteriological relapse after discontinuation of antibiotic therapy (Sande and Irvin, 1974; reprinted with permission of The University of Chicago Press).

combination of penicillin and streptomycin with only one relapse, suggesting that the addition of the aminoglycoside may allow a safe

TABLE 1

Relapse Rate of Penicillin Sensitive Non-Enterococcal Endocarditis

Regimen	No. of patients	Relapse rate	Authors
Penicillin and Streptomycin (2 weeks) then Penicillin (2 weeks)	≃ 300	0%	Wolfe and Johnson (1974) and others
Penicillin (4 weeks)	100	1%	Karchmer *et al.* (1979)
Penicillin and Streptomycin (2 weeks)	99	1%	Wilson *et al.* (1978)

reduction in the duration of treatment of this disease. These data are consistent with the observations made *in vitro* and in the animal model of endocarditis.

Similar observations have been made with *Staphylococcus aureus.* Sande and Courtney (1976) have demonstrated in broth that the combination of nafcillin plus gentamicin is more rapidly bactericidal than either drug alone, (see Fig. 5) and likewise more rapidly effective in sterilising cardiac vegetations in the animal model of endocarditis (see Fig. 6). We have recently studied the relevance of this observation in man, and have completed a comparative clinical study of addicts with *S. aureus* endocarditis treated with either nafcillin alone or in combination with gentamicin. There was no difference in mortality or relapse rate between the two regimens, but in infections involving the tricuspid valve, there was a more rapid clearing of bacteraemia in patients receiving a combination versus nafcillin alone. This is consistent with the observations made *in vitro* and in the animal model.

The model has also been used to study the relevance of bactericidal titres in serum. We have learned that a peak serum bactericidal dilution equal to (or greater than) $\frac{1}{8}$ correlates with therapeutic success in streptococcal endocarditis and that a bactericidal regimen is necessary for cure. Carrizosa and Kaye (1977) clearly demonstrated this principle by treating animals with experimental streptococcal endocarditis with various doses of procaine penicillin. Animals with a mean peak serum bactericidal dilution (taken one hour after injection) of less than $\frac{1}{8}$ had ineffective therapy, with more than 10^5 c.f.u./gram in the vegetations after 5 days. Animals receiving higher doses that achieved peak bactericidal dilution greater than $\frac{1}{8}$ had effective therapy, with a marked reduction of c.f.u./gram in vegetations. Most animals in these latter two groups had sterile vegetations.

Thus, studies with this model have helped, to: (a) establish the clinical relevance and credibility of dynamic killing curves in broth

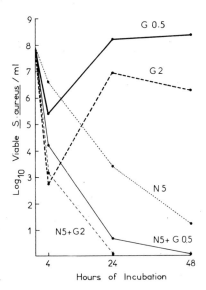

FIG. 5   Rate of killing of a strain of *S. aureus*, isolated from a patient with endocarditis, by various concentrations (0.5, 2, 5 μg/ml) of gentamicin (G) and nafcillin (N) alone or in combination, in broth (Sande and Courtney, 1976; reprinted with permission).

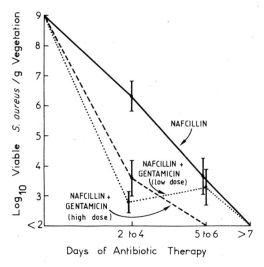

FIG. 6   Results of cultures of vegetations from rabbits treated with nafcillin and the combination of nafcillin plus gentamicin for three treatment periods (Sande and Courtney, 1976; reprinted with permission).

for predicting the relative rapidity with which antibiotics alone or in combination eradicate bacteria from cardiac vegetations *in vivo*, (b) confirm the potential value of measurements of serum bactericidal titres for monitoring maximally effective therapy.

Rabbit Meningitis

The second model to be discussed is a rabbit model of bacterial meningitis designed by Dr. Ralph Dacey and used in our laboratory for the last 6 years (Dacey and Sande, 1974).

The animal is suspended in a stereotaxic frame which allows a traumatic placement of a spinal needle into the *cisterna magna*. Continuous or intermittent sampling of clear cerebrospinal fluid (CSF) is thus possible during the treatment period. Arterial blood is sampled sequentially through an arterial line and a constant intravenous infusion pump is used to administer antibiotics. The 10^7 pneumonococci inocula are injected intracisternally and 16 hours later the animals have meningitis with clinical and bacteriological features similar to the disease in man. The treatment, which may be varied according to experimental design, is then initiated. Mortality of the untreated disease is 100% in 4 to 5 days.

This model has many advantages:

1) it is reproducible and allows for continuous or intermittent CSF sampling under controlled conditions;
2) the end-points are well defined and include CSF drug concentrations under steady state conditions, CSF bacterial counts and cure/relapse of the disease;
3) the clinical, pathological, biochemical and microbiological parameters are similar to that found in the human disease.

But it has also several disadvantages:

1) the pathogenesis of the disease varies from most natural infections in man since the organisms are directly injected into the CSF rather than finding their way via the bloodstream;
2) the pharmacokinetics and host defenses vary between species;
3) the response to therapy may therefore differ significantly from man.

Therapeutic lessons learned from the meningitis model are listed below:

1) The rate of bacterial killing by antimicrobials in broth is predictive of the relative rate at which the organisms are killed in CSF *in vivo*. The following studies illustrate this point (Stransbaugh and Sande, 1978). Utilising a rabbit model of *Proteus mirabilis* meningitis, we were able to achieve a rapid bactericidal effect using intravenously large dosages of gentamicin (Fig. 7). Chloramphenicol,

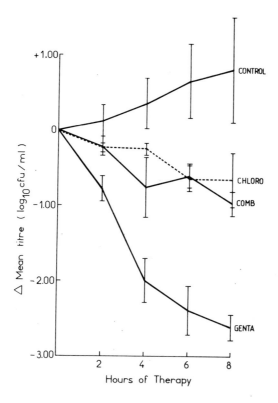

FIG. 7 Antagonism between chloramphenicol and gentamicin *in vivo*. Change in mean titres in cerebrospinal fluid (CSF) during therapy with gentamicin (30 mg/kg per hr) and chloramphenicol (5 mg/kg per hr) alone and in combination is shown. There were five rabbits in each group. Standard deviation is indicated by bars. chloro = chloramphenicol; genta = gentamicin; and comb = gentamicin plus chloramphenicol (Stransbaugh and Sande, 1978; reprinted with permission of The University of Chicago Press).

on the other hand, was bacteriostatic both *in vitro* and in the animal model. The bacterial counts increased slowly in control untreated animals. The addition of chloramphenicol to gentamicin *in vitro* demonstrated antimicrobial antagonism and elimination of the gentamicin bactericidal effect. The same phenomenon was observed *in vivo*. The combination produced a bacteriostatic effect similar to that of chloramphenicol alone.

Likewise (Scheld *et al.*, 1979a), *in vitro*, when 0.1 μg/ml of mecillinam was added to *E. coli* in broth, a bacteriostatic effect was demonstrated after 48 h of incubation. Ampicillin was ineffective at this concentration. The combination of the two drugs, however, produced a synergistic effect and produced sterility after 24 h (Fig. 8). When examined *in vivo*, in an *E. coli* model of

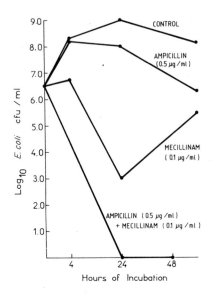

FIG. 8   Rate of killing of *E. coli* by antibiotics in broth (Schald *et al.*, 1979a, reprinted with permission of American Society for Microbiology).

meningitis, a similar response was demonstrated (see Table 2). Mecillinam alone reduced the bacterial titre over 8 h by 1.5 log. Ampicillin was bacteriostatic and the combination of mecillinam plus ampicillin achieved a more complete and rapid bactericidal effect, an example of *in vivo* antibiotic synergism. The same phenomenon has been demonstrated with *Listeria meningitidis* utilising gentamicin and ampicillin (Scheld *et al.*, 1979b).

TABLE 2

Bacterial Killing by Antibiotics in Experimental *E. coli* Meningitis

Antibiotic	No. of animals	Evolution of bacterial titre after 8 h therapy (a)
None	7	+ 0.12 (± 0.54)
Mecillinam	9	− 1.59 (± 0.54)
Ampicillin	11	− 0.08 (± 0.86)
Mecillinam + ampicillin	9	− 3.66 (± 1.03)

(a) Expressed by $\log_{10}$ of the number of colony forming units (CFU) per ml of CSF after 8 h of therapy versus the initial number. Standard deviation in brackets (Schald *et al.*, 1979a; reprinted with permission of American Society for Microbiology).

2) A second important therapeutic lesson learned from this model is that the drug concentration required to kill organisms in broth

may differ significantly from the concentration required to initiate bacterial killing in CSF *in vivo.* An illustration of this was demonstrated in the *Proteus* model of meningitis (Stransbaugh and Sande, 1978). In this series of studies (Fig. 9) the experimental strain of

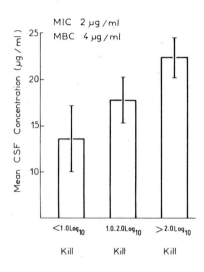

FIG. 9   Bacterial killing by gentamicin in experimental meningitis in 8 h.

Proteus mirabilis had a minimum bactericidal concentration (MBC) of 4 μg/ml of gentamicin. However, in order to achieve at least one log of bacterial killing in CSF *in vivo* over an 8 h period, a concentration of 17 μg/ml was necessary. Over 20 μg/ml were required to reduce the bacterial population by 2 logs, a phenomenon that was achieved with 4 μg/ml in broth. The explanation for this difference has not been completely resolved; however, it is interesting that, when the pH of the incubating medium is varied, a marked effect on the MBC of gentamicin results. At pH 7.4, the MBC was 1 μg/ml but at 6.8 the median MBC was 8 μg/ml. The pH of the CSF in bacterial meningitis was found to be 6.98. Thus, the environment in which the drug is asked to produce the therapeutic effect may significantly alter its ability to inhibit or kill the infecting microorganism.

3) The cure of experimental pneumococcal meningitis correlated directly with obtaining a bactericidal effect in CSF.

A large number of rabbits with pneumococcal meningitis were treated with either ampicillin, chloramphenicol or both drugs administered together. The experimental organism had a minimal inhibitory concentration (m.i.c.) of approximately 1 μg/ml of chloramphenicol and an MBC of approximately 8 μg/ml. Ampicillin alone in dosages that produced CSF concentrations considerably above the MBC were rapidly bactericidal, and in 24 h most of the animals had sterile CSF. However, with chloramphenicol given intramuscularly 3 times a day, in a dose that achieved a peak CSF levels of 3 μg/ml, only a bacteriostatic effect was demonstrated. When the dosage was markedly increased to achieve peak CSF concentrations above the MBC, a bactericidal effect was produced in the CSF, similar to ampicillin.

In therapeutic studies, the animals were treated for 5 days. Ampicillin therapy cured 14 out of 19 animals .(75%), results similar to those found in pneumococcal meningitis in man. None of the animals that received 5 days of therapy relapsed. Chloramphenicol therapy, with the doses that produced only a static CSF effect, cured only 3 out of 18 animals and most of the animals relapsed. When very high doses of chloramphenicol were used, a similar cure rate was achieved as found with ampicillin alone, and relapses were uncommon.

When the study was repeated using a more sensitive strain of *Pneumococcus* (MBC to chloramphenicol of 2 μg/ml), a bactericidal effect was demonstrated with the low dose of chloramphenicol and the cure rate was similar to that achieved with high dosages of chloramphenicol or ampicillin. Thus, these studies suggest that a bactericidal effect in CSF is a rational goal to achieve in the therapy of meningitis and that a milder effect might be detrimental.

Conclusion

We have tried to point out some of the advantages and disadvantages of two animal models of infection, and to articulate several of the therapeutic lessons learned from the utilisation of these two models. We would like to reiterate that it is always dangerous to directly extrapolate data from these models or any model to the therapy of man. However, we think that important lessons can be learned and that the controversial points can be examined. Finally, and perhaps most important, rational innovative therapeutic techniques can then be constructed, that can lead to controlled prospective clinical trials in man.

References

Calderone, R.A., Rotondo, M.F. and Sande, M.A. (1978). *Infect. Immun.* **20**, 279–289.

Carrizosa, J. and Kaye, D. (1977). *Antimicrob. Agents Chemother.* **12**, 479–483.

Dacey, R.G. and Sande, M.A. (1974). *Antimicrob. Agents Chemother.* **6**, 437–441.

Garrison, P.K. and Freedman, L.R. (1970). *Yale J. Biol. Med.* **42**, 394–410.
Karchmer, A.W., Moellering, R.C., Jr., Maki, D.G. and Swartz, M.N. (1979). *J. Am. Med. Assoc.* **241**, 1801–1806.
Sande, M.A. and Courtney, K.B. (1976). *J. Lab. Clin. Med.* **88**, 118–124.
Sande, M.A. and Irvin, R.G. (1974). *J. Infect. Dis.* **129**, 572–576.
Scheld, W.M., Fink, F.N., Fletcher, D.D. and Sande, M.A. (1979a). *Antimicrob. Agents Chemother.* **16**, 271–276.
Scheld, W.M., Fletcher, D.D., Fink, F.N. and Sande, M.A. (1979b). *J. Infect. Dis.* **140**, 287–294.
Stransbaugh, L.J. and Sande, M.A. (1978). *J. Infect. Dis.* **137**, 251–260.
Wilson, W.R., Geraci, J.E., Wilkowski, C.J. and Washington, J.A. (1978). *Circulation* **57**, 1158–1161.
Wolfe, J.C. and Johnson, W.D., Jr. (1974). *Ann. Intern. Med.* **81**, 178–181.

Discussion

Professor Davies: Taking the position of Devil's advocate, I can see that animal models are very interesting and can provide nice ways of studying certain diseases and certain effects of antibiotics under certain very specific sets of conditions. But I am slightly unsure about whether animal models are *useful* in the evaluation of new antibiotics. Could Professor Sande comment on that?

Professor Sande: I would be very careful in extrapolating directly from results with treatment of infection with a new agent in an animal model to the human experience. I think the value of animal models lies in taking an observation with a new agent. For example, mecillinam is an agent which looks extremely good *in vitro* against many of the Enterobacteriaceae when it is combined with other β–lactam antibiotics. *In vitro*, with both the *Escherichia coli* that I have shown today and also a *Klebsiella*, we found a dramatic synergism, particularly when the checkerboard techniques were used. When time-kill curves were used, however, there was synergism only against the *Escherichia coli* but not against the *Klebsiella*. We did not know what this meant. So, in order to try to resolve it to our satisfaction, we went to the animal model and discovered that it was only against the *Escherichia coli* that there was any synergism *in vivo*. There was no synergistic effect *in vivo* against the *Klebsiella*, against which there had been synergism demonstrated with the checkerboard techniques but not with the time-kill curves.

I would use the animal model to try to clarify our thinking on the significance of these various *in vitro* phenomena. I would not take it much further than that.

We have also examined cefamandole in the therapy of bacterial meningitis in humans, only after it had proved possible to demonstrate that it worked extremely well in the animal model. I am given confidence to go ahead with a clinical study if I am able to reproduce the *in vitro* phenomena in the animal model.

Professor Tomasz: Professor Sande demonstrated that ampicillin was bacteriostatic for *E. coli* in the meningitis model. He also showed that *E. coli* was inhibited but not killed by ampicillin when the bacteria were grown in broth culture. I have two comments or questions: first, I am surprised that ampicillin was bacteriostatic for the broth-cultivated cells. In a vigorously growing culture, ampicillin ought to be highly bactericidal for this bacterium and the lack of the bactericidal effects suggests that the culture medium was lacking some component needed for growth. Is the CSF a poor growth medium for *E. coli*? The second question is related to the observations reported in the literature according to which at least some bacteria may be more susceptible to antibiotics *in the infected host* (because of the presence of collaborating host factors) than they are *in vitro*. Is there any evidence for such synergistic effects in the meningitis model?

Professor Sande: But what happens in meningitis? Are the organisms rapidly dividing? It turns out in this model that the organisms grow extremely slowly. It is possible to demonstrate that a bacteriostatic effect of ampicillin can become a bactericidal effect if the concentration is much higher than would be expected from the kill curves obtained *in vitro* with rapidly dividing organisms. I think that the meningitis model has tried to bring us slightly closer to reality, because in meningitis these organisms are not rapidly dividing; a different phenomenon occurs *in vitro*. We have not studied the so-called "sub-m.i.c." effect in the meningitis model.

I agree that there is need to be cautious, and perhaps we are underestimating the value of the drug, but what happens in the animal model is closer to what is occurring in man than to what happens *in vitro*. That is where I think that the contribution is made from the animal model.

Professor Sabath: First, concerning the value of the animal model in differentiating the mecillinam/ampicillin synergy between *Klebsiella* and *Escherichia coli*, are there some data showing that the synergy was due in part to β–lactamase inhibition with one of those organisms and not the other? Is that a possible explanation?

Secondly, related to Professor Sande's answer to Professor Tomasz, in which he described obtaining a bactericidal activity by greatly increasing the ampicillin concentration, I would like to know what was the bacterial species. There is the paradoxical effect of decreased killing at very high concentrations.

Professor Sande: It was an *Escherichia coli*.

In answer to the first question, all that was demonstrated was a difference, a separation of the two methods of studying synergism. We did not examine whether it was β–lactamase-related. The demonstrated point was that the time-kill curves did not correlate with the checkerboard technique in the expression of synergism. Synergism has many different meanings, and clearly there was a separation between the types here.

Professor Videau: I would like to ask you if the experimental model is not essentially interesting to compare antibiotics of the same family and in particular to show the effect of serum protein bindings which are sometimes very similar for cephalosporins or beta-lactamines.

Professor Sande: With regard to the correlation of the protein binding, the penetration of the drug into the CSF correlates inversely with protein binding in a general way, and it certainly could lead to a whole host of other experiments in terms of inhibition of the binding.

It could be useful in comparing two antibiotics of the same class. Almost anything can be done with these models, including to compare drugs of the same class. I am sure that it would provide useful information. I cannot, however, answer the question specifically.

Pharmacokinetics as Criteria for Selecting and Assessing Antimicrobial Drugs

T. BERGAN

*Departments of Microbiology, Institute of
Pharmacy and Aker Hospital, University of Oslo,
Oslo, Norway*

Introduction

The question to be considered in this contribution is the basic elements of pharmacokinetics relative to antimicrobial agents and how this science may contribute to the assessment and selection of such agents. We are constantly improving our understanding of the key criteria required for appropriate assessment of antimicrobials, although the data are sketchy for many of those introduced before the last decade. Physiological variables influencing pharmacokinetics appear in Table 1. Still, there is great awareness of the significant contribution of descriptive and analytical pharmacokinetics and the number of new reports within this field is increasing ever faster.

TABLE 1

Physiological Variables Influencing Pharmacokinetics

Physiological factors	Influencing factors
Blood supply at absorption site	Rubbing, drugs, food, age, disease, posture, stress
Gastric emptying, gastro-intestinal motility	Food, drugs, liquids, age, disease
Binding to serum proteins and tissues	Affinity, lipid solubility, albumin concentration, drug level, binding competing drugs, disease
Hepatorenal blood flow	Cardiac output, drugs, disease
Hepatorenal extraction	Drugs (inducers, inhibitors), age, disease
Urine pH	Food, time of day, drugs, disease
Urine flow	Fluids, food, sweating, drugs

By pharmacokinetics we understand the science describing the fate of substances introduced into the body. It is composed of many factors, principally absorption, distribution, and elimination, but also encompasses protein binding, metabolism, and the ability of the agents to penetrate to extravascular compartments of the body. Absorption is characterised by rate and extent, distribution by apparent volume, rate and route of elimination, and whether dose dependent kinetics exists. One facet for which pharmacokinetics may be employed is the proposal of correct dosage schemas leading to optimal therapy without accumulation of the drug and toxic manifestations. This applies both to persons with normal rates of elimination and to diseased individuals. Healthy volunteers are required for basic studies of new agents e.g. comparisons of different pharmaceutical formulations. I shall in the following deal with experimental design, the basic pharmacokinetic elements to be assessed, and discuss interpretation of key pharmacokinetic criteria.

Experimental Design

Pharmacokinetic analyses are subject to considerable systematic errors and adequately sophisticated comparative and controlled experimental designs must be allowed. For pharmacokinetic studies, cross-over designs in which several doses are examined in randomised order in the same subjects are preferable.

Comparisons between different doses and dose schedules of the same drug are more valid when the data are derived from studies on the same individuals. An interval of 1–2 weeks should elapse between single dose studies in the same individuals, up to a month if multiple dose or steady state studies with different doses are to be compared. The concerns are that interference or induction of enzymes or mutual interaction between doses or dose schedules must be avoided. Choice and inclusion of proper experimental control doses are in general important. The details of protocol design obviously depend upon the purposes of the studies. The elements to be appropriately fulfilled for proper experimental designs have been described in detail e.g. by Westlake (1973).

Pharmacokinetic Models

Initially, the tool of the pharmacokineticist must be briefly outlined. Analyses are dependent upon presumptions that mathematical models can be used to adequately describe the dynamic changes of concentration within the body. If agreement between theoretically predicted and experimental observations is within acceptable limits, then the hypothesis can be accepted.

Basically, curves after absorption from e.g. the gastrointestinal tract or intramuscular (i.m.) injection often have a shape as illustrated in Fig. 1. The initial portion of the curve is called the absorption

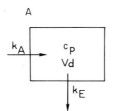

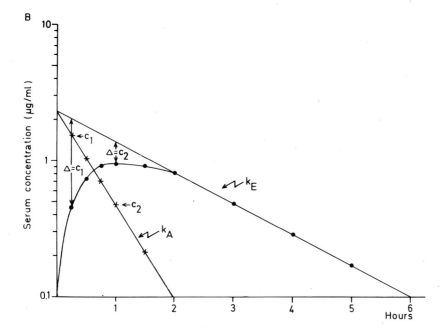

FIG. 1   Schematic representation of the first order one-compartment open model and corresponding pattern of serum curve after extravascular administration of antibiotics: (A) c_p represents the concentration in the central compartment (equalling the serum level), and V_d the distribution volume. The slopes k_A and k_E represent the absorption and elimination rates respectively. (B) The differences c_1 and c_2 indicated by feathering between serum curve and extrapolated elimination curve are plotted (in log scale) from the X-axis to render a straight line with a slope corresponding to the absorption rate.

phase, the final part the elimination phase. The basic question in pharmacokinetics is to determine the characteristics enabling prediction of concentrations in serum or other parts of the body relative to time. This particular curve is describable by a simple, one-compartment open model as shown diagrammatically in Fig. 1. With first order rates of both absorption and elimination, the serum concentration (c_p) curve follows the equation:

$$c_p = \frac{c_0 k_A}{k_A - k_E} (e^{-k_E t} - e^{-k_A t})$$

The symbols are defined in Appendix II.

In the case of the one-compartment open model, when the entire dose is given intravenously and the elimination rate follows a monoexponential course, the serum concentration curve appears as a straight line from the zero time, in a semilogarithmic plot (curve like that related to k_E in Fig. 1). In practice, such curves are only observable after infusions of long duration which generate a steady state level with balance between extravascular and intravascular levels. Another serum course pattern follows rapid intravenous injections.

Then concentrations are also constantly diminishing, but after rapid intravenous administration the course is at least biphasic as shown in Fig. 2. There is an initial faster disposition and a final slower slope. The former is referred to as the distribution phase or the α–phase, the latter as the elimination phase or β–phase. During the first part, drug is not only eliminated, but also penetrates simultaneously into the extravascular compartment until levels are in balance between both compartments. During the β–phase drug is transported only in the direction from the peripherical to the central compartment. By central compartment is understood the blood and those parts of the body which immediately exhibit equal concentrations. Since two isodirectional events occur in parallel and each is monoexponential, two compartments are required for mathematical modelling. This is illustrated in Fig. 2. The resultant curve is described by the equation

$$c_p = A \cdot e^{-\alpha t} + B \cdot e^{-\beta t}.$$

If absorption is completed before the distribution phase is finished, the serum curve assumes a different shape with a nose-like pattern as indicated in principle by Fig. 3. This is described by a two-compartment model also, and the curve expressed by the equation

$$c_p = A \cdot e^{-\alpha t} + B \cdot e^{-\beta t} - c_0 \cdot e^{-k_A t}$$

in which $c_0 = A + B$.

As a general operational rule, the model which presumes the least number of compartments, but still generates theoretical curves corresponding to the physiological realities, i.e. the observed data, is

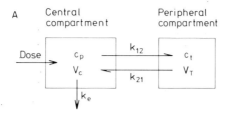

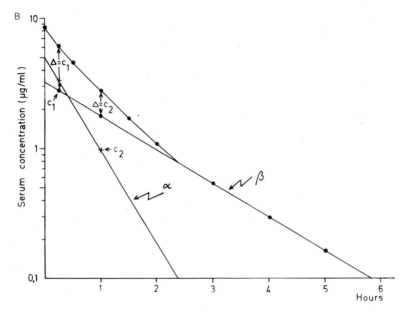

FIG. 2 Schematic representation of the first order two-compartment open model and corresponding pattern of serum curve after a rapid intravascular administration of antibiotics: (A) c_p and c_t are the concentrations in central and peripheral compartments respectively, V_c and V_t the corresponding distribution volumes, k_{12} and k_{21} the rates of transport in opposite directions between the two compartments. (B) The slopes α and β respectively represent the rates of apparent disposition during the distribution and elimination phases. Feathering is demonstrated as in Fig. 1.

preferred. It is assumed that choice of models with more compartments do not necessarily better represent the biological processes responsible for the course of the concentrations in serum or other parts of the body, unless information on additional rate processes is available.

The operational tool of pharmacokinetics is the computer. Refined curve fitting uses iterative programme procedures to obtain the best correspondance between the theoretical curve and the observed data. These values and their derived metrics constitute the basic pharmacokinetic characteristics. These results can and should be controlled

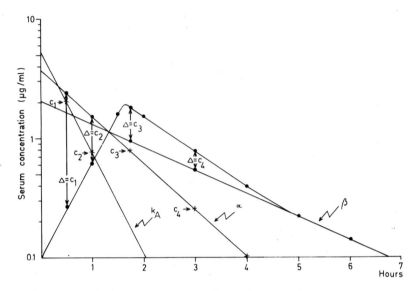

FIG. 3   Pattern of serum curve corresponding to the first order two-compartment open model after extravascular administration of antibiotics. See Figs 1 and 2 for explanation of symbols and feathering.

by the procedure of residuals or more simply by graphical feathering as demonstrated in Figs 1 and 2 and in Appendix I, which also indicates the derived parameters most commonly used in various pharmacokinetic models.

Absorption

Absorption implies the uptake of a substance introduced to the body by any route other than direct intravascular injections. The factors influencing absorption are listed in Table 2. Absorption is characterised

TABLE 2

Factors Influencing Absorption

Pharmaceutical variables (rate)	Formulation, salt form, esterification, water solubility, polymorphism
Physiological variables (rate + extent)	State of mucosal health, vascularity and blood flow, gastric emptying time, acid production, gastro-intestinal motility, hepatocellular bioconversion.

by the rate with which it occurs and the percentage of the dose absorbed. The model usually presumes that first order absorption occurs. The possibility of zero order absorption rates for penicillins have been assessed (Ehrnebo *et al.*, 1979). However, it is difficult to differentiate between zero order and first order, because the number of specimens per time interval must be very high to establish with sufficient statistical confidence that a regression fit is better to zero order than to a first order process. Also, parallel data from intravenous administrations in the same subjects are needed. In the paper of Ehrnebo *et al.* (1979), statistical assessment of the alternatives was not reported. Only diagrams were used to give visual impressions. For all practical purposes first order absorption processes may be assumed for all known antimicrobial agents (Wagner, 1975).

To establish optimal absorption from tablets, capsules, or oral suspensions, comparisons should be made with equimolar doses of aqueous solutions. Phenoxymethylpenicillins, for instance, are faster and more completely absorbed from aqueous solutions than from either tablets or suspensions (Bergan *et al.*, 1976). An aqueous solution circumvents the influence of properties related to the pharmaceutical preparations. Tablets of oxytetracycline, chloramphenicol, or phenoxymethylpenicillin with slow dissolution rates give lower serum levels (Aguiar *et al.*, 1968; Barr *et al.*, 1972; Bell *et al.*, 1971; Bergan *et al.*, 1973, 1976; Blair *et al.*, 1971). This is why generically equivalent drugs have given widely different concentrations. The situation has been rectified in many countries, where all marketed products now are optimally absorbed.

The problems involved in equivalence of oral dosage of different forms of one drug with the same amount of active ingredient per dose unit have been related to particle size, solubility, stability under the low pH of stomach content, and rate of tablet dissolution.

Effect of particle size on absorption has been demonstrated e.g. for sulphaethylthiadiazole (Kakemi *et al.*, 1962) and sulphadiazine (Reinhold *et al.*, 1945). For the latter, a suspension of fine particles is better absorbed than when larger particles are given. The serum peak was ca. 40% higher and the area under the serum curves some 20% higher with. the smaller particles. Better absorption of smaller particles has also been seen with griseofulvin for which micronisation of the particles has allowed a reduction of the dose to 50% of the originally marketed formulations (Atkinson *et al.*, 1962). Smaller crystals do not only raise the total amount absorbed, but also increase the absorption rate of e.g. griseofulvin (Goldberg *et al.*, 1966). Amorphous preparations of chloramphenicol and novobiocin have given better absorption than crystalline substances (Almirante *et al.*, 1960; Mullins and Macek, 1960). The amorphous form is more quickly dissolved. Improved absorption for the more water soluble forms of the same compounds has also been demonstrated for novobiocin (of which the acid, Na and Ca salts have been compared) (Furesz, 1958), for phenoxymethylpenicillin (of which acid, Na, Ca and benzathine salts have been compared) (Juncher and Raaschou, 1957), and ampicillin (of which the more soluble anhydrous form produces higher serum concentrations than the trihydrate form) (Poole et al., 1968).

In some instances, the agents may be susceptible to destruction in the acid stomach content. Esterification, or formation of salts or complexes with poor water solubility may be needed to protect the compounds, as it has been done with e.g. erythromycin and benzyl-penicillin. Protection from stomach acid is also achieved by tablets with enteric coating or capsules dissolving only in alkaline duodenal content. Another method of improving absorption is by formation of ester prodrugs. Esters like bacampicillin and pivampicillin with improved rates and extent of ampicillin absorption have been developed (Sjövall et al., 1978). Analogous is talampicillin (Bergan, 1978d). Bacmecillinam and pivmecillinam make the non-absorbable mecillinam suitable for tablet formulation (Bergan, 1978d). Carfecillin is an ester modification which has enabled gastrointestinal absorption of carbenicillin (Bergan, 1978d).

Bioavailability

The extent of absorption is expressed by the term bioavailability. It is the fraction of the dose which reaches the vascular biophase, i.e. the systemic circulation calculated from total area under the serum curves (AUC or F). The bioavailability f is preferably determined by comparison with intravenous injections (i.v.) and traditionally the total AUC referring to equal doses given extravascularly and intravenously are compared. Thus f = F (extravascularly given drug)/F (i.v. given drug).

If 1 g of a substance results in an F = 100 μg.h/ml after an i.v. dose and 85 μg.h/ml after a tablet, then the bioavailability is 85%. Percentages absorbed from oral antibiotics are shown in Table 3. It is worthwhile determining bioavailability also after intramuscular (i.m.) injections, since this, contrary to common belief, is below 100%. For instance, ampicillin has a bioavailability of 71% (Bergan, 1978b).

It is worthwhile pointing out that bioavailability depends upon experimental design. For instance, the area under the serum curve is smaller after rapid intravascular injection than after an infusion. This has been demonstrated for both gentamicin and mezlocillin (Mendelson et al., 1976; Ohlsson and Bergan, 1980), but is probably generally applicable. With mezlocillin, a bolus injection gave a total area of

TABLE 3

Absorption of Antibiotics from Oral Doses

Absorption %	Antibiotic
20–40	Fosfomycin (30–40), fusidic acid (30–40), griseofulvin (30).
40–60	Ampicillin (40–60), erythromycin (50), flucloxacillin (50–60), josamycin (50), lincomycin (40–50), novobiocin (50–60), phenoxymethylpenicillin (50).
60–80	Dicloxacillin (70), sulphonamides (50–90), classical tetracyclines (60–80).
80–100	Amoxycillin (85–95), ampicillin esters (85–95), cephalexin (80–95), chloramphenicol (80–90), clindamycin (90), cycloserin (80–90), doxycyclin and minocyclin (90–97), nalidixic acid (80–90), nitrofurantoin (90), rifampicin (90–95).

References: Bergan (1978d); Nauman (1975); Otten *et al.* (1975).

273 ± 66 µg.h/ml and a 30 min infusion resulted in 435 ± 58 µg. h/ml. The explanation for this phenomenon is that the entire non-protein bound intravascular portion of the drugs is eliminated rapidly e.g. by glomerular filtration. When the entire dose is disposed suddenly into the blood, almost all is initially available for renal elimination. It takes some time to transport the drug into extravascular body compartments such as tissues where the agent becomes protected from elimination by blood clearance. With proportionately more direct and initial disappearance into the urine, the area under the serum curve becomes smaller. Consequently, bioavailability figures are higher if extravascular doses are compared to bolus injections rather than to infusions over e.g. 0.5 to 2.0 h.

Bioavailability should primarily be determined in healthy individuals. Extravascular and direct intravenous administration ought to be studied in the same individuals. Plasma data assessment is preferred, but results should be supplemented by urine data. These also allow bioavailability estimates if renal elimination is substantial and the method of analysis is accurate and sensitive. Then, by analogy with the formula using serum data, the formula for urine is: $f_R = M_u$ (extravascularly given drug)/M_u (i.v. given drug). In practice, bioavailability determinations from urine data are more variable and are preferable mainly for internal controls of serum data estimates. Also, they are most suitable for agents without biotransformation.

The term bioavailability implies determination of the entire amount absorbed. In gastrointestinal absorption, though, the drug first passes the enzymatically active liver. Drugs which are actively metabolised may be partially transformed during liver passage, which reduces the AUC of unchanged substance. In serum, unchanged plus metabolised agent is a better indicator of absorption. Part of the substances may also disappear via the bile. Hepatobiliary elimination during absorption is referred to as the first pass effect.

The consequences of food, other drugs, for instance those acting on non-striated muscles and the autonomous nervous system, and impacts of disease on gastrointestinal absorption should be studied for new preparations. Lack of interference from food on absorption is a practically relevant asset, since oral doses are regularly taken with meals.

Descriptive pharmacokinetic analyses are necessary for internal studies to ensure that the formulations of e.g. tablets are optimal. The recipes must usually be modified from one drug to another. Dissolution should be rapid upon arrival of the tablets in the duodenum.

Serum Peaks

The peak concentrations are described as the maximum levels (c_{max}) and the time of their occurrence (t_{max}). The time of occurrence is an inaccurate measure. It depends to some degree upon the time intervals chosen during sampling and is thus necessarily inaccurately determined by direct assay data, unless very frequently sampled. Equations enabling calculation of c_{max} and t_{max} from basic pharmacokinetic characteristics are given in Appendix I. In general, an earlier peak is obtained if the absorption rate is high. Serum peaks occur when equal amounts are absorbed and excreted per time unit. Accordingly, the t_{max} is also related to the rate of elimination from serum. For instance, substances eliminated chiefly by the kidney have later peak occurrence in patients with renal dysfunction.

Distribution

Transport to extravascular parts of the body is subject to theoretical and practical problems. The kinetics of tissue penetration have been detailed elsewhere (Bergan, 1978c). Rates of transport differ from one site to another, but important is the fact that the area under the serum curve per time unit is proportional to the amount of antibiotic reaching extravascular sites. Smaller molecules penetrate better than larger ones. High lipid solubility is associated with better penetration through lipoprotein cell membranes. The actual concentrations may be determined on material from various body sites, e.g. urine, bile, cerebrospinal fluid (CSF), fluids collected in other body cavities, secretions (bronchia, sinus, middle ear, sputum, saliva, prostate exprimate), wound exsudate, or tissue homogenates. The therapeutic implications of concentrations in body fluids are obvious. Tissue homogenates, though, are associated with a series of theoretical and practical difficulties. The theoretical problems derive from the circumstance that homogenates contain everything in the tissue without regard to source. In kidney tissue homogenates, for instance, substances concentrated in the urine achieve high levels, although levels in renal lymph may be relatively low. Blood is a major constituent of e.g. lung and bone marrow tissues. The question is what relevance apparent tissue levels may have for tissue fluid concentrations, where the bacteria are most likely located at least during the initial phases of an infection.

A few approaches have been used to arrive at therapeutically relevant concentrations. Levels have been measured in tissue fluid collected after surgery (Alexander *et al.*, 1973; Baker and Hunt, 1968) (Fig. 4), in fluid from skin chambers mounted on superficially

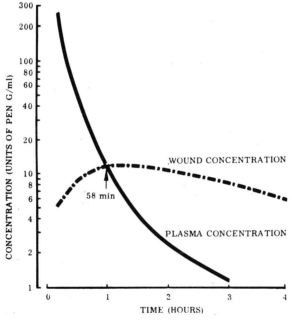

FIG. 4   Mean concentrations of benzylpenicillin in plasma and wound fluid after 100.000 IU intravenously (Baker and Hunt, 1968; reprinted with permission of authors and of American Journal of Surgery).

scarified skin (Tan *et al.*, 1972), skin blisters (Simon, 1976), and tissue chambers implanted subcutaneously (Bergan and Versland, 1978; Chisholm *et al.*, 1973; Schreiner *et al.*, 1978), in kidney or other tissues (Eickenberg, 1978). The usefulness of data from such sources is constrained by the fact that the tissues have been manipulated. Accordingly, perhaps lymph fluid better reflects tissue levels. As an example, Fig. 5 shows the levels of ampicillin and mecillinam

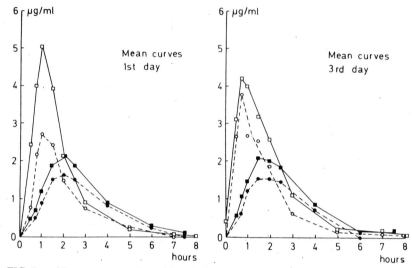

FIG. 5   Mean serum and peripheral (leg) lymph concentrations of ampicillin and mecillinam in 5 healthy volunteers after the first and seventh doses of 500 mg tablets with equimolar portions of bacampicillin and bacmecillinam. Ampicillin: —□—, serum, —■—, lymph; mecillinam: . . . ○ . . ., serum, . . . ● . . ., lymph. (Bergan *et al.*, 1979; reprinted with permission of Georg Thieme Verlag).

in serum and lymph collected from the legs of healthy volunteers in our laboratory (Bergan *et al.*, 1979). Fibrin clots and abscess fluid have also been studied (Barza and Weinstein, 1974; Barza *et al.*, 1974) (Fig. 6). These are certainly relevant to the conditions within an inflammatory process.

Generally, peak concentrations at extravascular loci are lower and occur later than in serum. Substances which are eliminated fairly rapidly from the serum, with a half-life less than 1–2 h, have repeatedly been shown to produce higher concentrations outside serum than in the intravascular compartment towards the end of the dosage intervals. For agents with a half-life of more than 9–12 h, on the other hand, more equivalence can be expected between non-protein bound levels in serum and outside the vascular compartment.

Serum protein binding is also relevant. Only the non-protein bound portion of the antibiotics are available for transport from the intravascular compartment. The degree of protein binding of antimicrobial agents is shown in Table 4. The binding restrict transport, distribution, elimination and antimicrobial activity. For practical purposes, the serum protein binding appears only to significantly

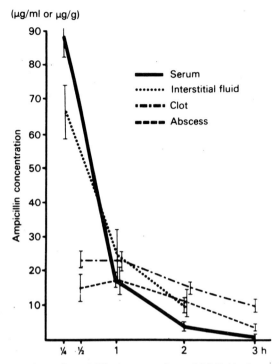

FIG. 6   Concentrations of ampicillin in serum, interstitial fluid, abscess fluid, and fibrin clot after intravenous doses of 50 mg/kg body weight to rabbits (Barza and Weinstein, 1974; reprinted with permission of authors and of The University of Chicago Press).

TABLE 4

Degree of Serum Protein Binding of Antibiotics

% binding	Antibiotics
0–25	Aminoglycosides (0)*, amoxycillin, ampicillin (15–20), cephacetril, cephradine (0–20), cephaloridine, cephalexin (15–30), polymyxin B, colistin (10–20), thiamphenicol (10–20), vancomycin (10).
30–75	Benzylpenicillin (50–65), carbenicillin (50), cefamandole, cefazolin (68–75), cephalothin (50–75), cephanone (30–70), chloramphenicol (40–50), clindamycin (40), demethylchlortetracycline (60–75), ethambutol (40), lincomycin (70), methicillin (30–50), minocycline (75), nalidixic acid (75), nitrofurantoin (50), para-aminosalicylic acid (50), phenoxymethylpenicillin (50–75), rifampicin (75), sulphamethoxazole (68), tetracyclines (classical) (20–50), trimethoprim (45–50).
80–98	Amphotericin, azidocillin (80–85), doxycycline (80–90), erythromycin (80–85), fusidic acid (90), griseofulvin (80), methacycline (80), novo-biocin (95–98), oxacillin, cloxacillin, dicloxacillin, flucloxacillin (90–96), sulphonamides (long acting).

* Approximate binding (%) at therapeutic levels.
References: Nauman (1975); Otten *et al.* (1975).

reduce free levels of drugs in the body when the protein binding is above 80% (Craig and Suh, 1978a). There are different protein binding levels in normal individuals, but variation is particularly pronounced in disease states. Reduced protein binding follows reduced serum concentrations of free fatty acids, accumulation of endogenous compounds such as bilirubin or free fatty acids, and pharmaceutical agents as occurs in reduced renal function (Craig and Suh, 1978b).

The over-all disappearance of agents from serum is expressed as distribution volumes. They are to be interpreted only as proportionality factors showing the ratio between serum levels and amounts within the body. They are without anatomical correlates. For example, we may consider the central distribution volume applicable to the one-compartment open model: $V_c = D/c_0$, where the D is the dose. A number of distribution volume estimates have been defined for the two-compartment model as indicated in Appendix I. The area distribution volume ($V_{d,area}$) is applicable to both the one and the two-compartment models. The β—phase distribution volume ($V_{d,\beta}$) is conceptually similar to the V_d of the one-compartment model and relates serum concentration and amounts in the body during the β—phase.

These distribution metrics are useful mainly for the comparison of chemically related agents. The isoxazolylpenicillins can be used to illustrate the point. Modr and Dvoracek (1970) found that equal intravenous doses of 0.5 g gave the lowest serum levels for oxacillin, intermediate ones for cloxacillin, and the highest ones for dicloxacillin (Fig. 7). The total area under the curve reflects the serum levels through their course, which are 7.5, 17.6 and 56.2 μg.h/ml respectively for oxacillin, cloxacillin and dicloxacillin; the respective distribution volumes are 26.2, 23.2 and 16.1 litres. This is a consequence not necessarily of a better penetration, as the distribution volume would imply, but follows the difference in serum levels alone, disregarding the loci to which the substances disappear. It is due to the fact that oxacillin is more rapidly excreted in the urine. The longer maintenance of higher serum levels is a characteristic which makes dicloxacillin more favourable. Another finding indicating favourable properties of dicloxacillin is its higher bioavailability after oral dosage: 80.4% instead of 66.8 and 77.4 respectively for oxacillin and cloxacillin.

Cephalosporins represent another example where much significance has been ascribed to the distribution volumes. Higher distribution volume has been claimed to imply preferable properties. Such rough generalities should be avoided. Cephalosporins with a high distribution volume disappear more quickly from serum as illustrated in

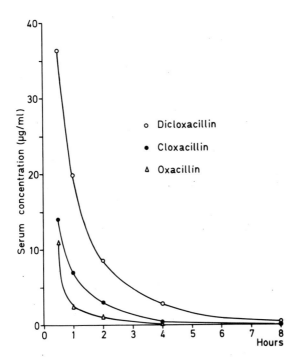

FIG. 7   Serum concentrations of isoxazolylpenicillins after 0.5 g intravenously (Modr and Dvoracek, 1970; reprinted with permission of authors and of Pergamon Press).

TABLE 5

Pharmacokinetic Properties and Non-Protein Bound Fraction of Cephalosporins.
Dose: 1.0 g intramuscularly.

Characteristic	Cephalothin	Cephaloridine	Cefazolin
V_d (l/kg)	23.2	19.2	10.4
t ½ (min)	41	84	126
Prot. binding (%)	62	23	69
Unbound concentration (μg/ml)			
at 4 h	0.5	4.8	7.6
at 8 h	0.1	0.8	2.0

Reference: Seydel, 1977.

Table 5. Cephalothin has the highest distribution volume and cefazolin the lowest one. The latter, though, has a longer half-life. Although the serum protein binding is highest for cefazolin, it has the highest levels during a substantial part of the dosage intervals. Analogously, substances like nitrofurantoin and nalidixic acid have high distribution volume metrics, but due to rapid renal excretion, therapeutic concentrations are not reached in e.g. tissues and they are useless for anything but urinary tract infections. The distribution volume only indicates how much has disappeared from the intravascular or central pharmacokinetic compartment.

Elimination

Elimination rates of the antimicrobial agents have received perhaps more attention than other pharmacokinetic aspects. The reason is its particular relevance to drug accumulation and estimation of dosage schedules. In Table 6 commonly used antimicrobial agents are grouped according to serum half-life.

TABLE 6

Grouping of Antibiotics According to Serum Half-Life

Serum half-life (hours)	Antibiotics
1–2	Penicillins, cephalosporins, erythromycin, nalidixic acid, nitrofurantoin
2–3	Aminoglycosides, cephradine, clindamycin, chloramphenicol, rifampicin, thiamphenicol
3–6	Fusidic acid, lincomycin, polymyxin, sulphisoxazole, sulphathiazole, vancomycin
7–12	Cycloserine, sulphadiazine, sulphamethizole, sulphamethoxazole, tetracyclines (classical), trimethoprim
13–24	Amphotericin, doxycycline, methacycline, minocycline, sulphonamides
> 24	Long term sulphonamides

References: Bergan, 1978d; Nauman, 1975; Otten *et al.*, 1975.

Serum half-life is estimated from the slope of the serum curve after completion of absorption and distribution. The serum half-life ($t\frac{1}{2}$) during monoexponential elimination equals $\ln2/k_E$ for the one-compartment model and $\ln2/\beta$ for the two-compartment model.

It may be pointed out that the total body clearance, $Cl_B = D/F$, is a model independent means of expressing elimination capacities.

In relation to repeated dosage, situations occasionally arise where the serum half-life changes with the number of doses. Agents may inhibit or enhance their own metabolisation or damage organs responsible for elimination. Accordingly, it is of paramount importance that pharmacokinetics are determined both after one dose and after achievement of steady state conditions, i.e. after 5–9 doses, depending upon serum half-life. Only by repeated dosage can multiple dose kinetics relevant to therapeutic situations be assessed.

The two-compartment model has occasionally been inadequate.

In addition to the fast distribution phase, and a slower β–phase, there is occasionally an even slower gamma-phase. Radioimmunoassay or enzyme linked immunosorbent assay techniques, which are much more sensitive than microbiological methods, have enabled the detection of a gamma-phase of e.g. aminoglycosides. The serum levels must then be followed for several days after the final dose (Kahlmeter *et al.*, 1978a and b; Schentag *et al.*, 1977a and b). It has been suggested that the slow final phase of the aminoglycosides correlates with binding to tissues, e.g. to kidney tissue, and thus may have important toxicological implications.

A slower final portion of the curve may be undetected after a single dose. Consequently several doses may be required for increased amounts in the peripheral compartment. This probably explains observations with serum levels of tetracycline (Dolusio and Dittert, 1969).

The relative contribution of each pharmacokinetic compartment may be determined from the areas under the drug concentration curves which are related to each of the disposition phases. Examples of relative contributions of areas and serum half-life of the respective pharmacokinetic compartments are shown in Table 7 for aminoglycosides, cephalosporins, and ethambutol: each phase has a separate

TABLE 7

Serum Half-Life (t½) and Fractional Areas (F%) of Pharmacokinetic Phases in Healthy Subjects

Antibiotic	α–phase		β–phase		γ–phase	
	t½α (min)	Fα (%)	t½β (h)	Fβ (%)	t½γ (h)	Fγ (%)
Cefamandole	5	14	0.4	55	1.2	31
Cephalothin	5	34	0.3	40	1.7	26
Ethambutol	5	26	3.1	47	10.2	27
Gentamicin			3.6	86	53	14
Netilmicin	23	15	2.0	72	37	13
Sisomicin	25	17	1.9	72	17	11

apparent half-life. The t½β is customarily the reported half-life for the two-compartment model because it usually associates with the dominant portion of the curves. The area under the serum curve of each phase is directly proportional to the fraction of the steady state concentration attributable to each. The final gamma-portion contributes 10–15% for the aminoglycosides. If this portion is omitted in estimations of steady state concentrations relevant to therapeutic effect, the error is not great. However, the error in determining total amount in the body at the end of the dosage intervals may be large if the gamma-phase is ignored. This may be relevant for toxicity considerations.

A number of points require special attention during half-life determinations. Basically, healthy individuals must primarily be studied, but also neonates, children, and pregnant women. Prolonged elimination in newborn children is well documented for most agents. Pregnant women have lower serum levels during the final trimester because of a larger distribution volume (Philipson, 1977; Philipson *et al.*, 1976). The influence of disease states also requires elucidation.

Patients with cystic fibrosis have lower serum concentrations of penicillins and perhaps aminoglycosides than normal persons. This follows a higher body clearance, in part due to different distribution and in part to faster renal elimination in cystic fibrosis (Bergan and Michalsen, 1980; Jusko *et al.*, 1975; Yaffe *et al.*, 1977). Agents which are especially directed against *Pseudomonas aeruginosa* or *Staphylococcus aureus*, should be studied in cystic fibrosis where such substances are important.

Gastrointestinal diseases may reduce absorption, if associated with increased passage or steatorrhoea (Davis and Pinola, 1968). Increased absorption may also occur. The latter applies to metronidazole which reaches higher serum levels during ulcerous colitis, Crohn's disease, and enterostomy (Bergan *et al.*, unpub. results). For other agents, chronic enteropathies have no effect on serum levels (Parsons *et al.*, 1976a and b).

Elimination occurs mainly through renal or hepatobiliary routes. The over-all first order elimination constant (k_E) equals the sum of the rates of the renal elimination (k_R) and of the metabolism and extra-renal elimination (k_M): $k_E = k_M + k_R$. Renal elimination is assessed by comparing the clearance of the substances to the renal

TABLE 8

Degree of Renal Elimination of Antimicrobial Drugs*

---

1. RENAL CLEARANCE BELOW CREATININE CLEARANCE
   Cephanone, cefazolin, chloramphenicol, clindamycin, colistin, erythromycin, lincomycin, novobiocin, rifampicin, sulphisoxazole, sulphamethoxazole, sulphadiazine, long and medium term sulphonamides, trimethoprim, vancomycin

2. RENAL CLEARANCE SIMILAR TO CREATININE CLEARANCE
   Aminoglycosides, amoxycillin, carbenicillin, cephaloridine, cephapirin, dicloxacillin, flucloxacillin, oxytetracycline, ristocetin, thiamphenicol, vancomycin

3. RENAL CLEARANCE 2–10 TIMES THE CREATININE CLEARANCE
   Ampicillin, azidocillin, benzylpenicillin, cephalosporins, cloxacillin, methicillin, oxacillin, nalidixic acid, nitrofurantoin, phenoxymethylpenicillin, short term sulphonamides (serum half-life less than 7 h)

---

* Aminoglycosides, cephalosporins, penicillins, polymyxins, sulphonamides, tetracyclines and thiamphenicol are eliminated mainly via the kidney and consequently need dosage modification in cases of renal insufficiency when their elimination is prolonged.
References: Bergan, 1978d; Nauman, 1975; Otten *et al.*, 1975.

clearances (Table 8). The degree of biliary elimination is illustrated by bile concentrations relative to serum levels (Table 9).

TABLE 9

Degree of Biliary Elimination of Antibiotics

Degree of biliary elimination	Antibiotics
MINIMAL, bile concentrations below serum levels	Aminoglycosides, cephalosporins, chloramphenicol*, isoxazolylpenicillins, polymyxin B, colistin
MEDIUM, bile concentrations close to serum levels	Clindamycin*, tetracyclines (classical)*, trimethoprim, thiamphenicol
HIGH, bile concentrations 10–15 times serum levels	Amoxycillin, ampicillin, erythromycin*, fusidic acid*, lincomycin*, novobiocin*
VERY HIGH, bile concentrations up to 100 times above serum levels	Methampicillin, rifampicin*

*   These drugs need dosage modification in case of hepatobiliary insufficiency in cases of prolonged elimination.
References: Nauman, 1975; Otten *et al.*, 1975.

Reduced renal or hepatic excretory capacity raises the serum half-life of agents eliminated through the respective organs. Many data have been already collected on the relationship between serum half-life and renal function for agents eliminated chiefly via the kidneys (Table 10). The first studies from Kunin and his group (Kunin and Finland, 1959; Kunin, 1967) may be regarded as pioneering work in this regard since they have started a whole school of studies relating elimination rates to reduced renal function (Dettli, 1977). Such investigations have now rightly become mandatory for new agents.

The renal function should be determined by creatinine clearance for clinical purposes, or preferably by inulin clearance, which more accurately determines renal function. In the case of lower functions, too high renal function values may be obtained when creatinine clearance is used instead of the true values of glomerular filtration rate as inuline clearance. Relating the serum half-life to only serum creatinine is misleading, although such a correlation has often been presented in the literature. The practice deserves criticism because the creatinine level may be within normal limits even in patients with distinctly reduced renal function. Nomograms relating serum creatinine and age demonstrate this clearly (Kampmann *et al.*, 1971). Serum creatinine as reference is therefore not acceptable even though a statistically satisfactory relationship can be determined between creatinine levels and t½. The consequent errors in estimating serum half-life are larger when serum creatinine is employed than when clearance determinations are carried out.

TABLE 10

Serum Half-Life (t½, Hours)* of Antibiotics at Different Renal Functions

Antibiotic	t½0	t½10	t½30	t½60	t½norm
Cephalothin	11.7	3.5	1.5	0.8	0.5
Cephaloridine	23.3	9.3	4.8	2.7	1.8
Benzylpenicillin	23.3	4.1	1.6	0.8	0.5
Ampicillin	6.4	4.4	2.8	1.8	1.2
Oxacillin	2.0	1.5	1.0	0.7	0.5
Carbenicillin	23.3	3.7	1.9	1.2	0.8
Erythromycin	5.4	4.2	3.0	2.0	1.4
Lincomycin	11.7	10.0	8.2	6.4	4.7
Vancomycin	233.0	41.2	17.2	9.3	5.8
Kanamycin	70.0	15.5	6.1	3.2	2.0
Streptomycin	70.0	17.5	7.8	4.2	2.6
Colistin	35.0	14.0	6.7	3.6	2.3
Polymyxin B	35.0	14.0	11.7	6.7	4.4
Gentamicin	70.0	15.5	7.0	3.7	2.3
Rolitetracycline	35.0	28.0	23.3	15.5	11.6
Chloramphenicol	3.5	3.3	3.0	2.7	2.3

*   t½0, t½10, t½30, t½60, and t½norm: serum half-life values at creatinine clearances of
0, 10, 30, 60 ml/min and normal renal functions.
Reference: Lüthy and Siegenthaler, 1973.

It should perhaps be stressed, though, that the spread is considerable even around regressions of t½ vs. clearance, so that extrapolations from such data should only function as presumptive indicators. This, unfortunately, applies particularly to low renal functions. Determination of ultimate serum half-life after a few days of therapy is recommended in each patient for e.g. aminoglycosides which have only a narrow margin between toxic and therapeutically effective serum levels. The t½ of aminoglycosides have a tendency to rise during the course of administration.

One point which has been sparsely emphasized is the fact that relationships between renal function as expressed by creatinine clearance and t½ are not necessarily log linear throughout the range of all the renal function, as it has been presumed in most cases. In low renal function, alternate routes of elimination may become important. This applies, for instance, to cefazolin (Fig. 8) (Bergan et al., 1977). In renal failure, hepatobiliary elimination prevents the t½ from rising above 30–40 h. This low capacity route of elimination can be neglected when the renal function is normal and when the renal route is considerably more efficient than any other route to eliminate the agent. The hepatobiliary route becomes important only when the renal capacity is relatively minor.

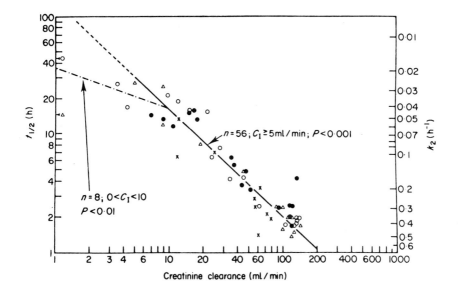

FIG. 8   Relationship between serum half-life of cefazolin and creatinine clearance as established by different experimenters (from Bergan *et al.*, 1977).

A final point which recently has become evident is the desirability of monitoring anti-infectious agents by both microbiological methods and chemical procedures. The former gives therapeutically relevant information in cases when biotransformation products are antimicrobially active. For instance, metronidazole has a longer t½ when assayed by a bacterial technique than when unchanged metronidazole is determined chromatographically (Bergan and Arnold, 1980). Chemical methods, such as high pressure liquid chromatography or gas liquid chromatography, allow assay of metabolites in addition to unchanged compounds and thus enable monitoring of parent substance plus biotransformation products. This enables detection of accumulation of metabolites in patients with renal insufficiency, even though the products may be present in minute amounts in normal individuals.

Capacity Limited Kinetics

One point requiring attention is the relationship between dose sizes and area under the serum curve (AUC), t½, and Cl_B. If higher AUC per dose unit results for higher doses, dose dependent elimination occurs (Fig. 9). A likely explanation then is the presence of saturable

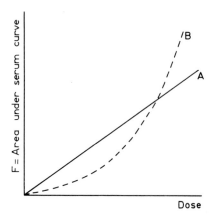

FIG. 9   Relationship between dose and area under serum curve in cases of dose independent (A) and dose dependent (B) pharmacokinetics. Substance B is subject to Michaelis–Menten kinetics.

processes, since enzymatic processes have an upper capacity limit. Elimination curves then follow the usual pattern of saturable enzymatic activity described by the Michaelis–Menten formula (Appendix I). Consequently, the phenomenon is referred to as Michaelis–Menten kinetics.

A high degree of metabolisation is not automatically associated with Michaelis–Menten kinetics. For instance, only 5–10% metronidazole appear unchanged in the urine. Yet, dose dependence does not occur with either tablets or suppositories up to 1.0 and 2.0 g respectively (Bergan and Arnold, 1980).

In general, the question of capacity limitation should preferably be studied after intravenous (i.v.) doses, if such preparations are available. This avoids interference from impacts of absorption and biopharmaceutical factors.

Lack of Michaelis–Menten kinetics is valid only up to the doses studied. Higher doses could surpass a threshold transformation capacity. Accordingly, licensing of higher doses should be backed by pharmacokinetic evaluations.

Capacity restricted pharmacokinetics can occur quite unexpected. Even penicillins, for instance, have now exhibited dose dependent pharmacokinetics. This was first demonstrated for mezlocillin (Bergan, 1978a), but subsequently for the chemically closely related azlocillin (Leroy et al., 1980). A similar pattern has not yet been demonstrated for other compounds in this group, but since dose dependence is often associated with enzymatic processes and biotransformation occurs for a number of commonly used penicillins (Thijssen and Mattie, 1976; Ullmann and Wurst, 1979) (Table 11),

TABLE 11

Number of Antibacterially Active Biotransformation Products of Penicillins
Excreted in Urine

No. of products	Antibiotics
0	Amoxycillin, mezlocillin
1	Ampicillin and its prodrugs (bacampicillin, pivampicillin, talampicillin), azidocillin, carbenicillin, epicillin, ticarcillin
2	Carfecillin

Reference: Ullmann and Wurst, 1979.

the possibility that dose dependence might apply to other penicillins as well should be evaluated.

Biotransformation commonly occurs with antimicrobial agents (Table 12). Both antimicrobially active and inactive products are

TABLE 12

Degree of Metabolisation of Antimicrobial Agents and Activity of Their Metabolites

Per cent metabolised	Antibiotics and activity* of their metabolites
Less than 25%	Aminoglycosides (0), cephalosporins, ethambutol, 5–fluorocytosine, fosfomycin, isoniacine, penicillins (mostly ± or 0), sulphonamides (with half-life below 8 h, 0), thiamphenicol.
30–60%	Cephalosporins [acetylated, cephalothin, cephapirin, (±), cefotaxime (+)], cycloserine (0), erythromycin (+), doxycycline (0), isoniazide, isoxazolylpenicillins, lincomycin, minocycline (0), nitrofurantoin, sulphonamides (of medium half-life, 0), trimethoprim (0).
Above 80%	Chloramphenicol (0), chlortetracycline (0), clindamycin, clotrimazole (0), fusidic acid (0), griseofulvin (+), nalidixic acid (+), novobiocin (0), para-aminosalicylic acid, rifampicin (+).

* When indicated between brackets, antimicrobial activity of metabolites: (+) active; (±) weakly active; (0) inactive or no metabolite (aminoglycosides).
References: Bergan and Arnold (1980); Nauman (1975); Otten *et al.* (1975).

formed. Accordingly, the possibility of capacity limitation should now be investigated for several antibiotics marketed before such evaluations became an integral part of the basic data. I am referring particularly to e.g. chloramphenicol, thiamphenicol, classical tetracyclines, and isoxazolylpenicillins, but also erythromycin, lincomycin, clindamycin, rifampicin.

Dosage Recommendations

All pharmacokinetic data, descriptive as well as analytical, may be utilised to formulate dosage recommendations. Initially, these should be based on pharmacokinetics of various dose sizes in healthy volunteers supplemented by studies in various disease states. Extravascular levels are particularly valuable in this regard. A minimum concentration likely to be therapeutically effective may be defined from knowledge of microbial sensitivity to the agent. The *in vivo* data can indicate what doses are necessary to obtain adequate levels for a sufficient portion of each dosage interval. However, the problems of extrapolating directly from *in vitro* sensitivity data are considerable, in that minimum inhibitory concentrations (m.i.c.) *in vitro* and in various body fluids may be different (Helm, 1977; Helm *et al.*, 1976; Shah *et al.*, 1976). Our data (Bergan and Carlsen, 1980) obtained from cultures exposed to exponentially diminishing concentrations of antibiotics, indicate that bacteria resume their growth once the agent levels are reduced below m.i.c. This implicates uncertainty as to whether there is really a period of cellular rest before post antibiotic recovery, as it has been suggested from experiments with microbes exposed *in vitro* to stable levels followed by rapid removal (McDonald *et al.*, 1976, 1977).

To stipulate dosage with sufficient accuracy, the formula $D = c_{min} \cdot (2^\epsilon - 1) \cdot V_d$ may be employed for one-compartment data (symbols explained in Appendix II). For the two-compartment model, $V_{d,\beta}$ applies.

What level to select for c_{min} is obviously open to discussion. It might preferably be deduced from experimental animal infections allowing determination of the relationship between minimum serum levels and the bacterial m.i.c.'s. Responses *in vitro* to exponentially reduced concentrations of antibiotics may also furnish valuable basic data. For all practical purposes, the levels of antimicrobials at a site of infection should exceed the m.i.c. during the major part of the dosage intervals. The peripheral levels are certainly dependent upon the extensiveness and place of the infectious process. Blister fluid or lymph levels are relevant to estimating extravascular level. Tissue chambers or concentrations in fibrin clots are certainly relevant. For agents with relatively longer $t\frac{1}{2}$, above 8–12 h, trough serum levels approach the minimum extravascular concentrations.

Successive therapeutic responses should depend on the minimum concentration at the foci of infection and not on the frequency of dosing. The realisation of this point is important now that our knowledge of better patient compliance with fewer daily doses has stimulated exploration of the possibility of employing fewer doses per 24 h. Each dose then must be higher as implied by the above formula. Drug toxicity may exclude the use of high single doses. The higher doses have the advantage that good penetration can be assumed. With the same total dose, infusions have given lower peripheral concentrations than those achieved by pulse dosing (Barza *et al.*, 1974).

Agents with a t½ above 6–8 h should be given with higher initial doses than the maintenance doses. Half-life values of 9–15 h necessitate initial doses (D*) at twice the maintenance doses (D). The initial doses necessary to give serum concentrations at the steady state levels from the very first dose may be calculated from the following equation:

$$D^* = \frac{D}{(1 - e^{-kE})(1 - e^{-kA})}$$

which applies to the one-compartment model (Krüger-Thiemer, 1960). In the two compartment model, β may be substituted for k_E, under the presumption that the β–phase contributes a dominant portion of the total AUC.

When dealing with newborns and smaller children, we have a problem in addition to a possibly slower rate of elimination. Doses cannot be prescribed simply in terms of body weight relative to adult because the distribution volumes in children and adults may be different. Aminoglycosides, for instance, have distribution volumes in newborns and infants which are 2–4 times higher than those found in adults. Consequently, the serum levels after adult doses per kg body weight would render therapeutically inadequate body levels in the children. A point of particular concern for pediatric dosage is the practice employing surface area as a reference. Such a practice has more error associated with it in younger children. Less serum level scattering is obtained if the doses are related to body weight, rather than to body surface area as that has been determined for e.g. netilmicin (Bergan and Michalsen, unpub. results).

The question is what doses to give patients with slower rates of drug elimination. This question has been dealt with elsewhere (Dettli, 1977), but the general rule of thumb is that the same mean or minimum serum levels should be reached in the diseased as in normal persons.

By mean serum concentration ($\bar{c}_p$) we understand the AUC during each dosage interval divided by the length of that period ($\tilde{f}$): $\bar{c}_p = F/\tilde{f}$. The average steady state blood level was defined by Wagner *et al.* (1965). If a given dose results in a AUC of 48 $\mu g.h/ml$, during a dosage interval of 8 h, then the mean concentration is 6 $\mu g/ml$.

The general formula is:

$$\bar{c}_p = \frac{1}{\tau} \cdot \int_0^\infty c_p \cdot dt$$

For the one-compartment model,

$$\bar{c}_p = \frac{D \cdot f}{V_d \cdot k_E \cdot \tau}$$

and for the two-compartment model:

$$\bar{c}_p = \frac{D \cdot f}{V_{d,\beta} \cdot \beta \cdot \tau} = \frac{D \cdot f}{V_c \cdot k_E \cdot \tau} = \frac{D \cdot f}{Cl_B \cdot \tau}$$

where f is the fraction of a dose absorbed (f = 1.0 for intravenous dosage).

For antimicrobial therapy, perhaps the mean serum level is significant, since body levels have to be maintained above a m.i.c. The formula for the mean serum level in the one-compartment open model is approximately $c_{min} = c_o/(2^\epsilon - 1)$ where ϵ is the ratio between the dosage interval τ and $t\frac{1}{2}$. When ϵ is maintained at the same value, the same minimal level is obtained in normal subjects as in patients with impaired elimination. Accordingly, the dosage interval must be extended in proportion to increases in serum half-life, although it takes more doses to reach steady state conditions in patients with prolonged rates of elimination (Fig. 10). For the

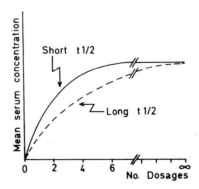

FIG. 10   Accumulation of a drug after repeated doses in individuals with normal serum half-life (———) or with prolonged elimination (— — —). Although the dose intervals have been adjusted to give the same ultimate mean serum level, a longer time elapses before the steady state is reached when the rate of elimination is reduced, due to renal or hepatic function impairment.

two- or three-compartment models, evaluation must be based on the pharmacokinetic compartment contributing the major portion of the AUC. The area under the curve contributed by each compartment equals the ratio between its Y–intercept and respective hybrid disposition constant.

Conclusion

There is no doubt that pharmacokinetics is a necessary adjunct to the development of new antimicrobial agents. This discipline may be used simply as a descriptive science. However, the great potential of pharmacokinetics is to be used as a powerful analytical tool enabling the clarification of relationships to physiological processes and disease states.

The aim of this book is to focus on criteria suitable for the selection of new antimicrobial agents or preference among available ones. In this chapter, the central question is what pharmacokinetic properties can be considered optimal. To some extent this may seem self-explanatory. Preferable are drugs with a quick and complete absorption from the gastrointestinal tract. A serum half-life of 4–10 h may be optimal; this renders sufficient stability in persistence of antimicrobial activity combined with sufficiently quick elimination to avoid the serious reactions in cases of allergy development during therapy for which long acting sulphonamides are notorious. Longer elimination also implies better economy and has the practical consequence that fewer doses are needed per day. The distribution volume as such is of little importance, since it does not indicate other characters than how much the antibiotic disappears from the serum compartment. More significant is the amount calculated for remaining extravascular drug still within the body. The protein binding ought to be low to achieve a high fraction of unbound drug whereby penetration within the body is facilitated. Agents should preferably not be metabolised, unless the metabolites are at least as active antimicrobially as the parent compound. Serum levels should be widely uninfluenced from disease states or concomitant intake of food or other drugs and dynamic effect should not be interfered with by other pharmaceuticals.

Pharmacokinetics represents a challenge to complete and detailed characterisation of new drugs during the development and later use of new antimicrobial drugs.

Appendix I

In this appendix, the pharmacokinetic models will be summarised and determination of pharmacokinetic properties from serum data by simple calculation and graphic procedures demonstrated. Appendix II defines the pharmacokinetic symbols used.

One-Compartment Open Model

Intravenous injection followed by only constant, first order elimination results in curves with a pattern shown in principle by Fig. 1. In a semilogarithmic plot, the curve of decreasing concentrations follows a straight line with the slope k_E which is the rate of elimination. The Y–axis intercept c_0 and k_E are the two parameters required to completely describe the model. To be noted is the point that the term k_E denotes relative amount removed from the body. If $k_E = 0.2\,h^{-1}$, 20% of the amount remaining in the body is removed per hour. The total absolute amount (in weight units) eliminated during the initial phase is higher than during the later phases.

Serum concentration curves follow the equation: $c_p = c_0 \cdot e^{-k_E t}$.

Derived pharmacokinetic parameters are:

Serum half-life:	$t\frac{1}{2} = \ln 2 / k_E$
Distribution volume:	$V_d = D / c_0$
Area distribution volume:	$V_{d,area} = D / k_E \cdot F$
Relative distribution volume:	$\Delta_d = V_d / W$
Total body clearance:	$Cl_B = D/F = k_E \cdot V_d$
Total area under serum curve (till infinity):	$F = (c_p) \cdot dt = c_0 / k_E$
Mean serum concentration:	$\bar{c}_p = F / \bar{t} = D / V_d \cdot k_E \cdot \bar{t}$

The slope of the final, declining portion of the curve corresponds to k_E and is determined by linear regression of $\ln c_p$ vs. time.

A plot of urinary excretion rate (mg/h) against time on a semilogarithmic scale gives a profile with the same slope as the disposition phase of the serum curve if only renally eliminated, and can be used as a control for the serum data if a major part of the drug is eliminated in the urine.

Serum half-life ($t\frac{1}{2}$) is the time required for the serum concentration to be decreased to one half of its original value. With monoexponential elimination (which gives a straight line in semilogarithmic plot), the $t\frac{1}{2}$ is constant without regard to the initial serum level. The serum half-life can be simply determined from two points on the semilogarithmically straight branch of the elimination phase of the serum curve. If serum concentrations are c_A and c_B at the times t_A and t_B, the half-life is

$$t\frac{1}{2} = \frac{\ln 2 / (t_A - t_B)}{\ln c_A - \ln c_B}$$

First order absorption from any extravascular site (gastro-intestinal, intramuscular and others) followed by first order elimination results in concentration curves as illustrated in principle by Fig. 1. The serum concentration curves then follow the formula:

$$c_p = \left| \frac{c_0 \cdot k_A}{k_A - k_E} \right| \cdot (e^{-k_E t} - e^{-k_A t})$$

Serum doubling-time due to absorption: $t\frac{1}{2}(a) = \ln 2 / k_A$.

The $t\frac{1}{2}$, V_d, Cl_B, F, and $\bar{c}$ are as defined above, except that adjustment must be made for amount absorbed. In the above formulas D must accordingly be substituted by $D \cdot f$ where f is the fraction of dose absorbed. The f is determined by comparisons of areas under serum curves after absorption from extravascular site and intravenous dosage, i.e. bioavailability assessment.

The straight line of a semilogarithmic plot of serum concentrations during the phase of elimination is extended towards the Y–axis and the difference between the corresponding regression and the actual observations during the absorption phase is extrapolated from the plot or calculated by a desk computer from the equation of the regression line. The differences are plotted at each point in time along the Y–axis. When the data are perfect, a straight line emerges in semilogarithmic plots. A linear regression of the logarithm to the base *e* for these concentration differences has a slope corresponding to k_A. This procedure is called the method of residuals, or commonly feathering. It demonstrates that the complex curvilinear serum curve may be interpreted as a composite of two straight lines (in semilogarithmic plots), each related to the separate monoexponential components of the corresponding equation. In perfect data, the line with slope k_A should intersect with the elimination line at $t=0$ if the drug is absorbed without any lag. If intersecting to the right of the origin, the corresponding time interval equals the lag time before apparent absorption.

The maximum concentration after the nth dose may be estimated from:

$$c_{n,max} = c_0 \left(\frac{k_A}{k_E}\right)^{-k_E(k_A - k_E)} \cdot \left(\frac{1 - e^{-nk_E \tilde{\jmath}}}{1 - e^{-k_E \tilde{\jmath}}}\right)$$

The corresponding minimum serum concentration is:

$$c_{n,min} = c_0 \frac{k_A}{k_A - k_E} \cdot \left[e^{-k_E \tilde{\jmath}} - e^{-k_A \tilde{\jmath}} \left(\frac{1 - e^{-nk_E \tilde{\jmath}}}{1 - e^{-k_E \tilde{\jmath}}}\right) \right]$$

The time of peak occurrence is:

$$t_{max} = \frac{\ln(k_A/k_E)}{k_A - k_E}$$

Two-Compartment Open Model

Intravenous injection of bolus doses is followed by a curve with at least two phases as demonstrated in Fig. 2. The initial part corresponds to the distribution phase, or α–phase, when the drug disappears from the circulation because of simultaneous penetration into extravascular parts of the body and elimination. The phase of slower disposition corresponds to mainly elimination and is called the elimination phase or β–phase. The serum curve follows the formula:

$$c_p = A \cdot e^{-\alpha t} + B \cdot e^{-\beta t}$$

where α and β are the disposition constants of the respective parts of the curve and A and B corresponding hybrid intercepts. From these, the basic parameters of the model, c_0, k_E, k_{12}, and k_{21} may be determined (defined in Appendix II). The curve may also be written as:

$$c_p = \frac{D(\alpha - k_{21})}{V_c(\alpha - \beta)} e^{-\alpha t} + \frac{D(k_{21} - \beta)}{V_c(\alpha - \beta)} e^{-\beta t}$$

By the method of residuals, commonly called feathering, on serum concentration plots, estimates of α and β, A, and B are obtained. Linear regression of $\ln c_p$ in respect to time of the terminal phase of the curve renders the slope β. The intercept of the line with the Y–axis corresponds to B. Extension of the straight final portion of the curve to the left and extrapolation of the difference between this straight line (semilogarithmic plot) and the observed points of the initial phase of rapid disposition, i.e. the distribution phase (α–phase), give values to be plotted at each time of observation on the Y–axis. With perfect data, a straight line results for which the slope corresponds to α, the disposition constant for the distributive process. This second line intersects the Y–axis at the point A.

The derived pharmacokinetic characteristics of the two-compartment model are:

Serum half-life: $t\frac{1}{2}\beta = \ln 2/\beta$

Serum disposition half-life during the distribution phase: $t\frac{1}{2}\alpha = \ln 2/\alpha$

Central compartment distribution volume: $V_c = D/c_0 = D/(A + B)$

Relative central compartment distribution volume: $\Delta_c = V_c/W$

β–phase distribution volume: $V_{d,\beta} = D/\beta \cdot F = D \cdot \alpha/(B\alpha + A\beta)$

Relative β–phase distribution volume: $\Delta_{d,\beta} = V_{d,\beta}/W$

Area distribution volume:

$V_{d,area} = D/k_E \cdot F = V_c k_E/\beta = V_{d,ss} + (k_E - \beta) V_c/k_{21}$

Extrapolated β–phase distribution volume:

$V_{d,extrap} = D/B = V_c(\alpha - \beta)/(k_{21} - \beta) = D/\beta F$

Steady state distribution volume: $V_{d,ss} = V_c + V_T = V_c(k_{12} + k_{21})/k_{21}$

Distribution volume of peripheral (tissue) compartment:

$V_T = V_c k_{12}/k_{21} = V_c k_{12} k_E/\alpha\beta$

Total body clearance: $Cl_B = D/F = k_E V_c = \beta V_{d,\beta} = \beta \cdot V_{d,extrap}$

Renal clearance: $Cl_R = M_u/F$

Total area under serum curve till infinity: $F = (A/\alpha) + (B/\beta) = D/V_c k_E$

Direct area estimation from the serum data by the trapezoidal rule:

$$F = \Sigma \frac{c_1 + c_2}{2} \cdot \Delta t$$

Rate constant (first order) for transfer from peripheral to central compartment: $k_{21} = (A\beta + B\alpha)/(A + B)$

Rate constant for elimination from central compartment:

$$k_E = \alpha\beta/k_{21} = \alpha\beta(A + B)/(A\beta + B\alpha)$$

Rate constant (first order) for transfer from central to peripheral compartment: $k_{12} = \alpha + \beta - k_E - k_{21} = AB(\beta - \alpha)^2/(A+B)(A\beta + B\alpha)$

Mean serum concentration: $\bar{c}_p = D/V_{d,\beta} \cdot \beta \cdot \bar{\gamma} = D/V_c \cdot k_E \cdot \bar{\gamma} = F/\bar{\gamma}$

Total amount in peripheral compartment after rapid i.v. injection:

$$X_T = D \cdot k_{12}(e^{-\beta t} - e^{-\alpha t})/(\alpha - \beta)$$

The distribution volumes are mathematical terms relating serum concentrations to total amount of drug in the body. $V_{d,ss}$ is only applicable for such an assessment at the time when total drug transport in both directions between compartment is zero. This corresponds to the peak of a curve describing the amount of drug in the peripheral compartment:

$$X_T = \frac{D \cdot k_{12}}{(\alpha - \beta)} (e^{-\beta t} - e^{-\alpha t})$$

Before this maximum, estimates of amounts in the body based on $V_{d,ss}$ are too high before the X_T maximum and too low after that point in time.

The $V_{d,\beta}$ describes the situation during flow equivalence when the phase of distribution is terminated, i.e. when the expression containing α becomes so small that it is neglectable. This occurs at the beginning of the β-phase. During this phase, the relationship between the amounts of substance in either compartment and the total amount in the body are constant and independent of time. During the β-phase, the ratio between the amount in the peripheral compartment and the amount in the central compartment remains constant. The $V_{d,\beta}$ and $V_{d,area}$ have the advantages that they are independent of the mode of drug administration, since the area under the serum curves are considered not to depend on it.

Yet another definition of distribution volume for the two-compartment model has been given (Riegelmann *et al.*, 1958), $V_{d,inf.eq} = X_T/c_{ss}$, which is the ratio between the amount of drug in the peripheral compartment and the serum level obtained during constant infusion over a period which is long enough to enable achievement of a stable serum level. Analysis of the expressions shows that this volume is equal to $V_{d,ss}$.

The distribution of the drug between the central and the extravascular compartment (also somewhat malconceptionally called tissue compartment) is important in the evaluation of antimicrobial agents. The fraction f_C of the original dose remaining within the central compartment at any time t is:

$$f_C = \frac{c_p}{c_o} = \frac{A \cdot e^{-\alpha t} + B \cdot e^{-\beta t}}{A + B}$$

The fraction f_T of the original dose in the peripheral compartment at any time t is:

$$f_T = 1 - \frac{F_t}{F} - \frac{c_p}{c_0} = \frac{AB\,(\alpha - \beta)}{(A+B)\,(A\beta + B\alpha)}\,(e^{-\beta t} - e^{-\alpha t}),$$

where F_t is the area under the serum curve till time t.

The fraction $f_{M,E}$ of the original dose lost from the central compartment by both metabolism and excretion at any time t is:

$$f_{M,E} = \frac{F_t}{F} = 1 - \frac{1}{A\beta + B\alpha}\,(\frac{A}{\beta}\,e^{-\alpha t} + \frac{B}{\alpha}\,e^{-\beta t})$$

Intravenous infusion data.   Pharmacokinetic parameters from post-infusion serum data must be derived by auxiliary equations (Gibaldi, 1969; Loo and Riegelman, 1970). The serum curves are in principle as shown in Fig. 11. Assessment according to the two-compartment open model enables estimation of α

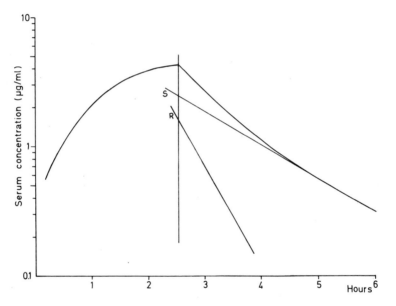

FIG. 11   Pattern of serum curve after infusion of antibiotics over a longer period. R and S are hybrid intercepts of α and β–phase disposition lines.

and β either through computer curve fitting or by feathering. An auxiliary Y–axis placed at the point of terminated infusion shows the auxiliary hybrid intercepts R and S for the post-infusion α and β–phases respectively. These adhere to the following equations:

$$R = \frac{k_0\,(\alpha - k_{21})}{V_c\,(\alpha - \beta)\alpha}$$

$$S = \frac{k_0\,(k_{21} - \beta)}{V_c\,(\alpha - \beta)\beta}$$

The above indicated formulas for the two-compartment model are applicable, but A and B in those equations are calculated from R and S according to the following equations:

$$A = RD\alpha/k_o$$
$$B = SD\beta/k_o$$

It may be difficult with limited serum data during the post-infusion period to differentiate between the two-compartment model and the one-compartment model. The more readily discerned the former one, the higher the ratio R/S, or A/B. As A approaches 0, a monoexponential course becomes increasingly appropriate with a one-compartment model at the extreme limit. The R/S ratio is always less than A/B, since $A/B = (\alpha - k_{21})/(k_{21} - \beta)$ and $R/S = (A/B)(\beta/\alpha)$ and β always is lesser than α. Accordingly, determination of two-compartment model characteristics may be difficult after infusion, if the A/B ratio after rapid intravascular injection is low. The two-compartment course even then may not be distinct.

Extravascular absorption in the two-compartment open model (first order absorption from the gastrointestinal tract, intramuscular injection or other extravascular site followed by first order elimination). A typical curve is shown in Fig. 3. The characteristic feature is a nose-shaped portion around the peak of the curve. This portion lies above a straight line drawn in semilogarithmic plots through the declining part of the curve. The main portion of the absorption in these instances is finished before the distribution phase is terminated.

Assessment by feathering starts with the final portion of the curve. A linear regression (r1) is made through $\ln c_p$ upon time. The straight line (semilogarithmic plot) is extended towards the Y–axis to give the intercept B. The differences between the observations within the period of faster disposition and the regression r1 are determined and plotted up the Y–axis. A straight line results with good data. The slope of this line corresponds to the rate constant of the distributive phase (α–phase) and is calculated by a linear regression (r2) on the ln concentration differences vs. time. The Y–axis intercept of this line corresponds to A. Evaluation of the absorption phase is achieved by determining the difference between the observations during absorption and the regression r2. The differences which thus in turn emerge are plotted and give rise to a separate regression (r3). When calculated with ln concentrations against time, the slope of r3 corresponds to the rate of absorption, k_A, and to an intercept $c_0 = A + B$ characterising the phase of absorption.

The formula for the curve is: $c_p = A' \cdot e^{-\alpha t} + B' \cdot e^{-\beta t} + C' \cdot e^{-k_A t}$, where A', B', and C' are as follows:

$$A' = \frac{k_A f D}{V_c} \cdot \frac{k_{12} - \alpha}{(k_A - \alpha)(\beta - \alpha)}$$
$$B' = \frac{k_A f D}{V_c} \cdot \frac{k_{21} - \beta}{(k_A - \beta)(\alpha - \beta)}$$
$$C' = \frac{k_A f D}{V_c} \cdot \frac{k_{21} - k_A}{(\alpha - k_A)(\beta - k_A)}$$

Under the presumptions that k_A is much larger than β and that there is no lag, $C' = -(A' + B')$ and for practical purposes, the following equation may be used:

$$c_p = A \cdot e^{-\alpha t} + B \cdot e^{-\beta t} + c_o \cdot e^{-k_A t}.$$

where A, B, and c_o are defined as above for intravenous injections. The equations for the derived pharmacokinetic parameters in this instance are also as defined for the two-compartment model and intravenous injection.

Multicompartment Models

The employment of pharmacokinetic models with more than two compartments have become widely explored. With the limited number of observations possible in most human studies, it is difficult to establish that e.g. a three-compartment open model gives a better fit than a two-compartment model, although better suitability of the former is possible. Levy *et al.* (1969) have pointed out the difficulties of differentiating between the two- and multicompartment models unless more than serum data are available.

Formulas for pharmacokinetic constants independent of model selection

Area distribution volume: $V_{d,\beta} = V_{d,area} = D / k_E \cdot F$

Total body clearance: $Cl_B = D/F = V_c \cdot k_E$

Mean serum level: $\overline{c}_p = F / \gamma$

Dose Dependent Pharmacokinetics

Dose dependent pharmacokinetics (also referred to as capacity limited kinetics or nonlinear kinetics) may be encountered when saturation of metabolic or transport processes occur, or when there is interference from saturation of binding to serum proteins or association to erythrocytes. Then the rate of elimination changes from K_m, which is the first order rate of metabolic elimination, to a constant and maximum rate (zero order) of V_{max} at the maximum level of biotransformation. The assumption is that change from K_m to V_{max} occurs abruptly at the point when the key enzyme involved becomes saturated. This is describable by Michaelis–Menten kinetics. The relationship between the rate of metabolism (V), the Michaelis–Menten constant (K_m), the maximum rate of metabolism (V_{max}), and the serum concentration of the drug (c_p) are given by the formula:

$$V = -\frac{dc_p}{dt} = \frac{V_{max} \cdot c_p}{K_m + c_p} \quad \text{or:} \quad \frac{1}{V} = \frac{K_m}{V_{max} \cdot c_p + 1/V_{max}}$$

When K_m is much higher than c_p, the formula simplifies to $1/V = K_m/V_{max} \cdot c_p$, which solved for V becomes: $V = -dc_p/dt = V_{max} \cdot c_p/K_m$. Then the process is essentially first order. The rate with serum concentrations above K_m is zero order: $V = dc_p/dt = V_{max}$. The approximate serum half-life equals $c_o/2V_{max}$, where c_o corresponds to the initial concentration.

The serum concentration equation in the one-compartment model is:

$$c_p = c_o \cdot e^{-(k_E + \frac{V_{max}}{K_m})t}$$

When the maximum rate is reached upon enzyme saturation and c_p is considerably above K_m, the $V = V_{max}$. The serum levels during the stage of saturation follow the equation:

$$c_p = \frac{1}{V_d} \cdot \left[(D + \frac{V_{max}}{K_m + k_E}) e^{-(K_m + k_E)t} \right] - \frac{V_{max}}{K_m - k_E}$$

This is a non-linear equation useful to describe serum concentration profiles during the saturation phase, when serum concentration reaches this level, immediately as it applies after rapid intravenous injections. The parameters of the Michaelis–Menten formula are derivable from Lineweaver–Burk plots (1974) of $1/V$ against $1/c_p$. The slope of the drived line equals k_m/V_{max} and the intercept $1/V_{max}$.

If in a one-compartment model a drug is eliminated by first order process(es) with the rate k_f in addition to a dose limited process, the change in serum concentrations follow the equation:

$$-\frac{dc_p}{dt} = \frac{k_f \cdot c_p \cdot (K_m + c_p)}{K_m + c_p}$$

which gives an equation not explicitly solvable for c_p.

The characteristics of non-linear pharmacokinetics are more difficult to determine in detail than first order kinetics. In order to detect dose dependent elimination pharmacokinetics, at least 2, preferably 3–4, intravenous doses must be given to the same individuals. The upper dose must give c_p exceeding the K_m. The serum data may suffice for determination of the Michaelis–Menten characteristics for drugs with rapid elimination. However, one may be limited to only suggest the existence of dose dependent pharmacokinetics by determining that total area under the serum curve per unit dose increases with higher doses, without full elucidation of K_m or V_{max}. This is the case, for instance, when only a modest dose limitation applies as e.g. for ureidopenicillins up to i.v. doses of 5.0 g (Bergan, 1978a).

Appendix II: Symbols

α	Slope of monoexponential line of serum disposition during the distribution, i.e. α–phase, of two-compartment model. This is an apparent, first order, disposition constant.
β	Slope of monoexponential line of serum disposition during slower second phase, elimination phase or β–phase, of two-compartment model. This is an apparent, first order, disposition constant.
ϵ	Relative dosing interval = $\tilde{\jmath} / t\frac{1}{2}$
$\tilde{\jmath}$	Dosing interval
A	Intercept with ordinate of back-extrapolated line of first monoexponential phase of serum disposition of two-compartment model, i.e. of α–line

AUC	Area under serum concentration vs. time curve, see F
B	Intercept with ordinate of back-extrapolated line of second mono-exponential phase of serum disposition of two-compartment model, i.e. of β–line
c_{max}	Maximum serum concentration
c_{min}	Minimum serum concentration
c_0	Sum of hybrid intercepts of disposition. $c_0 = A + B$ in two-compartment model, both after intravenous and after extravascular administration. It is notable that the latter does not include an expression (i.e. intercept) related to the process of absorption. In the one-compartment model this hypothetical drug concentration at $t = 0$ is obtained by back-extrapolation of a curve parallel to the monoexponential declining curve of the elimination phase placed such that the area under the line equals that under the observed serum curve
c_p	Serum concentration
$\bar{c}_p$	Average serum concentration
c_{ss}	Serum concentration at steady state following continuous zero order infusion
Cl_B	Total body clearance
Cl_R	Renal clearance
D	Dose, also used for maintenance dose
D*	Loading dose
F	Area under serum curve. Single letter symbols are preferable in mathematical equations. F consequently used in lieu of AUC which would imply three factors; the latter is often used in English literature; F is frequent in Continental works and has presedence by the circumstance that it was first used in pharmacokinetics
f	Fraction ($\leqslant 1.0$) of dose absorbed, i.e. that reaches the blood
f_R	Fraction eliminated renally
k_A	Absorption rate constant (first order)
k_E	Elimination rate constant from central compartment (first order). In one-compartment model also referred to as overall elimination rate constant
k_M	Metabolism rate constant (first order)
K_m	Michaelis–Menten constant
k_{NR}	Rate constant (first order) of transfer from central compartment by other than renal elimination
k_0	Rate of drug infusion (zero order)
k_R	Rate constant (first order) of renal elimination
k_{12}	Transfer rate constant (first order) for transport directed from central to peripheral compartment
k_{21}	Transfer rate constant (first order) for transport directed from peripheral to central compartment
ln	Natural logarithm (base e)
log	Common Brigg's logarithm (base 10)
Mu	Amount of drug eliminated in urine
R	Accumulation factor ($= D*/D$) (equals the R*, dose fraction, of Krüger-Thiemer, 1960)

t_0	Lag time preceding apparent initiated absorption after extravascular administration
t	Time after dosage
$t\frac{1}{2}$	Serum half-life
$t\frac{1}{2}\alpha$	Half-life of serum disposition during phase of distribution, i.e. α–phase
$t\frac{1}{2}\beta$	Half-life of serum disposition during phase of elimination, i.e. β–phase. Occasionally referred to as biological half-life
$\tilde{\jmath}$	Dosing interval
V	Initial rate of drug metabolism
V_c	Distribution volume of central compartment (two-compartment model)
V_d	Distribution volume of one-compartment model
$V_{d,\beta}$	Distribution volume of β–phase, two-compartment model
$V_{d,area}$	Distribution volume calculated from F, one- or two-compartment model
$V_{d,extrap}$	Distribution volume calculated for second compartment of two-compartment model
$V_{d,inf.eq.}$	Distribution volume of steady state calculated from serum concentrations achieved during constant infusion to stable serum levels
$V_{d,ss}$	Distribution volume at steady state calculated from k_{12}, k_{21}, and V_c (two-compartment model)
V_m	Theoretical maximum rate of process described by Michaelis–Menten kinetics = V_{max}. Also used to denote distribution volume of metabolite
V_{max}	Maximum rate of metabolism
V_T	Distribution volume of peripheral ("tissue") compartment
W	Body weight
X_T	Amount of drug in peripheral compartment

References

Aguiar, A.J., Wheeler, L.M., Fusari, S. and Zeiner, J.E. (1968). *J. Pharm. Sci.* **57**, 1844–1850.

Alexander, J.W., Sykes, N.S., Mitchell, M.M. and Fischer, M.W. (1973). *J. Trauma* **13**, 423–434.

Almirante, L., De Carneri, I. and Coppi, G. (1960). *Farmaco, Ed. Prat.* **15**, 471–482.

Atkinson, R.M., Bedford, C., Chiold, K.J. and Tomich, E.G. (1962). *Nature* (London) **193**, 588–589.

Baker, G. and Hunt, T.K. (1968). *Am. J. Surg.* **115**, 531–534.

Barr, W.H., Gerbracht, L.M., Letcher, K., Plaut, M. and Strahl, N. (1972). *Clin. Pharmacol. Ther.* **13**, 97–108.

Barza, M. and Weinstein, L. (1974). *J. Infect. Dis.* **129**, 59–65.

Barza, M., Brusch, J., Bergeron, M.G. and Weinstein, L. (1974). *J. Infect. Dis.* **129**, 73–78.

Bell, H., Johansen, H., Lunde, P.K.M., Andersgaard, H.A., Finholt, P., Midtvedt, T., Holum, E., Martinussen, B. and Aarnes, E.D. (1971). *Pharmacology* **5**, 108–120.

Bergan, T. (1978a). *Antimicrob. Agents Chemother.* **14**, 801–806.

Bergan, T. (1978b). *Antimicrob. Agents Chemother.* **13**, 971–974.

Bergan, T. (1978c). *Scand. J. Infect. Dis., Suppl.* **14**, 36–46.

Bergan, T. (1978d). *Antibiot. Chemother.* **25**, 1–122.

Bergan, T. and Arnold, E. (1980). Chemotherapy 26, 231–241.
Bergan, T. and Carlsen, I. (1980). Infection 8 (Suppl.), S103–S108.
Bergan, T. and Michalsen, H. (1980). Arzneim. Forsch. 29 (Suppl. 12a), 1955–1957.
Bergan, T. and Versland, I. (1978). Scand. J. Infect. Dis., Suppl. 14, 135–142.
Bergan, T., Berdal, B.P. and Holm, V. (1976). Acta Pharm. Tox. 38, 308–320.
Bergan, T., Brodwall, E.K. and Ørjavik, O. (1977). J. Antimicrob. Chemother. 3, 435–443.
Bergan, T., Engeset, A., Olszewski, W. and Solberg, R. (1979). Lymphology 12, 85–94.
Bergan, T., Øydvin, B. and Lunde, I. (1973). Acta Pharm. Tox. 33, 138–156.
Blair, D.C., Barnes, R.W., Wildner, E.L. and Murray, W.J. (1971). J. Am. Med. Assoc. 215, 251–254.
Chisholm, G.D., Waterworth, P.M., Calnan, J.S. and Garrod, L.P. (1973). Brit. Med. J. 1, 569–573.
Craig, W.A. and Suh, B. (1978a). Scand. J. Infect. Dis., Suppl. 14, 92–99.
Craig, W.A. and Suh, B. (1978b). Scand. J. Infect. Dis., Suppl. 14, 239–244.
Davis, E. and Pinola, R.C. (1968). Australas. Ann. Med. 17, 63–65.
Dettli, L. (1977). Prog. Pharmacol. 1, 1–34.
Dolusio, J.T. and Dittert, L.W. (1969). Clin. Pharmacol. Ther. 10, 690–701.
Ehrnebo, M., Nilsson, S.-O. and Boréus, L.O. (1979). J. Pharmacokinet. Biopharm. 7, 429–451.
Eickenberg, H.-U. (1978). Scand. J. Infect. Dis., Suppl. 14, 166–170.
Furesz, S. (1958). Antimicrob. Chemother. 8, 446–449.
Gibaldi, M. (1969). J. Pharm. Sci. 58, 1133–1135.
Goldberg, A.H., Gibaldi, M. and Kanig, J.L. (1966). J. Pharm. Sci. 55, 487–492.
Helm, E.B. (1977). "Antibakterielle Aktivität von Antibiotika in Körperflüssigkeiten". Johann A. Wülfing. Neuss, West-Germany.
Helm, E.B., Paulus, I., Shah, P.M. and Stille, W. (1976). Infection 4, 94–101.
Juncher, H. and Raaschou, F. (1957). Antibiot. Med. Clin. Ther. 4, 497–507.
Jusko, W.J., Mosovich, L.L., Gerbracht, L.M., Mattar, M.E. and Yaffe, S.J. (1975). Pediatrics 56, 1038–1044.
Kahlmeter, G., Jonsson, S. and Kamme, C. (1978a). J. Antimicrob. Chemother. 4, 143–152.
Kahlmeter, G., Jonsson, S. and Kamme, C. (1978b). J. Antimicrob. Chemother. 4, (Suppl. A), 5–11.
Kakemi, K., Arita, T. and Koizumi, T. (1962). J. Pharm. Soc. Jap. 82, 261–269.
Kampmann, J.P., Siersbæk-Nielsen, K., Kristensen, M. and Hansen, J.M. (1971). Ugeskr. Læg 133, 1269–1274.
Krüger-Thiemer, E. (1960). J. Am. Pharm. Assoc., Sci. Ed. 49, 311–313.
Kunin, C.M. (1967). Ann. Intern. Med. 67, 151–158.
Kunin, C.M. and Finland, M. (1959). Arch. Intern. Med. 104, 1030–1050.
Leroy, A., Humbert, G., Godin, M. and Fillastre, J.P. (1980). Antimicrob. Agents Chemother. 17, 344–349.
Levy, G., Gibaldi, M. and Jusko, W.J. (1969). J. Pharm. Sci. 58, 422–424.
Lineweaver, H. and Burk, D. (1974). J. Am. Chem. Soc. 56, 658–666.
Loo, J.C.K. and Riegelman, S. (1970). J. Pharm. Sci. 59, 53–55.
Lüthy, R. and Siegenthaler, W. (1973). Schweiz. Med. Wochenschr. 103, 740–743.
McDonald, P.J., Craig, W.A. and Kunin, C.M. (1976). In "Chemother.; Proc. 9th Int. Congr. Chemother., Vol. 2, Laboratory Aspects in Infections". (J.D. Williams and A.M. Geddes, eds), pp. 95–102. Plenum Press, New York.
McDonald, P.J., Craig, W.A. and Kunin, C.M. (1977). J. Infect. Dis. 135, 217–223.

Mendelson, J., Portnoy, J., Dick, V. and Black, M. (1976). *Antimicrob. Agents Chemother.* **9**, 633–638.

Modr, Z. and Dvoracek, K. (1970). *Adv. Biosci.* **5**, 219–230.

Mullins, J.D. and Macek, T.J. (1960). *J. Am. Pharm. Assoc., Sci. Ed.* **49**, 245–248.

Nauman, M. (1975). *Ars Medici* **30**, 1285–1312.

Ohlsson, H. and Bergan, T. (1980). *Arzneim. Forsch.* **29** (Suppl. 12a), 1958–1959.

Otten, H., Plempel, M. and Siegenthaler, W. (1975). Antibiotika-Fibel. Georg Thieme Verlag, Stuttgart.

Parsons, R.L., Jusko, W.J. and Young, J.M. (1976a). *J. Antimicrob. Chemother.* **2**, 214–215.

Parsons, R.L., Paddock, G.M., Hossack, G.A. and Hailey, D.M. (1976b). *In* "Chemother., Proc. 9th Int. Congr. Chemother., Vol. 4, Pharmacology of Antibiotics". (J.D. Williams and A.M. Geddes, eds), pp. 219–229. Plenum Press, New York.

Philipson, A. (1977). *J. Infect. Dis.* **136**, 370–376.

Philipson, A., Sabath, L.D. and Charles, D. (1976). *Clin. Pharmacol. Ther.* **19**, 68–77.

Poole, J.W., Owen, G., Silverio, J., Freyhof, J.N. and Rosenman, S.B. (1968). *Curr. Ther. Res. Clin. Exp.* **10**, 292–303.

Reinhold, J.G., Phillips, F.J. and Flippin, H.F. (1945). *Am. J. Med. Sci.* **210**, 141–147.

Riegelman, S., Loo, J. and Rowland, M. (1968). *J. Pharm. Sci.* **57**, 128–133.

Schentag, J.J., Jusko, W.J., Plaut, M.E., Lumbo, T.J., Vance, J.W. and Abrutyn, E. (1977a). *J. Am. Med. Assoc.* **238**, 327–329.

Schentag, J.J., Jusko, W.J., Vance, J.W., Cumbo, T.J., Abrutyn, E., DeLattre, M. and Gerbracht, L.M. (1977b). *J. Pharmacokinet. Biopharm.* **5**, 559–577.

Schreiner, A., Hellum, K.B., Digranes, A. and Bergman, I. (1978). *Scand. J. Infect. Dis., Suppl.* **14**, 233–237.

Seydel, J.K. (1977). *Adv. Clin. Pharmacol.* **14**, 3–20.

Shah, P.M., Schirmer, K.P., Helm, E.B. and Stille, W. (1976). *Arzneim. Forsch.* **26**, 1636–1638.

Simon, C. (1976). *Infection* **4**, (Suppl. 2), S91–S94.

Sjövall, J., Magni, L. and Bergan, T. (1978). *Antimicrob. Agents Chemother.* **13**, 90–96.

Tan, J.S., Trott, A., Phair, J.P. and Watanakunakorn, C. (1972). *J. Infect. Dis.* **126**, 492–497.

Thijssen, H.H.W. and Mattie, H. (1976). *Antimicrob. Agents Chemother.* **10**, 441–446.

Ullmann, U. and Wurst, W. (1979). *Infection* **7**, 187–189.

Wagner, J.G. (1975). "Fundamentals of Clinical Pharmacokinetics", pp. 173–202. Drug Intelligence Publications, Hamilton (Ill.).

Wagner, J.G., Northam, J.L., Alway, C.D. and Carpenter, O.S. (1965). *Nature* (London) **207**, 1391–1402.

Westlake, W.J. (1973). *In* "Current Concepts in the Pharmaceutical Sciences. Dosage Form, Design and Bioavailability". (J. Swarbrick, ed.), pp. 149–179. Lea Febiger, Philadelphia.

Yaffe, S.J., Gerbracht, L.M., Mosovich, L.L., Mattar, M.E., Danish, M. and Jusko, W.J. (1977). *J. Infect. Dis.* **135**, 828–831.

Discussion

Professor Fillastre: It was a pity that Professor Bergan did not have more time to comment on pharmacokinetics and renal function. I would just like to add this: it is known that drugs can modify drug absorption, particularly in patients with renal failure. It is often forgotten that uraemic patients have to absorb many drugs, such as iron, calcium or magnesium salts. In the presence of serious renal failure there is also an increased cardiac output, a very low renal blood flow and there is an increased blood flow in the liver and/or the gut. Such changes have to be accounted for in order to understand the modification of the pharmacokinetics in uraemic patients.

Pharmacokinetics may also be used to study tissue distribution in animals and in man. For example in excellent studies with aminoglycosides, Schentag and Fabre, in Switzerland, were able to demonstrate a shallow compartment. These studies were confirmed by autoradiography or measurement of tissue concentrations.

I would like also to comment on some other aspects of the relationships between drug distribution and kidney function and say that it is very important to look on the modifications of subcellular structures for instance in liver and kidney: this point should be seriously considered in a joint study between university and industrial laboratories. When a new molecule is synthesised it is essential to know whether it is potentially toxic for the subcellular elements like mitochondria and lysosomes. Such studies have led to substantial progresses in the understanding of the nephrotoxicity of old and new cephalosporins as well as of aminoglycosides. As you mentioned before, it is worth while to recall Kunin's excellent study recently published in Antimicrobial Agents and Chemotherapy, which stresses the toxic effects on subcellular structures. This kind of studies will perhaps allow in the future to avoid some hepatic or renal impairments by choosing the more appropriate antibiotic.

I am particularly concerned by aminoglycosides, and since we speak about the future, the relationship between the number of free amino groups in aminoglycosides and the renal toxicity must be regarded as unquestionable. Now there are some products, like sorbistin, not yet extensively studied, with 3 amino groups and without any nephrotoxicity. This is a good lead for the future.

Variation in the Antimicrobial Effects of β-lactam Antibiotics

A. TOMASZ

The Rockefeller University, New York, N.Y., U.S.A.

Introduction

Professor Williams, in his chapter (see page 117), has referred to the "beta-lactam tree": the tremendous multiplication in the number of available beta-lactams, fermentation products, semi-synthetic and synthetic compounds, which have been produced with an accelerating rate by the pharmaceutical industry. Often these compounds have considerable overlap in their antibacterial spectra and one wonders about the usefulness of the effort. To be sure, these beta-lactams are not produced in a completely blind search for anti-bacterial activity. There are several criteria that enter both into the search and design of the new beta-lactams, such as resistance to various beta-lactamases, improved pharmacokinetic properties, potency against species that represent the contemporary threat to health, e.g. *Pseudomonas*. In addition, there came the third-generation beta-lactams, exemplified, for instance, by thienamycin, representing a combination of wide antibacterial spectrum and an as yet unsurpassed specific activity. This unexpected discovery rekindled hope that it might be possible to find or to construct the "ultimate" beta-lactam, a kind of neutron bomb capable of annihilating any bacterial pathogen.

While isolation and production of new drugs is becoming increasingly expensive, the continued proliferation of beta-lactams in itself is reassuring if one keeps in mind that every successful improvement in drug design is bound to provoke sooner or later a "successful" countermove on the part of bacteria, as the spread of mechanistically diverse bacterial drug resistances demonstrates. The confusing and bewildering aspect of the beta-lactam tree originates from the fact that much of the search and design of new beta-lactams is still based on trial and error, and the reason for this is our prevailing ignorance concerning the mode of action of these fantastically powerful and selective antibiotics. Recent reviews give a more detailed account of the reasons why, after several decades of intensive and successful studies, the mode of action of beta-lactams still appears elusive (Tomasz, 1979). In this brief treatise I would simply like to point to what I believe are the three main types of puzzles that were brought into sharp focus by recent experiments and that require solution before the better understanding of the mode of antibacterial action of beta-lactams could be reached.

Interactions of Beta-Lactams with Bacteria

The first of these puzzles is the recognition that the same bacterium may respond to structurally different beta-lactams in very different manners. In fact, it is conceivable that classes of various beta-lactams achieve the reversible or irreversible inhibition of a bacterial cell by different mechanisms. The best illustration of this is provided by *E. coli*, in which various beta-lactams were shown to cause radically different morphological and antibacterial effects (Spratt, 1975).

The second puzzle is, in a way, the converse of the first one: different species of bacteria may respond quite differently to the very same beta-lactam. A good illustration has been provided by Dr. Horne's work in our laboratory in the case of the penicillin responses of three species of streptococci: group H, group A streptococci and pneumococci. Each of these species has comparable minimal inhibitory concentration values (m.i.c.) for penicillin, but beyond this, their responses to penicillin treatment differ drastically. Penicillin causes primarily a reversible growth inhibition in group H streptococci; rapid loss of viability occurs in penicillin-treated group A streptococci; and pneumococci not only die rapidly but also physically disintegrate during penicillin treatment (Horne and Tomasz, 1977). The growth inhibiting ("tolerant") response of group H streptococci is reminiscent of the response of murein hydrolase defective bacterial mutants (Tomasz and Holtje, 1977).

A third type of puzzle is emerging with the recognition, pioneered by George Warren and his associates, that within an infected host some beta-lactams may inhibit bacterial pathogens not on their own but in cooperation with components of the host (immune) defense system (Warren and Gray, 1967; Friedman and Warren, 1976).

These three puzzles reflect the mechanistic complexity of beta-lactam action. The diverse effects of different beta-lactams on a single bacterium most likely are due to the presence of multiple, functionally different beta-lactam "targets" (Penicillin Binding Proteins, PBP's, corresponding to beta-lactam sensitive synthetic enzymes or regulatory proteins in bacterial cell wall assembly). Species-specific variation in beta-lactam response is likely to be caused by differences in the mode and organization of cell wall assembly and by differences in the regulation of autolytic (murein hydrolase) activities in various bacterial species. The third type of variation in beta-lactam action has to do, presumably, with the sensitization of bacteria (that have suffered sublethal surface damage by the beta-lactam treatment) to host (immune) factors. I would like to illustrate each one of the variabilities with examples from our laboratory's work.

The drug-to-drug variability of physiological effect may be illustrated by the tremendous differences in the specific activities of beta-lactams as inducers ("triggers") of suicidal murein hydrolase activity in *E. coli* (Kitano and Tomasz, 1979). Dr. Kitano has exposed growing bacteria (containing radioactive label in their cell walls) to various concentrations of beta-lactams for brief time periods (5–10 min); these bacteria were then incubated in drug-free buffers and the rate with which they degraded their cell walls was measured. Beta-

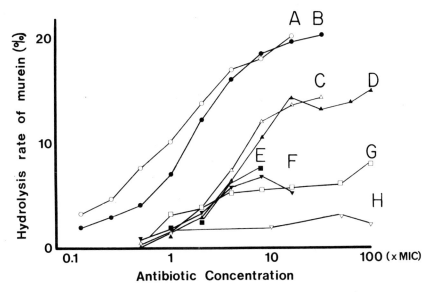

FIG. 1   Autolysin triggering efficiency of various beta-lactams. The activity of triggered autolysin is shown as the degradation rate (per cent) of murein after 2 h incubation. Antibiotics: cephaloridine (A), cephalothin (B), benzylpenicillin (C), ampicillin (D), dicloxacillin (E), cephalexin (F), 6–APA (G) and mecillinam (H). Replotted from data of Kitano and Tomasz (1979).

lactams were found to differ very significantly from one another in their specific activities in this assay (Fig. 1). Similar types of variabilities have been observed in our laboratory in gonococci, in group B streptococci and in pneumococci.

Bacterium to bacterium variation in the response to the same beta-lactam (penicillin) is illustrated by the example of streptococci quoted earlier. Figure 2 shows the spectrum of antibacterial effects

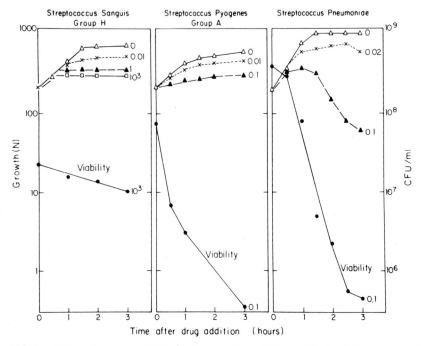

FIG. 2   Effect of benzylpenicillin on the growth, viability, and lysis of three species of streptococci. Exponentially growing cultures received benzylpenicillin at the concentrations (units/ml) indicated. Growth and lysis were monitored by nephelometry (Coleman nephelometer). Viability was determined as described in the text. CFU, Colony-forming units (Horne and Tomasz, 1977; reprinted with permission of American Society for Microbiology).

from growth inhibition through bactericidal activity to lysis (Horne and Tomasz, 1977).

The third type of variation may be illustrated by *S. sanguis*. This is a typical tolerant bacterium that does not lyse and loses viability only slowly during penicillin treatment. However, as Dr. Horne in our laboratory has shown, it is sufficient to make the environment of the drug-treated cells somewhat more complex by adding a heterologous murein hydrolase to the medium, and these bacteria will show sensitivity to the exogenous hydrolase by loss of viability

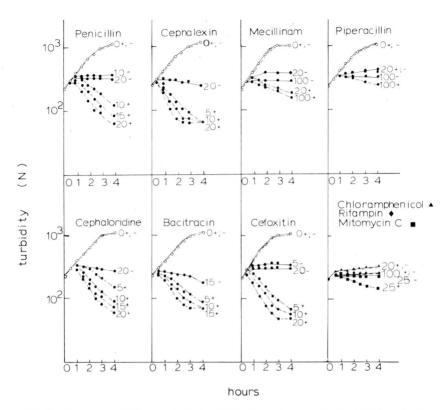

FIG. 3   Response of *S. sanguis* strain Wicky to various metabolic inhibitors in the presence of C–phage associated lysin. Numbers represent the concentrations of the drugs expressed in multiples of the m.i.c. values. The m.i.c.'s for the antibiotics were as follows: benzylpenicillin, 0.05 μg/ml; cephalexin, 10 μg/ml; mecillinam, 8 μg/ml; piperacillin, 0.05 μg/ml; cephaloridine, 0.02 μg/ml; bacitracin, 25 μg/ml; cefoxitin, 3 μg/ml; chloramphenicol, 3 μg/ml; rifampin, 0.1 μg/ml; and mitomycin C, 0.1 μg/ml. Symbols: (———,–) control samples minus enzyme; (– – –, +) plus enzyme (1.5 U/ml). (Horne and Tomasz, 1980a; reprinted with permission of American Society for Microbiology.)

and lysis (Fig. 3) (Horne and Tomasz, 1980a). Individual beta-lactams differ substantially in their specific activities as "sensitizers". Warren and his colleagues have pioneered this work by demonstrating similar sensitization of various bacterial strains to a variety of immune or host-defense mechanisms and various beta-lactams again have differed in their specific activities (Warren and Gray, 1967; Friedman and Warren, 1976). Sensitization of penicillin treated staphylococci or group B streptococci to the bactericidal activity of human polymorphonuclear leucocytes (PMN) have also been reported (Molavi *et al.*, 1978; Horne and Tomasz, 1980b).

Comparative Evaluation of Beta-Lactams

Besides documenting the variability in beta-lactam effects, these observations also have resulted in the development of experimental systems in which the specific activity of a given beta-lactam may be evaluated in a particular, highly specific assay. While, admittedly, the precise biochemical basis of these assays is not yet understood, they may provide a way to characterise beta-lactams by criteria that are more versatile and sophisticated than just m.i.c. values. One of my propositions would be to utilise these assays for introducing some kind of phenomenological classification into the tremendous number of available beta-lactams. This effort may produce clues from which a better understanding of a structure–function relationship might eventually be derived, which, in turn, could be fed back into drug design. Alternatively, it is also possible that at least some of the assay systems referred to may be introduced into a relatively early stage of the screening for new antibiotics. An ideal way of performing such an enormous task would seem to be through the close cooperation of academic and pharmaceutical laboratories that would have mutual interests in such an undertaking.

Beta-lactam molecules may encounter a variety of bacterial defense mechanisms at the outer boundaries of the target cells. Beta-lactamases and permeability barriers may represent such defenses and "successful" beta-lactams must have structural features to overcome these barriers in order to express their antibacterial effect. However, once beyond the bacterial barriers, beta-lactams will react with drug sensitive bacterial proteins which are likely to be the PBP's. Drug-to-drug variability of antibacterial potency and variation in the type of antibacterial effect (reversible of irreversible) are most likely to be consequences of the multiplicity and functional diversity of PBP's and the selective affinities of various beta-lactams for these PBP's.

Therefore, it would seem important to establish the selective affinities of various beta-lactams for bacterial PBP's as a way to provide answers to simple and basic questions such as why different beta-lactams have such widely varying antibacterial potencies (different m.i.c. values) for a given bacterium. Such work has been initiated in several laboratories. We have been using competition assays and a radioactive penicillin of high specific radioactivity for a screening of the PBP inhibitory patterns of various beta-lactams using pneumococcus as one of the test organisms. The advantage of this system is that it allows labelling of the PBP's in live, exponentially growing bacteria and thus a correlation between the m.i.c. value and the PBP-inhibitory pattern of a beta-lactam may be, at least in theory, established. Furthermore, a relatively small modification of the assay

TABLE 1

Effect of Pretreatment with β–Lactam Antibiotics on the Penicillin-Binding Proteins of *S. pneumoniae*

β–lactam antibiotic[a]	m.i.c. (nmoles/ml)	I_{50} binding concentration (nmoles/ml) for penicillin-binding protein[b]					Morphological response[c]
		1a	1b	2a	2b	3	
Benzylpenicillin (1)	0.017	0.115 (6.8)	0.14 (8.2)	0.195 (11.5)	0.22 (12.9)	0.034 (2.0)	None
Cefotaxime (2)	0.026	0.015 (0.6)	0.0072 (0.3)	0.0052 (0.2)	0.056 (2.2)	0.0086 (0.3)	None
Piperacillin (3)	0.046	0.94 (20.4)	0.62 (13.5)	0.185 (4.0)	0.051 (1.1)	0.042 (0.9)	Swollen (0.5)
Cephaloridine (4)	0.057	0.05 (0.9)	0.018 (0.3)	0.042 (0.7)	1.45 (25.4)	0.0066 (0.1)	Swollen (0.5)
Nafcillin (5)	0.061	0.27 (4.4)	0.061 (1.0)	0.19 (3.1)	0.42 (6.9)	0.32 (5.8)	Swollen (0.5)
Ampicillin (6)	0.070	0.06 (0.9)	0.0066 (0.1)	0.023 (0.3)	0.105 (1.5)	0.045 (0.6)	None
Dicloxacillin (7)	0.102	0.34 (3.3)	0.39 (3.8)	0.36 (3.5)	0.60 (5.9)	0.97 (9.5)	None
Methicillin (8)	0.48	9.2 (19.2)	5.2 (10.8)	0.54 (1.1)	1.15 (2.4)	2.05 (4.3)	Swollen (0.5)
Cephalothin (9)	0.49	<0.016 (<0.03)	<0.016 (<0.03)	0.19 (0.4)	0.86 (1.8)	0.08 (0.2)	None
Oxacillin (10)	0.63	1.75 (2.8)	1.6 (2.5)	0.42 (0.7)	1.45 (2.3)	0.17 (0.3)	None
Sulbenicillin (11)	0.87	4.6 (5.3)	1.55 (1.8)	4.9 (5.6)	3.7 (4.3)	0.66 (0.8)	None
Cefoxitin (12)	3.68	6.8 (1.9)	0.145 (0.04)	2.4 (0.7)	8.0 (2.2)	<0.037 (<0.01)	None
Cefadroxil (13)	4.3	4.6 (1.1)	8.0 (1.9)	1.3 (0.3)	12.0 (2.8)	<0.14 (<0.03)	None
Cephalexin (14)	8.75	7.2 (0.8)	4.5 (0.5)	2.2 (0.3)	28.0 (3.2)	0.29 (0.03)	None
Mecillinam (15)	8.8	1320.0 (150.0)	185.0 (21.0)	30.0 (3.4)	155.0 (17.6)	50.0 (5.7)	None
Cefsulodin (16)	22.2	23.0 (1.0)	37.0 (1.7)	6.7 (0.3)	52.0 (2.3)	1.55 (0.07)	None
6–APA (17)	105.0	2900.0 (27.6)	480.0 (4.6)	30.0 (0.3)	370.0 (3.5)	160.0 (1.5)	None
Cephalosporin C (18)	114.4	13.0 (0.1)	<1.14 (<0.01)	20.0 (0.2)	19.0 (0.2)	8.5 (0.07)	None

a Number in parentheses refers to plots of figure 4.

b Values indicate the concentration of antibiotic required to inhibit the subsequent binding of ([³H] benzylpenicillin) by 50%; underscoring indicates the minimal value of the series. Values in parentheses indicate multiples of the m.i.c. values.

c Values in parentheses indicate the lowest multiple of the m.i.c. value that resulted in the morphological effect.

(Williamson *et al.*, 1980; reprinted with permission of American Society for Microbiology) allows the recognition of crypticity (permeability barrier) also. Table 1 shows the results of such an *in vivo* PBP labelling assay as performed by Drs. Williamson and Hakenbeck. Each number in the table was derived by exposing live pneumococci to a series of concentrations of the corresponding beta-lactam in the radioactive penicillin competition assay (Williamson *et al.*, 1980). The fluorograms were scanned and the concentration of the beta-lactam needed to cause 50% inhibition of the various PBP's was established. It should be noted that, in pneumococci, intrinsic resistance to penicillin is known to be accompanied by gradual, cumulative changes in the affinities of several PBP's for penicillin (Zighelboim and Tomasz, 1980). Thus, at least two of the three groups of PBP'S of this bacterium appear to be physiologically important targets for penicillins. Table 1 documents the tremendous and selective changes (in affinity for the various PBP's) that accompany variation in beta-lactam structure. Figure 4 illustrates one type of information that

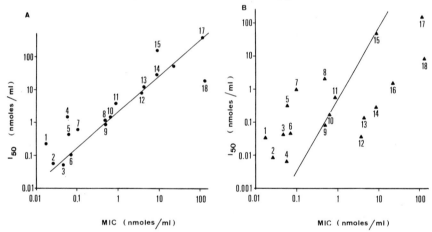

FIG. 4   Correlation between m.i.c. values of the antibiotics tested and their affinities (I_{50} values) for (A) PBP 2b and (B) PBP 3. The data were obtained directly from Table 1, and the line for PBP 3 plotted after linear regression analysis. (Williamson *et al.*, 1980; reprinted with permission of American Society for Microbiology.

one may derive from such data: an apparent correlation between affinity for PBP 2b and the log of the m.i.c. value (Williamson *et al.*, 1980). A similar approach has been used in *E. coli* by Dr. Nozaki and his colleagues (1979).

The three types of variabilities referred to earlier in this paper as the three "puzzles" of the field occur superimposed on one another and this fact can generate inhibitory responses that are specific both of the beta-lactam and of the species of bacterium. A beta-lactam like mecillinam may have very low m.i.c. value in one type of bacterium and very high m.i.c. values in others. Other lines of evidence indicate that a given beta-lactam may be a powerful inducer of irreversible effects in one species while remaining a relatively bacteriostatic agent in another bacterium. This type of variation in antibacterial potency may offer an alternative principle for the modification of beta-lactam structure, in which the aim would be the development of antibiotics of highly restricted (and thus highly selective) antibacterial spectrum. Clearly, this is the exact opposite of the approach I have referred to earlier as the antibacterial "neutron bomb" and, using another militaristic term, this alternative may be referred to as that of "limited warfare" against bacterial pathogens. Given the apparently inexhaustible ability of bacteria for designing counter-measures against antibiotics, as illustrated by the large variety of drug resistant mechanisms spread by plasmids and transposons through bacterial populations, one could argue in favour of selectivity and restraint in our warfare against bacteria. The undesirable and un-necessary side-effect of beta-lactams resistant to the beta-lactamases of *Bacteroides* illustrate the problems that antibacterial "overkill" may create. Clearly, the development of highly selective beta-lactams as effective chemotherapeutic agents would require a parallel development of fast diagnostic techniques. However, the develop-ment of highly specific, rapid diagnostic techniques would be well within the realm of possibilities and would present a stimulating challenge to both academic and industrial microbiologists and chemists.

Conclusion

During the past decades we have been witnessing the emergence of bacteria resistant to formerly effective chemotherapeutic drugs. Dr. Sande has mentioned during one of the discussions at this meeting the experience of U.S. hospitals with large infectious disease wards: infections by bacteria resistant to most commonly used antibiotics have been experienced and, in some cases, the number of usable chemotherapeutic agents was reduced to one or two drugs, i.e., uncomfortably close to none. One should also note the shift in hospital patient populations (at least in the more affluent Western countries) toward various types of "compromised" hosts (old patients or with primary disease affecting the immune system) who would increasingly depend on chemotherapy.

These changes in the nature of the pathogens and patients argue strongly for the continued development of antibacterial agents of matching inhibitory potencies and there is little doubt in my mind that beta-lactams will remain most useful among such agents.

In this brief treatise I suggested ways that may help in what Dr. Williams has referred to as the "trimming of the beta-lactam tree". One of the suggestions has to do with the introduction of more versatile functional assays (available in the academic research laboratories) for the characterisation of beta-lactams with the eventual aim of arriving at a more rational structure–function relationship. The other suggestion was that of strategy: I tried to make a case for exploiting and further developing already existing limitations in the antibacterial spectrum of groups of beta-lactams, with the aim of developing an arsenal of highly selective antibacterial agents capable of a limited warfare specifically against the pathogen in question. Effective work along these lines would require close cooperation between academic laboratories interested in mode-of-action studies and the industrial researchers engaged in the development of drugs that we hope will be effective against the pathogens of the near future.

References

Friedman, H. and Warren, G.H. (1976). *Proc. Soc. Exp. Biol. Med.* **153**, 301–304.

Horne, D. and Tomasz, A. (1977). *Antimicrob. Agents Chemother.* **11**, 888–896.

Horne, D. and Tomasz, A. (1980a). *Antimicrob. Agents Chemother.* **17**, 235–246.

Horne, D. and Tomasz, A. (1980b). *In* "Proc. 11th Int. Cong. Chemotherapy and 19th ICAAC, Boston, 1979". (J.D. Nelson and C. Grassi, eds), pp. 1127–1129. American Society for Microbiology. Washington, D.C.

Kitano, K. and Tomasz, A. (1979). *Antimicrob. Agents Chemother.* **16** 838–848.

Molavi, A., Metcalf, J. and Root, R. (1978). 18th ICAAC, Atlanta, Abstract n⁰ 203.

Nozaki, Y., Imada, A. and Yoneda, M. (1979). *Antimicrob. Agents Chemother.* **15**, 20–27.

Spratt, B.G. (1975). *Proc. Nat. Acad. Sci. US* **72**, 2999–3003.

Tomasz, A. (1979). *Ann. Rev. Microbiol.* **33**, 113–137.

Tomasz, A. and Höltje, J.V. (1977). *In* "Microbiology – 1977". (D. Schlessinger, ed.), pp. 209–215. American Society for Microbiology, Washington, D.C.

Warren, G.H. and Gray, J. (1967). *Can. J. Microbiol.* **13**, 321–328.

Williamson, R., Hakenbeck, R. and Tomasz, A. (1980). *Antimicrob. Agents Chemother.* **18**, 629–637.

Zighelboim, S. and Tomasz, A. (1980). *Antimicrob. Agents Chemother.* **17**, 434–442.

Discussion

Professor Sande: In his last series of experiments did Professor Tomasz demonstrate that, when the polymorphs were lysed and the lysozyme was released from the polymorphs, there was a synergistic effect on the tolerant *Streptococcus sanguis*? Is that what he was showing with penicillin?

Professor Tomasz: I showed – on a slide – how the bacteriostatic response of *S. sanguis* to penicillin treatment can be modified so that the penicillin inhibited cells will go on to lyse. This was achieved by adding a heterologous murein hydrolase (phage-associated lysozyme or human urinary lysozyme) to the growth medium. The interpretation was that treatment with the beta-lactam has sensitised the cells to the lytic action of the exogenous enzyme. I also mentioned – but did not document with slides – the similar case of Group B streptococci. Here, penicillin treatment has greatly stimulated the bactericidal action of human polymorphonuclear white blood cells (PMN) and this effect required specific antibody as well. The interesting – and potentially important – observation was that beta-lactams (and other cell wall inhibitors) differed considerably in their "specific activities" as sensitisers to lysozyme or human PMN. In this case specific activities are expressed in terms of growth inhibitory (m.i.c.) units of the inhibitors. These observations suggest that *in vivo* (i.e. in the infected host) the invading bacterium may be caught in the cross fire of antibiotic and immune factors – in contrast to the situation in the test tube, where the bacterium is inhibited or killed by the antibiotic alone. All this would support what Professor Sande said in his presentation about the importance of *in vivo* testing in the case of some antibacterial agents.

Professor Braun: The picture of the action of penicillins is rather complicated. Now there are tolerant mutants which apparently lack endopeptidase or transglycosylase. On the other hand, there are the binding proteins for which, in most cases, the functions are unknown – although they are known as "binding proteins". Would Professor Tomasz now say that it is possible to correlate the binding protein, PBP4, with the endopeptidase?

Professor Tomasz: I pointed out two correlations. First – in the highly beta-lactam tolerant mutants of *E. coli*, there is a decrease in the specific activity of endopeptidase and these mutants also appear to have substantially less PBP4 – as indicated by penicillin binding assays. The endopeptidase activity of the *E. coli* PBP4 has been already suggested by other workers. The second correlation is that beta-lactams with high affinity for the *E. coli* PBP1 also have the highest specific activity in triggering autolytic cell wall degradation.

Professor Waldvogel: It is well-known that Group A streptococci, pneumococci and penicillin-sensitive *Staphylococcus aureus* are more sensitive on a weight basis to penicillin G than to the semisynthetic penicillins. Has Professor Tomasz tried with his model, for instance in pneumococci, to find out whether the binding of methicillin occurs on different penicillin-binding proteins as does penicillin G, in order to explain this quite impressive difference in the sensitivity of the organism to penicillin G as opposed to the semisynthetic penicillins?

Professor Tomasz: We looked at the affinities of several beta-lactams for the various penicillin binding proteins (PBP) in a number of bacterial species, namely Groups A and B streptococci, gonococci, staphylococci and pneumococci. A detailed evaluation of such studies — for pneumococci — is part of my presentation. The general conclusion is that different beta-lactams show widely different patterns of binding to the various PBP's. The correlation between affinity for a specific group of PBP's and the antibacterial effectiveness (m.i.c.) is much less clear. In pneumococci, only about two thirds of the beta-lactams tested showed a straight line correlation when the log of drug concentration needed to inhibit PBP2b (to 50%) was plotted against the log of the m.i.c. values.

Professor Sabath: First, in Professor Tomasz' experiments with lysis, I presume that it was egg-white lysozyme?

Professor Tomasz: The first one was human urinary lysozyme, the second a phage-associated lysin.

Professor Sabath: Are there differences in the action of the lysozymes from different sources, or are they fairly similar in their relationship to bacterial lysis with antibiotics?

Professor Tomasz: In the case of *Streptococcus sanguis* it does not seem to make much difference whether a C—phage associated lysine, which is an amidase, is used, or human urinary lysozyme. With the pneumococcus, the pneumococcus' own autolysin has to be used.

Professor Sabath: The main part of my question is an attempt to integrate Professor Tomasz' and Professor Chabbert's presentations. In dealing with heterogeneity of strains with regard to their susceptibility to killing, Professor Tomasz' work suggests that at least one possible aspect would be the differences in their lytic enzymes. With such heterogeneous populations, does the presence of the lytic enzyme in the rapidly killed part act on the minority part of the population which may be deficient in these autolytic enzymes? Conversely, has he seen examples — this is something he did not mention much in his presentation — of inhibitors of those autolytic enzymes possibly dampening the killing effect on the cells which are otherwise competent, in terms of being killed in a rapid fashion?

Professor Tomasz: Yes, we have often seen this type of effect in experiments. A group of cells can release its murein hydrolase and attack the others from without. A group of bacteria may release the lipoteichoic acid, or lipid inhibitor and protect other bacteria in the environment.

Professor Demain: I think that there are two types of screening involved in the pharmaceutical activity. First, the one discussed by Professor Tomasz of how it is perhaps possible to predict from drugs already developed those that might be the most effective. There is also the problem of screening for new antibiotics. Many of us would like to see more mode of action studies in this type of research, rather than simply the ability to produce a clear zone on a plate. It is difficult to convince people involved in screening about this, because if modes of action were to be used at all, they would prefer to use it at a later stage after a number of activities have been isolated. About the only way in which to be convincing on this matter is by telling a group involved in screening that a mode of action test is available which may be more sensitive than the diffusion test producing a clear zone on a plate.

Concerning Professor Tomasz' suggested second and third methods, that is, activation of murein hydrolases or their deregulation, or sensitisation to PMN killing, do any of these activities show up at a concentration of drug lower than the one able to inhibit the growth of the intact organism?

Professor Tomasz: They are drugs which seem to begin to deregulate autolysins below their m.i.c. There are sensitisation phenomena: some drugs are extremely powerful in that regard, and they seem to act at sub-m.i.c. levels. I do not, however, advocate using these particular assays for initial screening. They are too complicated.

Dr. van Heijenoort: Is there a clear correlation of identity demonstrated between transglycosylase activity in the *Escherichia coli* mutants and the binding proteins, 1 A or 1 B, or is there nothing shown?

Professor Tomasz: The beta-lactam tolerant mutants of *E. coli* are defective in the activity of the murein hydrolase (the murein transglycosylase described by Joachim Höltje in 1975). Therefore, we suggested that this enzyme may be involved with the penicillin induced cell wall degradation and lysis of *E. coli*. The beta-lactams most effective in triggering this suicidal activity of transglycosylase seem to have high affinity for the PBP1b. However, we have no evidence that this binding protein has hydrolytic activity.

Screening of Inhibitors of Protein Biosynthesis

D. VÁZQUEZ

*Centro de Biología Molecular, Universidad
Autónoma de Madrid, Madrid, Spain*

Introduction

The process of protein synthesis can be arbitrarily divided, for didactic purposes, into (a) events taking place prior to translation and (b) those belonging to the translation mechanism that take place at the ribosome level.

Concerning the inhibitors acting prior to translation a number of compounds have been synthesised in the last twenty years which are now clinically used because they are very effective inhibitors of N^{10}–formyl–tetrahydrofolate formation. These compounds inhibit methylation and formylation and block f–Met–tRNA$_F$ synthesis by preventing N^{10}–formyl–tetrahydrofolate formation. In bacteria, f–Met-tRNA$_F$ is precisely the substrate required for initiation of the translation process and therefore a number of dihydrofolate analogues, specially trimethoprim, are very useful drugs in therapeutics since they prevent protein synthesis prior to the initiation of the translation process (Vázquez, 1974).

On the other hand, practically all the natural antibiotic inhibitors of protein biosynthesis in medical use specifically block the translation process. Antibiotic inhibitors of steps taking place prior to translation are of little relevance in therapeutical use mainly due to their lack of selective action. This is the case of borrelidin (an inhibitor of threonyl–tRNA synthesis) and furanomycin (an inhibitor of leucyl–tRNA synthesis) which are active on bacterial and mammalian cells. Therefore we will refer here only to antibiotic inhibitors of the translation process.

Process of Translation and Molecular Bases for the Selective Action of Antibiotic Inhibitors

Process of Translation

The overall reactions taking place in the process of translation in bacteria are shown in Fig. 1, where the sites of action of an ample group of antibacterial translation inhibitors as recently reviewed are indicated (Vázquez, 1979). There are at least two types of protein synthesis: procaryotic and eucaryotic. However, certain features are common to both types. Therefore, translation inhibitors acting on bacterial systems can be broadly classified according to their selectivity into those affecting (a) both procaryotic and eucaryotic systems (Table 1), and (b) only procaryotic systems (Table 2)

TABLE 1

Inhibitors of Translation Acting on Procaryotic and Eucaryotic Systems

Actinobolin	Hygromycin B
Adrenochrome	Nucleocidin
AHR–1911	Pactamycin
Amicetin group:	Polydextran sulphate
Amicetin	Polyvinyl sulphate
Bamicetin	Puromycin
Plicamicetin	Pyrochatechol violet
Anthelmycin	Showdomycin
Aurintricarboxylic acid	Sparsomycin
Blasticidin S	Tetracycline group:
Chartreusin	Chlortetracycline
Edeine A_1	Doxycycline
Fusidic acid	Oxytetracycline
Gougerotin	Tetracycline
Guanylyl–methylene–diphosphate	Tosylphenylalanylchloromethane
Guanylyl–imido–diphosphate	

(reprinted from Vázquez, 1979, with permission)

(Vázquez, 1979). Most of these inhibitors with only a few exceptions (fusidic acid and GTP analogues) interact directly with the ribosomes. In general, antibiotics affecting procaryotic-type systems are

FIG. 1 (opposite)   Translation process in bacteria. Site of action of translation inhibitors. * Do not interact with polysomes. Therefore bind to free ribosome subunits and prevent only the first few rounds of peptide bond formation. ** Is an inhibitor of aminoacyl–tRNA binding in intact cells or in integrated systems in which elongation is proceeding in the presence of EF–Tu and EF–G. Does not inhibit aminoacyl–tRNA binding in resolved systems in the absence of EF–G. Can inhibit translocation in cell-free systems. *** Can also inhibit translocation in cell-free systems. **** Does not inhibit peptide bond formation in resolved assays. However, it blocks this step in intact cells and integrated systems by preventing the release of EF–Tu–GDP bound to the ribosome. ***** Do not interact with polysomes. Do not inhibit translocation in many model systems. Bind to free ribosome subunits and prevent elongation of the nascent polypeptide chain when it reaches a certain size, before polysome formation (reprinted from Vázquez, 1979, with permission).

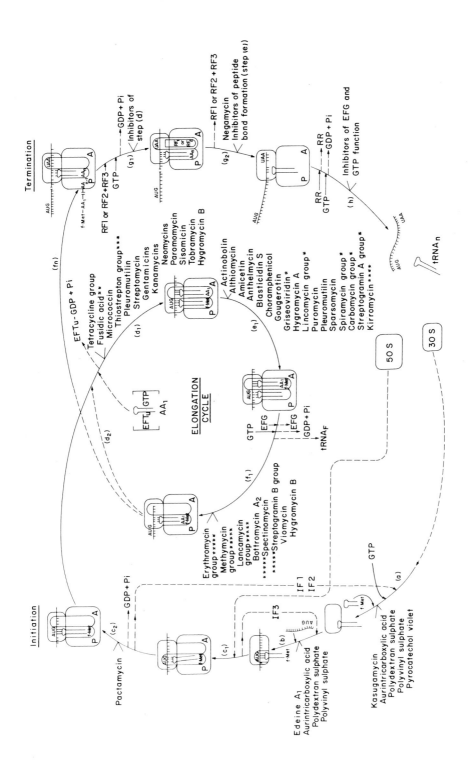

TABLE 2

Inhibitors of Translation Acting on Procaryotic Systems only

Althiomycin	Micrococcin
Avilamycin	Negamycin
Berninamycin	Rubradirin
Bottromycin A$_2$	Spectinomycin
Chloramphenicol group:	Streptogramin A group:
Chloramphenicol	Ostreogrycin G
D–AMP–3	Streptogramin A
D–Thiomycetin	Streptogramin B group:
D–Win–5094	Staphylomycin S
Cloacin DF13	Streptogramin B
Colicin E3	Viridogrisein
Griseoviridin	Streptomycin group:
Hygromycin A	Amikacin
Kasugamycin	Gentamicin
Lincomycin group:	Kanamycin
Celesticetin	Neomycin
Clindamycin	Paromomycin
Lincomycin	Sisomicin
Macrolide antibiotics:	Streptomycin
Carbomycin group:	Tobramycin
Carbomycins	Streptothricins
Josamycin	Thermorubin
Leucomycins	Thiostrepton group:
Niddamycins	Siomycin
Erythromycin group:	Sporangiomycin
Erythromycins	Thiopeptin
Neospiramycins	Thiostrepton
Oleandomycin	Viomycin group:
Lankamycin group:	Capreomycin
Chalcomycin	Viomycin
Kujimycin A	
Lankamycin	
Methymycin group:	
Forocidins	
Methymycin	
Narbomycin	
Neomethymycin	
Picromycin	
Spiramycin group:	
Angolamycin	
Relomycin	
Spiramycins	
Tylosin	

(reprinted from Vázquez, 1979, with permission)

active in bacteria, blue-green algae, mitochondria and chloroplasts, whereas those acting on eucaryotic–type systems are active in higher cells which are known to have 80S type cytoplasmic ribosomes. Therefore, most antibiotics included in Table 1 are not clinically used due to their toxicity, since they are active on cytoplasmic ribosomes from human cells. However, there are some interesting exceptions to this rule, since activities of fusidic acid and tetracyclines on mammalian cells are very weak (Contreras *et al.*, 1978), as compared with their activities on bacteria. The reason is that only bacteria have an active transport system for these antibiotics, which allows their concentration in the cytoplasm.

Therefore most translation inhibitors in medical use belong to the types of antibiotics included in Table 2. However, in general these antibiotics are also active on mitochondrial systems, as indicated above, and hence their selectivity as antibacterial agents is not absolute. Thus, in clinical use, the toxicity of chloramphenicol is undoubtedly due in most cases to its inhibitory action on mitochondrial ribosomes (Various contributors, 1974). In some cases this appears to be also the basis for the reported toxicity of a number of translation inhibitors. Furthermore, besides the mitochondrial system, another protein synthesising system which is as sensitive to chloramphenicol as the mitochondrial one has been reported to function in synaptosomes (Ramirez *et al.*, 1972).

Selective Action of Antibiotic Inhibitors

According to the view presented above it might appear that there are not enough bases for a selective action in clinical use of the antibacterial antibiotics that inhibit translation, since they are also inhibitors of protein synthesis in mitochondria and perhaps in some other organelles of mammalian cells. However, for the antibiotics to act on mitochondrial ribosomes in mammalian cells, they have to cross the cellular plasma membranes and also the mitochondrial membranes. Indeed there are important differences in the permeability barrier of bacteria and mitochondria.

Furthermore despite the broad scope of the inhibitors of translation indicated in Tables 1 and 2, it is now widely recognised that there is a low susceptibility of mitochondrial ribosomes to a number of translation inhibitors when compared with the sensitivity of bacterial ribosomes. Indeed sensitivity of mitochondrial ribosomes to fusidic acid, macrolides and antibiotics of the lincomycin, streptogramin and aminoglycoside groups, is rather low as compared to the susceptibility of bacterial ribosomes to the same antibiotics (Vázquez, 1979; Denslow and O'Brien, 1978). This is not surprising, since there are some important differences between bacterial and mitochondrial ribosomes. Indeed mitochondrial ribosomes lack the 5S ribosomal RNA of the larger ribosomal subunit. The precise role of this component in the ribosome is not well known but it has certainly an important structural role, and therefore it is obvious that there should be differences between bacterial and mitochondrial ribosomes. Furthermore, there are very significant differences within the mitochondrial ribosomes: their sedimentation coefficients range from 55S in the case of ribosomes from mammalian mitochondria to 80S in the case of those from protozoa (Borst and Grivell, 1971).

Therefore, the differences between bacteria and mitochondria in permeability and in ribosomal structure justify the selection of new antibacterial antibiotics that inhibit translation.

Design of New Screening Techniques for Inhibitors of Translation

Resolved systems adequate for screening of inhibitors of the peptide bond formation step (step e_1 in Fig. 1) have been devised. Peptide bond formation is only one step in the complex sequence of reactions involved in protein synthesis. It is possible, however, to resolve the reaction by using some well defined experimental systems. The antibiotic puromycin has been a very useful tool for the study of peptide bond formation. This antibiotic is known to be an analogue of the aminoacyl–adenosine moiety of aminoacyl–tRNA. This is precisely the part of the aminoacyl–tRNA which is involved in peptidyl transfer, and puromycin can replace aminoacyl–tRNA as a substrate for the reaction. However, puromycin lacks that part of the molecule responsible for interaction with the template and the 30S ribosome subunit. Consequently, the use of puromycin provides a simplified method to study peptide bond formation. In this system the $\alpha-NH_2$ group of puromycin can be linked to the C–terminal end of a f–Met- or peptidyl–group. The product of the puromycin reaction (f–Met–puromycin or peptidyl–puromycin) is unable to take part in the next step of protein synthesis. However, all the evidence indicates that formation of a peptide bond between puromycin and a f–Met or peptidyl–group takes place by the same mechanism as peptide bond formation in protein synthesis. Peptide bond formation between either f–Met or Ac–Leu and puromycin can be studied in an even more simplified system described as the "fragment reaction" (Fig. 2). Indeed the terminal fragments CAACCA–Met–f and CACCA–Leu–Ac can be prepared by enzymic digestion of f–Met–tRNA and Ac–Leu–tRNA respectively, followed by electrophoretic purification. The CAACCA–Met–f and CACCA–Leu–Ac fragments undergo a ribosome-catalysed reaction with puromycin in the presence of Mg^{++}, K^+ or NH_4^+ and methanol or ethanol (20 to 70%, v/v). Ribosomes can be replaced by their 50S ribosomal subunits, showing that the peptidyl transferase centre that catalyses peptide bond formation in the process of translation is integrated in the larger subunit of the bacterial ribosome (Monro et al., 1969).

However the peptidyl transferase centre of the larger ribosomal subunit catalyses not only peptide bond formation in protein

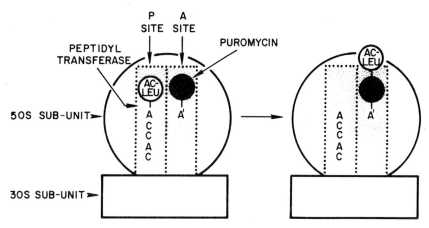

FIG. 2   Fragment reaction assay for peptide bond formation using CACCA–Leu–Ac as the donor substrate.

synthesis (step e_1 in Fig. 1) but also peptidyl–tRNA hydrolysis in the termination reactions (step g_2 in Fig. 1). These reactions can be studied by using a number of systems to test the activities of the peptidyl transferase center, which can therefore catalyse in very simplified systems not only peptide bond formation ("fragment reaction assay"), but also ester formation ("assay for f–Met–ethyl ester formation") and peptidyl–tRNA hydrolysis ("assay for f–methionine release") (Table 3) (Monro *et al.*, 1969; Scolnick *et al.*, 1970; Caskey *et al.*, 1971). The use of solvents might affect in some

TABLE 3

Resolved Systems for Peptidyl Transferase Activity

Assay system	Substrate	Additions	Product
Fragment reaction (Monro *et al.*, 1969)	CACCA–[³H]Leu-Ac | Ribosome	Puromycin and ethanol	Ac–[³H]Leu– puromycin
Ethyl ester reaction (Scolnick *et al.*, 1970)	f–[³H]Met–tRNA | Ribosome	Ethanol and tRNA or CCA	f–[³H]Met–ethyl ester
f–[³H]Met release (Caskey *et al.*, 1971)	f–[³H]Met–tRNA | Ribosome	Acetone and tRNA or CCA	f–[³H] Met

cases the strength of the inhibitory effects produced by some antibiotics, since it has clearly been shown that the solvents (methanol, ethanol and acetone) differentially affect the affinities of the substrates and of the antibiotics for the ribosome. However, these systems are very useful and valid since a wide range of peptide bond formation inhibitors have been tested in the three assays using bacterial ribosomes and shown to be very effective. There is only one interesting exception: the f–methionine release reaction induced by acetone is stimulated by lincomycin although it is a well known inhibitor of peptide bond formation. The reason for this result is not well understood but interestingly enough most of the antibiotics of the lincomycin group do not behave like lincomycin in this simplified release reaction, being very effective inhibitors of f–methionine release in the acetone assay (Caskey, pers. comm.).

When dealing with the screening techniques using the "fragment reaction", "f–Met–ethyl ester reaction" and the "f–methionine release" assays, it is important to carry out the reactions with ribosomes from both Gram-positive and Gram-negative bacteria. Indeed it has been shown that a number of antibiotics such as lincomycin, streptogramin A, streptogramin B and some macrolides present affinities for ribosomes of Gram-positive higher than those for ribosomes of Gram-negative bacteria. Therefore, the preferential susceptibility of Gram-positive bacteria to some antibiotic inhibitors of protein synthesis is not only due to a differential permeability to the antibiotics (Vázquez, 1979).

Discussion

As indicated above, a number of inhibitors of protein biosynthesis might present toxicity in their medical use due to their possible inhibitory effect on translation in mitochondria and perhaps in some other mammalian procaryotic organelles. However, it is well known that mitochondria widely differ from bacteria in their permeability barrier. Furthermore, ribosomes from mitochondria differ from those of bacteria in a number of structural features that frequently determine response to antibiotics different from that of the bacterial ribosomes. Therefore, the search for antibacterial inhibitors of protein biosynthesis is still potentially useful. Even in the case of inhibitors active on mitochondrial and mammalian ribosomes, such as the tetracyclines, differences in permeability might allow their clinical use.

The simplest way for screening protein synthesis inhibitors would be testing the incorporation into the protein fraction of intact bacteria of an amino acid which is not incorporated in the cell-wall fraction and is not a precursor of nucleic acids. However this sort of test will not provide information concerning the specific step(s) blocked by the inhibitor and this should be investigated in further standard assays using mainly cell-free systems (Vázquez, 1979).

On the other hand the simplified cell-free systems described above ("fragment reaction", "f–Met–ethyl ester reaction" and "f–methionine release") are potentially very useful tools for the screening of new inhibitors of translation which interact with the peptidyl transferase centre on the 50S ribosomal subunit and therefore block peptide bond formation and termination. Similar assays with mammalian ribosomes from mitochondria and cell cytoplasm will provide useful information concerning the selective action of the inhibitors. Unfortunately there are no such simple methods to study other steps of translation, therefore they cannot be tested so easily in cell-free systems.

Since most inhibitors of translation interact with the ribosome, investigation of the interaction of such antibiotics with the ribosome provides a means to analyse their modes of action. Indeed binding of even an unlabelled antibiotic to ribosomes can be studied by standard methods, such as equilibrium dialysis and sedimentation of the ribosomes by centrifugation, provided that it competes for binding with a suitable labelled antibiotic (Fernandez-Muñoz *et al.*, 1971). The information will be particularly useful when the mode of action of the labelled antibiotic is known. Hence these binding studies might be also useful as a complementary and simple screening technique.

From the observation of Fig. 1 and Tables 1 and 2 it is obvious that there is a wide range of inhibitors of elongation and termination acting selectively in procaryotic systems and hence useful as antibacterial agents. However, we do not know the reason for the very poor number of inhibitors of initiation with such a selective action on bacteria. It appears that the ribosomal sites involved in the initiation process have been maintained rather conservatively since most antibiotics and chemicals affecting initiation in bacteria are also effective in eucaryotes. However, the process is more complicated in eucaryotes which require a number of initiation factors which are absent in bacteria. Indeed an increasing number of natural compounds (interferon, double stranded RNA and the translational inhibitor) specifically control or inhibit initiation in eucaryotic systems.

References

Borst, P. and Grivell, L.A. (1971). *FEBS Letters* **13**, 73–88.

Caskey, C.T., Beaudet, A.L., Scolnick, E.M. and Rosman, M. (1971). *Proc. Nat. Acad. Sci. U.S.A.* **68**, 3163–3167.

Contreras, A., Vázquez, D. and Carrasco, L. (1978). *J. Antibiotics* **31**, 598–602.

Denslow, N.D. and O'Brien, T.W. (1978). *Eur. J. Biochem.* **91**, 441–448.

Fernandez-Muñoz, R., Monro, R.E. and Vázquez, D. (1971). *Methods Enzymol.* **20**, 481–490.

Monro, R.E., Staehelin, T., Celma, M.L. and Vázquez, D. (1969). *Cold Spring Harb. Symp. Quant. Biol.* **34**, 357–368.

Ramirez, G., Levitan, J.B. and Mushynski, W.E. (1972). *FEBS Lett.* **21**, 17–20.

Scolnick, E., Milman, G., Rosman, M. and Caskey, T. (1970). *Nature* **225**, 152–154.

Various contributors (1974). *In* "Chloramphenicol–thiamphenicol: Known and Unknown Aspects of Drug-host Interactions". *Postgrad. Med. J. Suppl.* **50**, 11–151.

Vázquez, D. (1974). *FEBS Lett.* **40**, (Suppl.) S63–S84.

Vázquez, D. (1979). "Inhibitors of Protein Biosynthesis". Springer-Verlag, Berlin, Heidelberg, New York.

Discussion

Professor Braun: I would like to comment on Professor Vázquez' statement that inhibitors against procaryotes should be selected and those that are active also against eucaryotes should be discarded. I agree completely that the general statement is true, but I want to emphasise, by means of an example, that something both interesting and surprising can be shown when the latter sort of inhibitors is not discarded. The example is pulvomycin which is like kirromycin, an inhibitor of the elongation step in protein synthesis, by interaction with the Tu-factor. This has been studied by Heinz Wolff and Bärbel Schmidt in our department. Pulvomycin inhibits protein synthesis of procaryotes and is also active against eucaryotic cells, but there it does not inhibit protein synthesis. Apparently it inhibits RNA synthesis, shown with Ehrlich carcinoma cells.

Professor Vázquez: In spite of its double mechanism, pulvomycin cannot be considered as a useful antitumour agent. I was restricting my talk today to anti-bacterial antibiotics.

Dr. Videau: We know that antibiotics which bind to the ribosomes have quite different affinities. You have shown that streptogramines for example had a very efficient binding. Do we begin to understand the structural features that account for this binding and don't you think it could be applied to screening methods?

Professor Vázquez: The ribosome is a very complicated structure, and very little is known about the precise sites of antibiotic interactions on the ribosome. For instance, within the peptidyl transferase centre, which is the most studied part of the ribosome, I have quoted a number of antibiotics because each one displaces the others, or competes with them in some way, i.e. they do not bind at the same site on the ribosomes. It is not possible to say much about the precise site of action of antibiotics. However, I am very much intrigued by the fact that if ribosomal proteins are studied, no protein is ever found which is common in bacteria and higher cells. The sequence is now being studied, and more will be known about this in the future.

It is interesting that these antibiotics which are not used clinically, gougerotin, blasticidin, amicetin, etc., which are derivatives of purine, pyrimidines or amino-sides, probably bind because the ribosomal RNAs facilitate their interactions with the ribosome. This also suggests that apparently there may be some common features in the RNA of the larger subunit of bacteria and eucaryotic cells. However, the antibiotics do not bind directly on to the RNA, but something else is required, which seems to be different kinds of proteins. But for the moment, studies on these proteins have shown some conflicting results.

Professor Richmond: When eucaryotic ribosomes are translating viral messages, is their sensitivity to antibiotics the same as when they are translating eucaryotic messages?

Professor Vázquez: There are very small differences. Interestingly, there are now some models which postulate some difference in intact cells. Apparently, permeability is drastically affected in infected cells, and some drugs which do not act in intact cells in the eucaryotes do act in virus-infected ones. For instance, the GTP analogue, GMP–PCP, and blasticidin or gougerotin, are inactive in intact mammalian cells, but they are very active in virus-infected cells because they are easily permeable.

Professor Davies: Although we are probably primarily interested in trying to do something about human infection, we are talking about antibiotics and there are many plant diseases against which antibiotics are extremely useful. Some of the inhibitors of protein synthesis that have been described are very good and effective protectors of plants, when those plants are infected in some way. In trying to consider our search for useful new compounds that may be used for the benefit of man, compounds of this type must also be considered. The inhibitors of eucaryotic protein synthesis must not always be thrown away because they may be useful.

Antimicrobial Treatment via Iron Metabolism

V. BRAUN and K. HANTKE

Mikrobiologie II, Universität Tübingen,
Tübingen, Germany

Introduction

Iron is an essential element for organisms since it is a constituent of haeme and non-haeme proteins of respiratory chains and of many enzymes. The solubility product constant of ferrous hydroxide at $25°C$ is 10^{-15}, the constant for ferric hydroxide is in the order of 10^{-38} (Sillen and Martell, 1964; Weinberg, 1978). The very low solubility of ferric iron under aerobic physiological (pH 7) conditions requires that organisms produce substances which bind iron ions.

The iron carriers are proteins or ligands of low molecular weight. Iron is bound in human milk to lactoferrin (Bullen, 1976; Schade, 1975) and in the serum to transferrin (Bullen *et al.*, 1974; Yancey *et al.*, 1979). Microbial invaders have to compete with their hosts for the elusive iron. They do so by producing highly efficient ligands with formation constants as high as 10^{52} (Raymond and Carrano, 1979). Human serum transferrin, with a formation constant of 10^{30}, is only 25–30% saturated with Fe^{3+}. This implies that the amount of free ionic iron is about $6 \times 10^{-9} \mu M$, which is eight orders of magnitude less than required for microbial growth (Weinberg, 1978). Therefore, serum does not support microbial growth unless the organisms release sufficient amounts of ligands with strong formation constants for iron to scavenge the rare metal and to transport it into the cell. In the following, host parasite interactions with regard to iron will be described with *Escherichia coli* as an example. After briefly reviewing the current knowledge, possible ways to defend microbial invaders by iron limitation will be discussed.

Iron Transport Systems of *Escherichia coli*

The known iron transport systems of *E. coli* are summarised in Table 1.

TABLE 1

Iron Uptake of *Escherichia coli*

Ferric iron ligands	Remarks	Log stability constant
1) enterochelin	induced by low iron concentration	52
2) ferrichrome	produced by certain fungi	29
3) citrate	induced by citrate	25*
4) low affinity system	ligand unknown, suppressible by nitrilotriacetate	—

* equilibrium constant of unprotonated form; the value for protonated complex is 12 (According to Raymond and Carrano, 1979; Sillen and Martell, 1964).

From the pharmaceutical point of view the most important transport system is that of ferric enterochelin (also called enterobactin) (Yancey *et al.*, 1979). Enterochelin is produced by *E. coli* and other Enterobacteriaceae in response to iron limitation in the growth medium (Rodgers and Neilands, 1973; Rosenberg and Young, 1974; Woodrow *et al.*, 1979). At the same time, the transport system is induced as the esterase which degrades the ligand after uptake of ferric enterochelin into the cell. In addition, a protein in the outer membrane is formed which strongly binds ferric enterochelin. Mutants which lack this receptor protein are unable to take up ferric enterochelin (Fig. 1) (Braun, 1977, 1978; Braun and Hantke, 1977; Hancock *et al.*, 1976; Wookey and Rosenberg, 1978).

The specific transport system for ferrichrome is peculiar since the ligand has been found as a product of certain fungi but not of *E. coli* or other bacteria (Byers and Arceneaux, 1977; Diekmann, 1973; Keller-Schierlein *et al.*, 1964; Neilands, 1977; Rodgers and Neilands, 1973). The ability to transport ferrichrome and to use iron may only be important when *E. coli* cells (and *Salmonella*) share a habitat with fungi. The known elements of the transport system are depicted in Fig. 2.

The ability of *E. coli* cells to induce a ferric citrate transport system when cultured in the presence of 100 μM citrate (Frost and Rosenberg, 1973, Rosenberg and Young, 1974) may only be relevant for strains which grow in an environment with high concentrations of citrate, for example on plant material. It has been found in *E. coli* K12, *E. coli* B and in *Aerobacter aerogenes* but not in *E. coli* W and in *Salmonella typhimurium*. Concomitant with the citrate transport

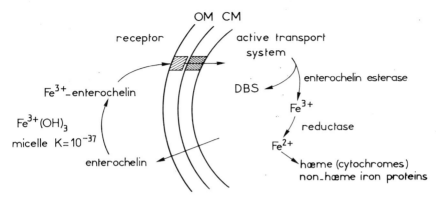

FIG. 1 Model of ferric enterochelin transport into cells of *E. coli*. Enterochelin is synthesised under iron limiting growth conditions and excreted. It solubilises polymeric forms of iron in the medium. Transport requires a receptor protein of the outer membrane specified by the *fepA* gene (formerly designated *feuB* or *cbr*), and an additional function of the cytoplasmic membrane, controlled by the *fepB* gene. Release of the iron probably involves reduction to the ferrous state and hydrolysis of enterochelin by an esterase. The hydrolysis products (dihydroxybenzoylserine, DBS) are excreted and not used for enterochelin synthesis (From Rosenberg and Young, 1974, with permission), (see Fig. 3).

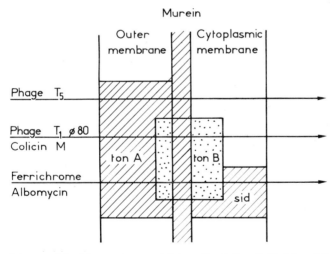

FIG. 2 Scheme of ferrichrome transport into cells of *E. coli*. Uptake of ferrichrome requires the activity of at least 3 genes (*tonA, tonB, sid*). The *sid* gene product is presumably the permease in the cytoplasmic membrane. The *tonA* and *tonB* gene products have been identified. Iron is released from the complex by reduction, the ligand is modified to a product with low iron affinity and excreted (A. Hartmann and V. Braun, submitted for publication). Components of the transport system are also used by phages T1, T5, φ80 and by colicin M to infect cells (Braun, 1977, 1978; Braun and Hantke, 1977; Neilands, 1977).

system appears a protein in the outer membrane which is absent in some ferric citrate transport mutants (Hancock *et al.*, 1976).

The low affinity system functions only in media with plentiful iron, it is poorly defined, no iron ligand is known, and it may just be passive diffusion of iron.

Possible Defense Mechanisms against Bacterial Infections based on Iron Limitation

For growth of microorganisms in most environments where they compete for nutrients with other cells, the iron supply is a decisive factor. Growth limitation by iron deficiency has amply been documented in many cases (Bullen, 1976; Bullen *et al.*, 1974; Kochan, 1975; Schade, 1975; Weinberg, 1978; Yancey *et al.*, 1979). The following discussion is mainly based on the assumption that treatments which create bacteriostatic conditions would be sufficient to allow the defense mechanisms of organisms to overcome microbial infections.

Interference with the Synthesis of Iron Ligands

Enterochelin   Starting from chorismate, the major branch point compound in aromatic biosynthesis, at least 6 steps are known which solely lead to the production of enterochelin (Fig. 3). These include the synthesis of dihydroxybenzoate, dihydroxybenzoyl serine and the polymerisation of the latter to the cyclic trimer. A screening programme could be devised for compounds which interfere with enterochelin synthesis by selecting for growth inhibition under iron limiting conditions. Furthermore, mutants which lack enterochelin esterase and therefore are unable to degrade the ligand were found to grow poorly on low–iron media (Rosenberg and Young, 1974). Compounds which inhibit enterochelin esterase would cause growth inhibition due to iron shortage.

Ferrichrome   The pathway of ferrichrome biosynthesis and of other iron ligands of the hydroxamate type is not known in all steps (Emery, 1974). Ferrichrome synthesis in *Ustilago sphaerogena* involves the following intermediates: ornithine, δ–N–hydroxyornithine, δ–N–acetyl–δ–N–hydroxyornithine which forms with 3 glycine residues a cyclic hexapeptide. One could screen for compounds which interfere somewhere in the pathway of ferrichrome biosynthesis. The most effective inhibitor would be one which interferes with the formation of the hydroxamate group of all iron

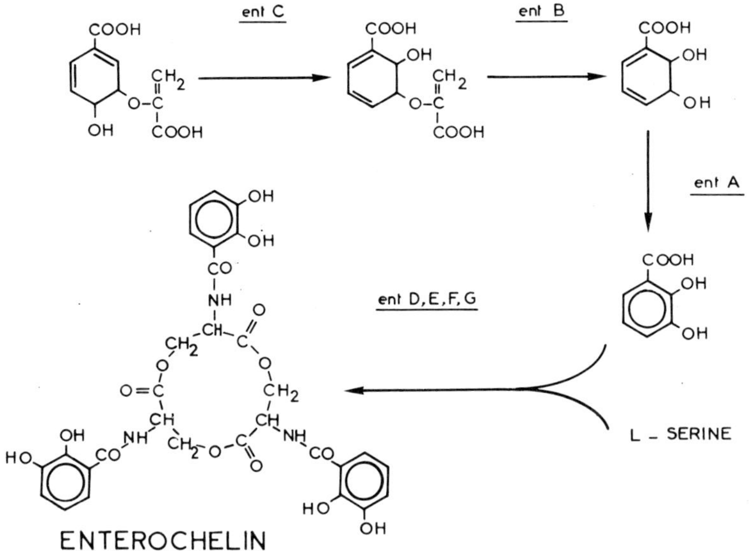

FIG. 3   Enterochelin biosynthesis as summarised by Rosenberg and Young (1974) (with permission). Starting from chorismic acid, isochorismic acid, dihydro-dihydroxybenzoic acid and finally dihydroxybenzoic acid are formed. Serine is linked to dihydroxybenzoic acid but does not appear as free dihydroxybenzoyl serine. It has been suggested that the final stages of enterochelin synthesis occurs at a membrane bound enzyme complex allowing immediate excretion of the ligand (Woodrow *et al.*, 1979). *ent* designates genes whose products are involved in enterochelin biosynthesis.

ligands of this type (Diekmann, 1973; Emery, 1974; Ernst and Winkelmann, 1974).

Inhibition of Transport

Inhibition of transport can be envisaged at various steps of the uptake process. The outer membrane receptor proteins at the cell surface could be blocked by ligands bound to macromolecules which prevent entry of the iron complex into the microbial cell. That such an approach is feasible was recently shown. Ferricrocin was chemically coupled to polyethylene glycol. The polymer-bound ferricrocin still supplied iron specifically via the *tonA, tonB, sid* dependent uptake system but with a rate below 10% of the rate of free ferricrocin (Coulton *et al.*, 1979). This reduction of the iron supply would probably be sufficient to prevent growth under natural conditions with low concentrations of available iron.

Iron ligands could be coupled to homologous proteins to use them as antigenic determinants for antibody production. In fact, naturally occurring antibodies which suppress bacterial growth in serum by interference with the iron supply have clearly been demonstrated. The bacteriostatic properties of human and horse sera, besides iron limitation by transferrin, were attributed to the presence of antibodies which either prevent synthesis or excretion of enterochelin. In our view, it is highly likely that antibodies against enterochelin may be present in the serum. They could inhibit excretion of enterochelin which presumably passes through the outer membrane by the pores formed by major proteins (porins) (Nikaido, 1979). Excreted enterochelin could be bound to antibody and would then be unavailable for iron transport. In fact, no catechol compounds were found in the serum infected with cells which were able to produce enterochelin. By addition of iron, bacterial growth was resumed. The production of naturally occurring antibodies could result from outer membrane components, most likely the receptor proteins which are released continuously during bacterial growth or cell lysis.

One could also think of synthetic compounds which are structurally similar to siderophores but poor iron carriers to paralyse the transport system. They could be thermodynamically weak iron complexes or kinetically very stable complexes. An isosteric equivalent of enterochelin has been synthesised (Fig. 4) with the aim to treat secondary hemochromatosis, an iron-overload disease with various causes (Venuti et al., 1979). This compound supported growth of a *Salmonella typhimurium* strain unable to synthesise enterochelin and failed to promote growth of an *E. coli* strain which lacked the outer membrane receptor protein of enterochelin. A synthetic design along this approach could yield a variety of compounds which could be tested as inhibitors of the ferric enterochelin transport system or which could be used as antigenic determinants to rise enterochelin specific antibodies.

Use of Microbial Iron Ligands as Carriers for Antibiotics

The use of antibiotics is often curtailed by their insufficient entry into cells. The ideal case would be the active transport of an antibiotic into microbial cells which would lower the therapeutic dose considerably (Braun, 1977; Franklin, 1973; Höltje, 1979; Kadner, 1978; Raymond and Carrano, 1979; Zähner et al., 1977). In the field of iron transport compounds, nature has shown how to bring antibiotics into cells. There are inhibitory compounds, called sideromycins, which are structurally analogous to growth supporting compounds, the sideramines.

The best understood pair is ferrichrome and albomycin (Fig. 5).

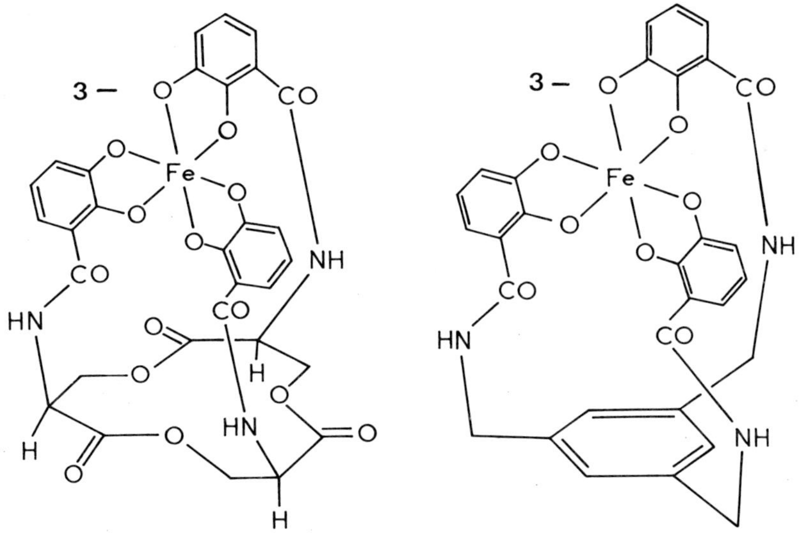

FIG. 4 Dreiding models of enterochelin (left) and of an analogous synthetic compound (1, 3, 5 – tris N, N', N" – 2,3 dihydroxybenzoyl) aminomethylbenzene (From Venuti *et al.*, 1979; with permission of the authors and of The American Chemical Society).

The antibiotic albomycin is transported into cells of *Escherichia coli* and *Salmonella typhimurium* by the same uptake system as the iron-supplying ferrichrome complex (Braun, 1977, 1978; Braun and Hantke, 1977; Coulton *et al.*, 1979; Hancock *et al.*, 1976; Hartmann *et al.*, 1979; Luckey *et al.*, 1972; Neilands, 1977). The ferrichrome-like portion of albomycin serves as a vehicle to bring the antibiotically active part into the cell. The latter is released by hydrolysis and is retained in the cell whereas the iron ligand is excreted like the iron-free deferri—ferrichrome (Hartmann *et al.*, 1979). The released compound can be concentrated 500 fold within the cell. The antagonistic action of other sideramines and sideromycins was noticed already when they were discovered (Keller-Schierlein *et al.*, 1964). In another case, ferrioxamine B and the related antibiotic A22765, it was clearly shown that the antagonism is caused by competition for the uptake system and not at the target site (Nüesch and Knüsel, 1967).

Following the design of naturally occurring sideromycins, attempts have been made with synthetic compounds in which antibiotics were coupled to sideramines to bring them into cells via the iron transport systems. The sulfanilamidonicotinic acid ferricrocinyl ester (Fig. 5) inhibited cells of *Staphylococcus aureus* at a concentration of 0.05 μM which was 1000 times lower than the minimal inhibitory concentration of the free sulfonamide (50 μM) (Diddens, 1979; Zähner *et*

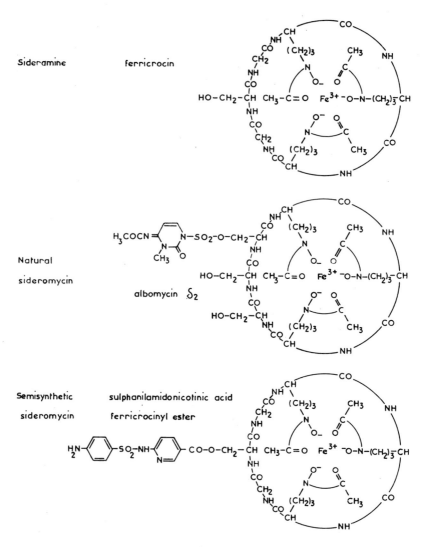

FIG. 5   Structure of ferricrocin, of albomycin and of the synthetic derivative sulfanila-midonicotinic acid ferricrocinyl ester (From Zähner *et al.*, 1977, with permission of authors and of Japan Antibiotics Research Association). The formula of albomycin is probably incorrect in the area between the hexapeptide ring and the pyrimidine derivative (W. Keller-Schierlein and H. Maehr, pers. comm.). In ferrichrome the serine residue of ferricrocin is replaced by a glycine residue. Both compounds transport iron into cells of *E. coli* with comparable rates.

al., 1977). The inhibition could be neutralised both by ferricrocin and by p—aminobenzoic acid showing that the semisynthetic compound facilitates the uptake and that the sulfonamide exerts its usual inhibition of the C1 metabolism. The same compound was also active against an *E. coli* K12 strain which cannot synthesise enterochelin. The inhibition of *E. coli* was only observed when the cells had been grown under iron limiting conditions by which the ferrichrome transport system is induced (Diddens, 1979). Ferrioxamine B was also an active carrier. In both cases, a spacer between the iron carrier and the antibiotic had to be introduced to obtain active compounds. The reason is unknown but could be sought in the possible requirement to release the antibiotic from the carrier in the cell.

Conclusion

The use of sideromycins as antimicrobial agents was mainly hampered by the high frequency of spontaneous resistant mutants with a defect in the transport system. However, no inhibitor of the enterochelin–type has been described. A search for an antagonist of the enterochelin transport system would be profitable since Enterobacteriaceae probably cannot grow without iron supply via enterochelin in most natural environments. For the near future, the rise of siderophore specific antibodies could lead to a rapid success because the defence by naturally occurring antibodies would be exaggerated. Such antibodies would function in two ways. They would trap the released siderophores in the growth environment and they would bind to the microbial receptors at the cell surface loaded with enterochelin and block the uptake. Moreover, the action of the immune system would be supported by the antibodies bound to microbial cells. Siderophores with chemically reactive side chains occur naturally and enterochelin analogues have been synthesised. It is important that the analogues are stable and lack the ester linkages of enterochelin. The transport system tolerates, to an astonishing degree, modification of the siderophores. A vast body of evidence has been collected which demonstrates that iron limitation is naturally applied to reduce microbial growth but only few trials can be found in the literature where this defence principle has been tested therapeutically.

Acknowledgements

The authors' work was supported by the Deutsche Forschungsgemeinschaft (SFB 76) and the Fonds der Chemischen Industrie.

References

Braun, V. (1977). *Naturwissenschaften* **64**, 126–132.
Braun, V. (1978). *In* "Relations between Structure and Function in the Prokaryotic Cell". (Y. Stanier, H.J. Rogers and B.J. Ward, eds), pp. 111–138. Cambridge University Press, London.

Braun, V. and Hantke, K. (1977). *In* "Microbial Interactions, Receptors and Recognition, Series B", Vol. 3. (J.L. Reissig, ed.), pp. 101-137. Chapman and Hall, London.

Bullen, J.J. (1976). *In* "Ciba Foundation Symposium 42". Elsevier North Holland Biomedical Press, Amsterdam, Holland.

Bullen, J.J., Rogers, H.J. and Griffiths, E. (1974). *In* "Microbial Iron Metabolism". (J.B. Neilands, ed.), pp. 517–551. Academic Press, New York.

Byers, B.R. and Arceneaux, E.L. (1977). *In* "Microorganisms and Minerals". (E.D. Weinberg, ed.), pp. 215–249. Marcel Dekker, New York.

Coulton, J.W., Naegeli, H.-U. and Braun, V. (1979). *Eur. J. Biochem.* **99**, 39–47.

Diddens, H. (1979). "Untersuchungen zum Transport von Antibiotika über die Aufnahmesysteme für Oligopeptide und Sideramine". Thesis, Universität Tübingen.

Diekmann, H. (1973). *In* "Handbook of Microbiology", Vol. 3. (A.J. Laskin and H.A. Lechevalier, eds), pp. 449–457. C.R.C. Press, Cleveland.

Emery, T. (1974). *In* "Microbial Iron Metabolism". (J.B. Neilands, ed.), pp. 107–123. Academic Press, New York.

Ernst, J. and Winkelmann, G. (1974). *Arch. Microbiol.* **100**, 271–282.

Franklin, T.J. (1973). *Crit. Rev. Microbiol.* **2**, 253–272.

Frost, G.E. and Rosenberg, H. (1973). *Biochim. Biophys. Acta* **330**, 90–101.

Hancock, R.E.W., Hantke, K. and Braun, V. (1976). *J. Bacteriol.* **127**, 1370–1375.

Hartmann, A., Fiedler, H.-P. and Braun, V. (1979). *Eur. J. Biochem.* **99**, 517–524.

Höltje, J.-V. (1979). *Forum Mikrobiologie* **2**, 249–255.

Kadner, R.J. (1978). *In* "Bacterial Transport". (B.P. Rosen, ed.), pp. 463–493. Marcel Dekker, New York.

Keller-Schierlein, W., Prelog, V. and Zähner, H. (1964). *Fortschr. Chem. Org. Naturst.* **22**, 279–322.

Kochan, J. (1975). *In* "Microbiology – 1974". (D. Schlessinger, ed.), pp. 273–288. American Society for Microbiology, Washington, D.C.

Luckey, M., Pollack, J.R., Wayne, R., Ames, B. and Neilands, J.B. (1972). *J. Bacteriol.* **111**, 731–738.

Neilands, J.B. (1977). *In* "Advances in Chemistry Series". (R.F. Gould, ed.), pp. 3–32. American Chemical Society, Washington, D.C.

Nikaido, H. (1979). *Angew. Chem.* **91**, 394–407.

Nüesch, J. and Knüsel, F. (1967). *In* "Antibiotics", Vol. 1. (D. Gottlieb and P.D. Shaw, eds), pp. 499–541. Springer Verlag, Heidelberg.

Raymond, K.N. and Carrano, C.J. (1979). *Acc. Chem. Res.* **12**, 183–190.

Rodgers, G. and Neilands, J.B. (1973). *In* "Handbook of Microbiology", Vol. 2. (A.J. Laskin and H.A. Lechevalier, eds), pp. 823–830. C.R.C. Press, Cleveland.

Rosenberg, H. and Young, J.G. (1974). *In* "Microbial Iron Metabolism", (J.B. Neilands, ed.), pp. 67–82. Academic Press, New York, London.

Schade, A.L. (1975). *In* "Microbiology – 1974". (D. Schlessinger, ed.), pp. 266–269. American Society for Microbiology, Washington, D.C.

Sillen, L.C. and Martell, A.E. (1964). "Stability Constants of Metal Ion Complexes". The Chemical Society, London.

Venuti, M.C., Rastetter, W.H. and Neilands, J.B. (1979). *J. Med. Chem.* **22**, 123–124.

Weinberg, E.D. (1978). *Microbiol. Rev.* **42**, 45–66.

Woodrow, G.C., Young, J.G. and Gibson, F. (1979). *Biochim. Biophys. Acta* **582**, 145–153.

Wookey, P. and Rosenberg, H. (1978). *J. Bacteriol.* **133**, 661–666.

Yancey, R.J., Breeding, S.A.L. and Lankford, C.E. (1979). *Infect. Immun.* **24**, 174–180.

Zähner, H., Diddens, H., Keller-Schierlein, W. and Naegeli, H.U. (1977). *Jap. J. Antibiot.* **30**, S201–S206.

Discussion

Professor Tomasz: The last strategy described by Professor Braun in building analogues of the siderochrome system raises some questions. First, these analogues would function only if the natural carrier concentration is low in the medium. Are they competitive with each other?

Professor Braun: This has not really been studied because the first compound was reported in late 1979. They are probably effective competitors because it appears that they transport iron into the cells or they can supply iron. This has not been demonstrated by transport studies, but by plate studies in which a growth zone is obtained under iron-limiting conditions. The first point I wanted to make is that it is fairly easy to obtain derivatives which still bind to the receptor but which are not taken up.

Secondly, it would be possible to raise antibodies against such compounds by covalently linking them to proteins, putting the proteins back into the animal or into human beings. This would give antibodies which recognise this kind of compounds.

Professor Tomasz: I understand that, but returning to the use of these carriers as transporting agents to "smuggle" into the bacteria sulphonamides, for instance, the liberation of the active antibiotic intracellularly requires enzyme activity. What enzyme is present?

Professor Braun: It is not known in this case. I think that Professor Gilvarg will probably comment on this later. It is clear with the peptide transport system because in that case there are peptidases, which release the active antibiotic.

Professor Tomasz: Is there not a limit to the maximum amount of the anti-metabolite that can be smuggled into the bacterium because it is coupled to the transport of a ligand, iron, of which little is needed for the bacterial cell?

Professor Braun: I can refer to only one *in vitro* study. It has not yet been tried *in vivo*. It is a completely new idea.

Professor Sabath: Professor Braun's comments about enterochelin are extremely fascinating. First, is it general among the Enterobacteriaceae, and possibly also *Pseudomonas*, to produce enterochelin or a similar compound?

Professor Braun: This has not really been studied on a large scale. There are some *Pseudomonas* which produce hydroxamate-type iron complexes, and this type of *Pseudomonas* probably does not produce an enterochelin. It is known only for *E. coli*, *Salmonella* and *Aerobacter aerogenes*.

Professor Sabath: Secondly, Professor Braun mentioned the possibility of antibodies to enterochelin as being a therapeutic approach. Have such experiments been done, or is it only theoretical at the moment?

Professor Braun: It is clear that there are specific antibodies against enterochelin in human serum in the normal situation.

Professor Rinehart: *Pseudomonas aeruginosa* produces something called a pyochelin, which is different from enterochelin. The structure of that compound is not yet complete, but it is hoped to have it in about two-week's time.

Professor Sande: About its practicability, are these various enterochelins antigenically distinct from species to species, or have they common antigenic determinants so that, if it were possible to harvest one of them, antibodies could be developed against an entire spectrum of organisms?

Professor Braun: The hydroxamate-type iron complexes are certainly different. The only approach on a broad basis would be to inhibit their synthesis. I do not know, however, whether this is always the same type of synthesis. That is one drawback. The enterochelin seems to be the same for all organisms where it is found.

Suppression of Resistance

J. DAVIES

*Department of Biochemistry, University of
Wisconsin, Madison, Wisconsin, U.S.A.*

Introduction

The objective of my paper is to try to describe how to create a
primeval state in which all antibiotics will work against all organisms,
that is, all organisms will be sensitive. I will try also to describe ways
in which we can perhaps create new antibiotics out of old ones. In
this respect, one should presume that antibiotic resistance is a major
clinical problem and that it will continue to increase as a problem,
although this can be debated.

To set the stage for my presentation we must discuss how resistance
is established. It will then be possible to discuss the resistance genes,
their dissemination among bacteria and their products. It is first
necessary to define the enemy, and then perhaps something can be
done against it.

Resistance Mechanisms and Acquisition of Resistance

Mechanisms of Resistance

The six standard mechanisms of resistance have been listed in Table 1.
Some are encountered more frequently than others in bacteria but all
of them have been detected in plasmid-carrying strains or in mutants.
One should immediately stress the problem of mutants: when the
cell becomes impermeable to an antibiotic and can no longer transport the drug, new types of antibiotics that can penetrate the cell by
another mechanism or by diffusion, will be required and this is where
biochemical studies of permeability will be very important.

TABLE 1

Mechanisms of Resistance

1. Cell becomes impermeable (transport–defective) to antimicrobial agent.
2. Target site for drug is altered – binds less well or not at all.
3. Overproduction of target – antimicrobial agent is "titrated-out".
4. Requirement for metabolite is reduced – exogenous source required.
5. Drug is detoxified – inactivated.
6. Cell can by-pass the blocked reaction – replacement enzyme or pathway.

Determinants of Resistance in Bacteria

If we consider the ways by which an organism might develop resistance (Table 2), it appears that all these systems have an equal

TABLE 2

Determinants of Resistance in Bacteria

1. Gene alteration (mutation)
2. Gene substitution
3. Gene inheritance — Plasmids — conjugative / non-conjugative — Transposons
4. Gene multiplication

opportunity to operate. Although gene alteration and mutation are likely to become increasingly important, I want to focus primarily on the mechanisms concerned with gene inheritance.

There are a number of different ways by which genes can be disseminated within microorganisms. The three ways (as shown in Table 3) by which a resistant population can develop may not be exclusive but are the main mechanisms of resistance spreading. The mechanisms by which these plasmid transfers occur (conjugation, transduction or transformation) are not really important for our purpose.

Possible Routes to Counteract Antibiotic Resistance

We now examine the possible ways to overcome or reduce antibiotic resistance, its development or expression (Table 4); most of them should be obvious approaches to everyone concerned, for example by controlled and reduced use of antibiotics, by better aseptic techniques or by research into new active structures. Clearly some of the mechanisms are not likely to be effective, and I will try to give examples of a non-useful mechanism as well as potential useful approaches to the problem.

TABLE 3

Mechanisms by which Antibiotic Resistance is Disseminated

1. Clonal Transfer:	Resistance due to single species of microorganism – with or without R–plasmid – spread by mechanical means
2. Single Plasmid:	Unique R–plasmid is spread throughout several bacterial families by variety of gene transfer mechanisms
3. Multiple Plasmid:	Several R–plasmids from single or multiple sources may be transferred coincidentally

TABLE 4

Possible Routes to Overcome or Reduce Antibiotic Resistance
(development or expression)

1. Controlled and reduced use of antibiotics
2. Aseptic techniques to prevent clonal transfer
3. New antibiotics (natural or semi-synthetic) refractory to resistance mechanism
4. Inhibition of determinants of antibiotic resistance
5. Interference with plasmid transfer
6. "Curing" of resistance plasmids
7. Antibiotic combinations

"Curing" Agents: the Useless Weapons

Curing of resistance plasmids has been suggested in the past on the assumption that it would be possible to invent a new kind of "magic bullet" which would shoot plasmids out of cells, and restore the latter to an antibiotic sensitive state; this approach is not feasible. Table 5 lists some of the agents that have been suggested for the

TABLE 5

"Curing" Agents: Interfere with Normal Segregation of Plasmid or Select Spontaneous Segregants

Intercalating agents:	Acridine orange, ethidium bromide
RNA polymerase inhibitors:	Rifampicin
Gyrase inhibitors:	Novobiocin, coumermycin
Surfactants:	Sodium dodecyl sulphate
Others:	Temperature shift

curing of plasmids. In spite of the fact that some of these compounds, like novobiocin or coumermycin are highly effective at removing plasmids or promoting the appearance of segregants, their use as prophylactic drugs is not conceivable. A toxicity problem is likely to be encountered with the many intercalating agents which are carcinogens or mutagens.

Considering the phenotypic properties conferred by plasmids

TABLE 6

Phenotypic Properties Conferred by Plasmids

Replication, Recombination
Repair, Restriction, Modification
Resistance to Toxic Ions, Antimicrobials and Bacteriophages
Metabolic Activities: Catabolism of Sugars and Aromatic Compounds, Biosynthesis of
    Secondary Metabolites
Altered Surface Structure (K 88, K 99)
Pathogenicity: Enterotoxin, Haemolysin
Conjugal Transfer, Transposition

(Table 6), it should be kept in mind that bacteria maintain these extrachromosomal elements for other purposes than to make themselves resistant. Many other characteristics are coded by resistance plasmids and provide a counterselection against the curing action of the drug. Besides, applying curing agents to bacteria may force many resistant determinants into an even more stable state since it is well-known that many resistance genes are transposable. The list of the "jumping genes" in Table 7 is frequently augmented, and recently,

TABLE 7

Plasmid – Associated Transposable Elements

RESISTANCE:	Neomycin, Kanamycin
	Chloramphenicol
	Penicillin, Cephalosporin
	Tetracycline
	Trimethoprim
	Sulphonamides
	Streptomycin
	Gentamicin
	Erythromycin, Lincomycin
	Mercuric Ion
	Methicillin
ENTEROTOXIN:	ST, SEB
CATABOLISM:	Lactose, Raffinose
	Sulphur Compounds
	Histidine

---

the capacity of being transposable has been demonstrated for gentamicin resistance genes. Consequently, the ability of transposons to jump into the chromosome would make them stable and more difficult to eliminate. Thus, rather than the rats leaving the sinking ship when a curing agent is applied, the rats, in this case the resistance determinants, will join an even bigger and better ship, sitting there in the chromosome.

Curing agents, therefore, are not effective. Similar arguments can be raised against agents which might affect transfer mechanisms. The other argument against the use of curing agents concerns their efficiency; they must be absolutely effective, otherwise the few remaining resistant bacteria will grow when antibiotic is re-introduced.

Interference with Enzymatic Modification of Antibiotics

We should now consider a successful approach when enzymes are involved in the determination of resistance by modification of antibiotics. Table 8 give some schemes of interference with enzymatic alteration of antibiotics, and other examples will be discussed.

TABLE 8

Interference with Enzymatic Modification

1. Antibiotic analogue is no longer a substrate, e.g. amikacin.
2. Antibiotic analogue is poor substrate (higher K_m), e.g. 5-*epi*-sisomicin.
3. Antibiotic analogue is enzyme inhibitor, e.g. clavulanic acid (may or may not retain antibiotic activity; may or may not be dead-end inhibitor).

Fluoramphenicols (see Fig. 1) Derivatives of chloramphenicol (*1*), such as (*2*), having a fluorine atom replacing the hydroxyl group in

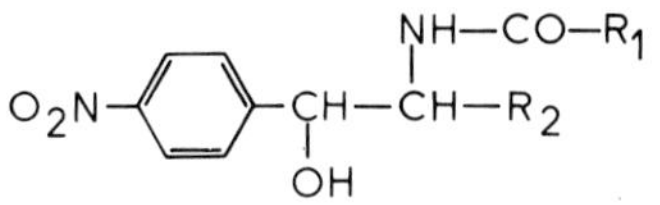

	- R_1	- R_2
1	- $CHCl_2$	- CH_2OH
2	- $CHCl_2$	- CH_2F
3	- CHF_2	- CH_2F

$$O_2N \underset{OH}{\overset{NH-CO-R_1}{- CH - CH - R_2}}$$

FIG. 1 Chloramphenicol derivatives that are not modified by acetyltransferase (CAT).

the 3-position, and (*3*), having moreover, in the side chain, two fluorine instead of the two chlorine atoms, have been recently described and seem to be very effective drugs. They are not modified by any chloramphenicol acetyltransferase (CAT), nor are they inhibitors of the enzyme, but these compounds bind effectively to ribosomes and behave in the same way as the parental compound.

Clavulanic and olivanic acids (see Fig. 2) These β-lactams belong to another class of compounds that interact with β-lactamase, according to a now well documented mechanism. These natural compounds are dead-end inhibitors of β-lactamases. Some of them are simultaneously antibiotics and enzyme inhibitors. Unfortunately,

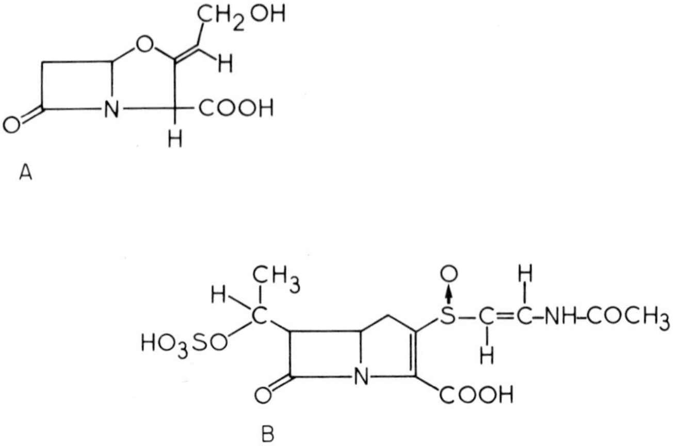

FIG. 2   (A) clavulanic and (B) olivanic acids, inhibitors of β–lactamases.

nature has anticipated that pharmaceutical companies and biochemists will try to develop antiresistance mechanisms at the enzyme level, and in many cases has provided isozymes that are refractory to inhibition. This is true for the β–lactamases, some of which are not as effectively inactivated by these inhibitors.

Aminoglycosides   With the aminoglycoside-modifying enzymes the situation is even worse, since there are some 10 or 12 different enzymes, each of which has isozymic forms varying in their substrate range (Table 9). For the chemist and the biochemist, it is hard to imagine how it would be possible to make a single derivative of an aminoglycoside and expect it to be effective against all strains carrying any one of these enzymes. It should be also pointed out that several of the aminoglycoside-modifying enzymes may be present in the same cell, so that an inhibitor would have to work against several enzymes at the same time.

   A good example of a single enzyme inhibitor is netilmicin, an analogue of sisomicin. Netilmicin is an inhibitor of one acetyltransferase, but unfortunately not of all of them. Figure 3 shows that netilmicin is a substrate but also a competitive inhibitor of this enzyme. After this first success in this area, other modifications have now appeared. Good examples are provided by the 5–*epi* derivatives of sisomicin and gentamicin B (see Fig. 4). The epimerisation of the 5–hydroxy group has a remarkable effect, since it changes completely the conformation of the molecule and affects its ability to be a substrate for several inactivating enzymes, as shown by a

TABLE 9

Aminoglycoside–Aminocyclitol Modifying Enzymes in Resistant Bacteria

Modification	Enzyme	Typical Substrates[a]
Acetylation	AAC (2')	Gentamicin, tobramycin
	AAC (6')	Tobramycin, kanamycin, amikacin, neomycin, gentamicin[b]
	AAC (3)	Gentamicin, tobramycin, kanamycin
Nucleotidylation	ANT (4')	Amikacin, tobramycin, kanamycin
	ANT (2")	Gentamicin, tobramycin, kanamycin
	ANT (3")	Streptomycin, spectinomycin
	ANT (6)	Streptomycin
Phosphorylation	APH (3')	Kanamycin, neomycin
	APH (3")	Streptomycin
	APH (2")	Gentamicin
	APH (5")	Ribostamycin

[a] Not all substrates are listed; each enzyme exists in a variety of forms with different substrate ranges.

[b] Gentamicin C_{1a} is a substrate for AAC (6'); another component of the gentamicin complex, gentamicin C_1, is not.

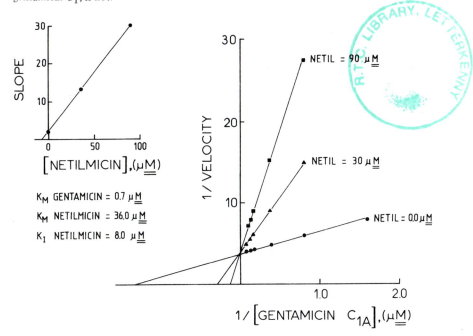

FIG. 3   Kinetics of action of the 3–N–acetyl–transferase from JR 88 strain on gentamicin and inhibition of gentamicin acetylation by netilmycin.

comparison of K_m values for sisomicin and gentamicin B, and their 5–*epi* derivatives for several enzymes (Table 10). Figure 5 shows the

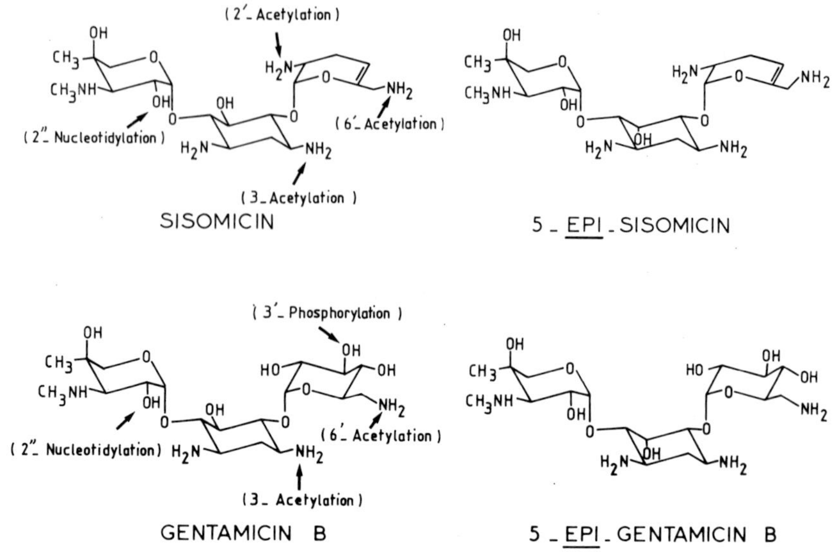

FIG. 4　Structures of sisomicin and gentamicin B and of their 5−*epi* derivatives [Vastola, A.P., Altschaefl, J. and Harford, S. (1980). Antimicrob. Agents Chemother. *17*, 798−802; reprinted with permission of American Society for Microbiology].

TABLE 10

Comparison of the K_m Values of the Aminoglycoside Modifying Enzymes for Antibiotic Substrates

ENZYME	K_m (μM)			
	Sisomicin	5−*epi*−sisomicin	Gentamicin B	5−*epi*−gentamicin B
ANT (2")	<1.0	8.5	<1.0	55.0
APH (3')		1.3		1.1
AAC (3)−I	0.7	94.7	2.1	83.3
AAC (6')	4.3	5.2	3.1	2.8
AAC (2')	0.8	40.0		

[Vastola *et al.*, 1980 (see Fig. 4); reprinted with permission of American Society for Microbiology.]

effect of 5−epimerisation on the kinetics of the enzymatic 3−acetylation of gentamicin B. Furthermore, it should be stressed that the 5−*epi* derivatives compare favourably with a compound presently on the market, amikacin (see Fig. 6), when their substrate activity is estimated for several enzymes as shown in Table 11. But 5−*epi*−sisomicin is only a competitive inhibitor and what is needed are dead-end inhibitors. Although 5−*epi*−sisomicin is not a perfect

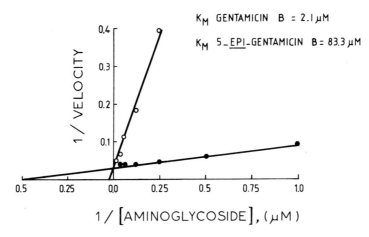

FIG. 5   Kinetics of the 3–acetylation of gentamicin B (−●−) and 5–*epi*–gentamicin B (−○−) by the enzyme AAC (3)–I [Vastola *et al.*, 1980 (see Fig. 4); reprinted with permission of American Society for Microbiology].

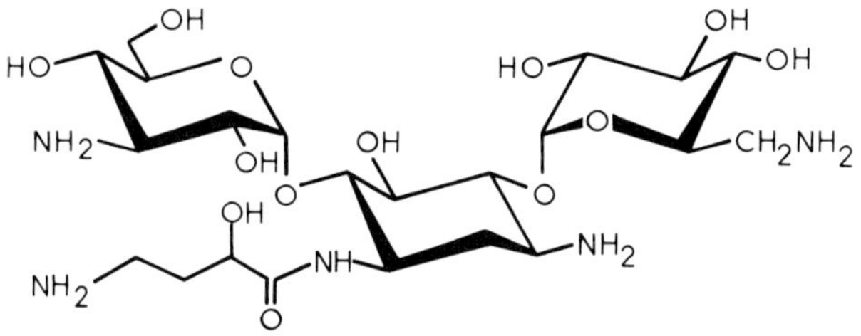

FIG. 6   Structure of amikacin.

antibiotic, it can provide us with a good lead towards overcoming the problem of multiple resistance enzymes.

Finally, there are a number of highly promising antibiotics including interesting new aminoglycosides on the market at the moment, and new natural aminoglycosides such as sorbistin and destomycin have been isolated and offer interesting prospects for the future.

Antibiotic Research Methodology

In future antibiotic research one of the first things to be considered about a new antibiotic will be the mechanism of resistance. There is good circumstantial evidence that models can be found for resistance mechanisms to almost all antibiotics in producing microorganisms, actinomycetes for example. Nearly all the aminoglycoside-modifying enzymes can be found in actinomycetes, either in producing or

TABLE 11

Substrate Activity of Various Inactivating Enzymes Towards Amikacin and 5−*epi*−sisomicin

	AAC(3)	APH(3')	ANT(2")	AAC(2')	AAC(6')	APH(2")
Amikacin (1−N−HABA−kanamycin)	0	+	0	0	++	+
5−*epi*−sisomicin	+	0	+	+	++	+

0 : not detectable or very low substrate activity
+ : weak substrate activity
++ : good substrate activity

non-producing strains. 15 years ago, with our present knowledge, by looking in actinomycetes we could have anticipated the problem of resistance to aminoglycosides and we might have begun to take steps to solve this difficulty earlier. In the future, when dealing with a new antibiotic, it will behove us to look for drug-modifying enzymes in the producing microorganisms and to consider them immediately as potential sources of resistance mechanisms in order to learn how to avoid them.

Conclusion

Although it is easy to paint a black picture about resistance, there are many antibiotics available and in clinical use, for which there is no plasmid-determined mechanism of resistance (Table 12). In the

TABLE 12

Some Antimicrobials in Clinical Use for which no R−Plasmid-Mediated Resistance
is Known

Rifamycins
Vancomycin
Nitrofurans
Nalidixic Acid
Bacitracin
Colistin
Phosphonic Acids (?)
Methicillin (?)

case of phosphonic acids and methicillin resistance, it is unclear whether or not plasmids are involved. But mutations have been found in some cases and, therefore, we have to concern ourselves with resistance by other mechanisms. With the appearance of new and exciting phosphonic acid derivatives which are 100-fold more active than the currently existing ones, chemists should be brought into the group to make these initially nice compounds even better for clinical use.

In this brief paper, I tried to stress the following points: if we are concerned about resistance, there are ways by which it ought to be possible to overcome it. It must be realised, however, that nature will continue to battle against us. In the particular cases where there is no known resistance in spite of much use of the antibiotics, by modifying these compounds and tailoring them to our use, it may still be possible to produce therapeutically useful compounds.

Discussion

Dr. Bost: Could Professor Davies comment on the interest in two compounds he mentioned, sorbistin and destomycin?

Professor Davies: They are two aminocyclitol antibiotics which only have low activity at their present stage of development. Sorbistin, in particular, has no resistance mechanism, as far as I am aware. Destomycin has a resistance mechanism that is present in the cells that make it, so it should be possible to protect against that. In these cases, it is a matter of taking a compound which is perhaps a poor antibiotic and making it into a good one. This is where the help of the chemists is needed.

Dr. Gero: In one case Professor Davies mentioned that the target site might be changed. With erythromycin and lincomycin the target site was altered by methylation or permethylation of the ribosome. Is such a target site alteration known among the aminocyclitol antibiotics?

Secondly, could methylase inhibitors be used to prevent the resistance?

Professor Davies: There are known alterations of target sites with the aminoglycosides, occurring as mutations, but none occurs by enzymatic modification, at least as far as is known.

With regard to methylase inhibitors, I would be concerned about them because the ribosome must be methylated in order to function. A highly specific methylase inhibitor would be required; the kind of specificity requested may be too great. The RNA of ribosomes must be methylated, not necessarily to protect it from antibiotics but in order to function. If the methylation which leads to resistance to erythromycin and lincomycin is blocked, it must be done in such a way that it does not also block methylations occurring in other parts of the RNA. In my view, a general methylase inhibitor will not be effective. Such an inhibitor would be an antibiotic because it would kill the cell, and probably also eukaryotic cells.

Professor Braun: In the case of resistances not conferred by plasmids, for example, phosphonic acids or nitrofurans, which target site might undergo mutation, or is there some way of determining it?

Professor Davies: The target site is known for the phosphonic acids, which are inhibitors of an enzyme used in cell wall synthesis. With the nitrofurans, it is apparently an effect on oxidation–reduction processes, and there are several mutations which can give rise to resistance to nitrofurans, which is one of the difficulties with this class of compounds. It is not clear whether resistance to nitrofurans is due to failure of transport.

Professor Richmond: The approach advocated by Professor Davies is splendid, but is it really practicable? I am worried that he is asking for site-directed irreversible inhibitors, in effect, and of course the whole of enzymology today is dominated by a great interest in them. In those instances in which they have been developed, they have tended to be toxic. The underlying problem here is that in order to have this reactivity there will inevitably be toxicity. Can this be avoided? For example, clavulanic acid is a more reactive β-lactam, it is an inhibitor of certain lactamases and some toxicity problems begin to appear.

Professor Davies: The problems cannot be belittled. There are site-directed enzyme inhibitors, some of which are antibiotics, so I do not think that the approach is so impracticable. But no matter what antibiotic or inhibitory substance is used, the problem of toxicity has to be faced.

Professor Braude: As a layman in this regard, may I ask how often can mutations occur? How frequently does one have to be prepared to deal with them?

Professor Davies: The problem is not so much one of when or how often a mutation occurs, but whether the selective pressure is there to expose it. Clearly, mutations are occurring all the time. Antibiotic-resistant organisms are being produced continually, and most of the time they do not set any problem, since they probably do not compete well with their sensitive relatives. But when a selection is applied — that is, an antibiotic — the resistance is seen, and in that circumstance the resistance is important. Mutations are only exposed when the selection pressure is present.

Professor Chabbert: It would be important to me to be able to discriminate between genes which might be transposable and those which might not. For instance, with the cephalosporins, after 20 years we apparently have no idea about the possible transposition of the genes. Those genes responsible for resistance to cephalosporins are apparently not transposable. Does Professor Davies think that in the future the situation will be the same, or may become clearer?

Professor Davies: That is asking me to make wild predictions! I am sure that any gene has the capacity to become transposable. In particular, when talking about resistance plasmids and about the selective pressure of antibiotics, the probability is much higher of a resistance determinant becoming transposable than is the probability of transposition of any structural gene. There are reasons for wanting to create new plasmids which will survive in different strains. The way to do this is by the selective pressure of antibiotics, followed by transposition.

Adhesive Properties of *E.coli* Strains Isolated from Urine: Presentation of an *"In Vivo"* Study Model

G. CHABANON

Laboratoire de Bactériologie et de Virologie,
C.H.U. Rangueil, Toulouse, France

Introduction

The very general term "bacterial adhesion" is defined as the ability of some microorganisms to bind firmly to surfaces of various types. Adhesion is not an exclusive property of one, or even a few, particular microbial species; the surfaces of either inert solid objects or living animal or plant cells can constitute the material support for adhesion.

The role of adhesion in the implantation and persistence of a bacterial population in a given area is often evoked, which emphasizes the important and very remarkable place that such a property holds in understanding the ecology of the microbial world. This property is not only found in the microbial species which normally make up the commensal flora in the natural cavities of man and animals, but also in pathogenic or potentially pathogenic bacteria for which adhesion is an important element of pathogenicity.

It has recently been demonstrated that some *E. coli* strains which are isolated from urine can bind to the surface of various cells and that, when this property exists, it can be an important factor in pathogenesis.

The present paper is divided into three parts. Firstly, I will describe an original model for *in vitro* detection of bacterial adhesive properties; I must emphasize that tests of this kind have only been made on *E. coli* strains isolated during urinary tract infection. Secondly, I will give the first results from a study on the various surface structures of bacteria which may be involved in adhesion and finally, I will discuss the role of *E. coli* adhesion in the clinical expression of urinary tract infection.

Study of Adhesive Properties

The first publications dealing with the systematic study of the adhesive properties of *E. coli* strains isolated from urine describe test models using a support of cells of human origin.

These cells can be:

1) desquamated cells from the urinary tract; found in the urine they are a handy source and serve as the basis of C. Svanborg's method for the detection of bacterial adhesion by collecting exfoliated epithelial cells which are normally found in urine (Svanborg-Eden, 1976). In general, most of these cells belong to one of two categories: they are either transitional epithelial cells from the urinary bladder, or squamous cells which, in women, originate on the surface of the external genital organs and on the trigone of the bladder;

2) vaginal cells collected for the same purpose by vaginal rinsing or scraping (Mardh and Weström, 1976; Fowler and Stamey, 1977);

3) finally, cells from the external urethral orifice or the urethral canal, collected by swabbing (Mardh *et al.*, 1979).

Two characteristics are common to all cells used in adhesion tests, whatever their origin. Firstly, the surface of the cells obtained may be covered with saprophytic flora; this is particularly frequent in vaginal and perimeatic cells and even repeated washing cannot eliminate such bacteria when they are well bound. The presence of these bacteria makes any adhesion test very difficult to perform, particularly in its final count. Secondly, the majority of these cells are already desquamated or are about to be; if the vitality of these cells is checked by staining at the time of testing, many are found to be dead. For this reason, we feel that it is essential to carefully check cell vitality before the test is conducted.

In our study of adhesion by *E. coli* strains isolated from urine, we chose a monolayer of cells cultured *in vitro* as the support (Hartley *et al.*, 1978; Chabanon *et al.*, 1979). Several considerations guided our choice. At first, cultured cells constitute an identical support from one experiment to another; it is not the case when cells are obtained from donors. In addition, this method is easy to carry out and the absence of endogenic bacteria offers a total guarantee in the quantitative assessment of adhesion. Above all, the vitality of the cells is preserved, a characteristic which is of highest value in all studies on interactions between the support cell and the bacteria during the process of adhesion.

The principal steps in the adhesion test are the following:

1) Preparation of the cell monolayer. We use an epithelial cell line of human origin which was initially obtained from human foetal intestine. It is marketed by Flow Laboratories under the reference: Intestine Cell Line 407, ATCC CCL6. The cells are grown on a glass cover slip surface for 2 days in individual tubes in 1.8 ml of BME medium containing, in addition, foetal calf serum, sodium bicarbonate and streptomycin.

2) Preparation of a culture of the bacterial strain to be tested. Bacteria are grown during 18 h at 37°C in stationary liquid medium containing yeast extract, then centrifuged and resuspended in phosphate-buffered saline (PBS) (pH 7.2) to give a final cell density of about 10^{10} bacteria/ml.

3) Incubation of bacteria and cells. The cell line monolayer is washed twice with PBS and then 10^9 bacteria are added to each tube. The test tubes are incubated at 37°C for 30 min. without any shaking. At the end of the bacteria/cell contact period, the monolayer is washed several times to eliminate unbound bacteria. Then, after fixing, the cells are Giemsa stained.

4) Interpretation of the adhesion test. The stained cells are examined under a microscope and the bacteria bound to the surface of 10 cells in one microscope field are counted; 20 microscope fields are examined in succession (Fig. 1). The adhesion index is given by the mean number of bacteria on the surface of one cell. The adhesion index is used to class the different bacterial strains as very adherent [20 bacteria or more per cell, (++)], adherent [less than 20 bacteria per cell, (+)] or non adherent [no bacteria, (−)] (Chabanon *et al.*, 1979).

Two remarks should be made concerning the actual adhesion test. First, the bacterial inoculum used for the test contains about 10^9 bacteria. A tenfold decrease in the inoculated bacterial population leads to a very marked fall in the number of bound bacteria. Secondly, the contact time between bacteria and cells is 30 min at 37°C. With our system, incubation for one hour does not significantly increase the number of bound bacteria; beyond this time, the bacteria have a direct toxic effect which results in progressive loosening of the cell monolayer.

Study of Bacterial Surface

Whatever the nature of the mechanisms involved in the adhesion process, all of them are related to the presence of compounds or particular structures on the surface of the adhering bacteria, but these "adhesion factors" can be very different according to the bacterium strain or species.

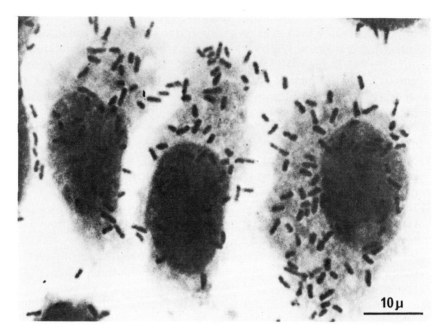

FIG. 1   Microscopic aspect of *E. coli* bacteria adherent to cell surface (bar = 10 μ).

In the present situation, what we want to know is whether fimbrial structures are eventually responsible for the adhesiveness of *E. coli* strains isolated from urine, as it has been described for strains causing acute diarrhoea in man and animals.

The morphology of fimbriae was first described during the 1950s; they are filamentary appendices, 8 to 10 nm wide, situated around the edges of the bacteria, but their appearence is radically different from that of the flagellae (Fig. 2). A close relationship was early established by Duguid (1955) between the ability of certain strains of *E. coli* to bind to and agglutinate red blood cells (RBC) and the presence of fimbriae on the surface of these bacteria. But the interest raised by haemagglutination properties of *E. coli*, which were recognised since the beginning of this century, was further aroused by the discovery of quite particular K antigen from enteropathogenic *E. coli* in man, piglets and calves. When this type of antigen, which is a protein rather than a polysaccharide, is present, it enables the bacteria to adhere to the surface of the intestinal epithelium and to colonise the upper part of the small intestine. This antigen is a haemagglutinin (HA) with a fimbrial structure. It is indexed according to the host from which such *E. coli* are isolated; for example, CFA I and II in human strains and K88 and K99 in animal strains are among

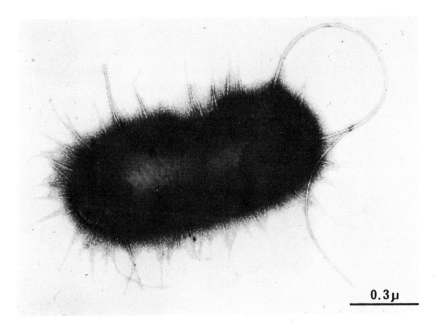

FIG. 2   Morphology of fimbriae in *E. coli* (bar = 0.3 μ).

the most well known. However, an important distinction must be made among *E. coli* haemagglutinins based on the fact that some of them cannot agglutinate red blood cells when D—mannose is present in the culture medium; they are called mannose-sensitive haemagglutinins (MS—HA). Other haemagglutinins are unaffected by the presence of D—mannose and are therefore said to be mannose-resistant (MR—HA). In addition, when the agglutinated bodies induced with these MR—HA are heated slightly, the bacteria come off the surface of the red blood cells and the agglutinated bodies dissociate. This type of reversible HA is called EMR—HA (E:eluting). In a recent general review, Duguid (1979) listed the various properties which characterise these two types of HA found in *E. coli*. We should add to his description by mentioning that the K antigens of enteropathogenic *E. coli* are HA of the EMR type.

What about the possible relationships between the presence of fimbriae and the adhesive property of *E. coli* isolated from urine? The first part of our study had three aims: (1) to systematically test the presence of haemagglutinins in adherent and non adherent *E. coli* isolated from urine; (2) to analyse the effect of culture temperature and heating on both HA activity and adhesion in *E. coli*; (3) to detect the presence of fimbriae in adherent *E. coli* with and without the ability to agglutinate red blood cells by using electron microscopy (E.M.).

I must make it especially clear that the same bacterial suspension was used for the haemagglutinin test and for visualisation of fimbriae and was prepared by culture in liquid medium until the stationary phase, as for the adhesion test.

Initially, RBCs from humans and various animals (guinea-pig, horse, rabbit, sheep and cow) were tested in parallel for HA. It became rapidly apparent that human and guinea-pig RBCs were the most frequently agglutinated and that agglutination rarely occurred with RBCs of the other species. In addition, *E. coli* strains which agglutinate human and guinea-pig RBCs also agglutinate RBCs from other animal species. The results reported in this paper therefore concern tests for HA using only human and guinea-pig RBCs. Our study revealed various phenomena:

1) HA is encountered almost as frequently in adherent *E. coli* as in non adherent *E. coli* (40% and 57.5% respectively), towards man and guinea-pig RBCs (Table 1).

TABLE 1

Haemagglutination by *E. coli* Strains Isolated from Urine

Erythrocytes from[a]		Number of active strains	
Man	Guinea-pig	Adherent	Non-adherent
+	−	2	5
−	+	1	15
+	+	5	3
Total active strains		8	23
Number of tested strains		20	40
Active strains %		40	57.5

[a] (+) agglutination   (−) no agglutination

2) The expression of HA activity does not depend on a specific blood group (A, B, AB and 0 group RBCs may or may not be agglutinated). The same is true for the Rh factor. However, *E. coli* strains which agglutinate guinea-pig erythrocytes most often belong to the non adherent group of bacteria.

3) There is usually no correlation between the amount of HA, when present, and the intensity of adhesion.

4) When HA in adherent strains is studied, it proves to be MR in 87.5% of cases and without associated elution, but it must be mentioned that our study did not provide the ideal conditions

recommended by Duguid (1979) for testing this last phenomenon; MR–HA is encountered less frequently in non adherent strains (34.7%). The HA from non adherent *E. coli* strains is most frequently MS and acts exclusively on guinea-pig RBCs. We found only one strain in which a MS–HA was present along with the adhesive property (Table 2).

TABLE 2

Sensitivity to Mannose of Haemagglutination by Active *E. coli* Strains

Erythrocytes[a] from		Number of agglutinating strains			
		Adherent		Non-adherent	
Man	Guinea-pig	MR[b]	MS[b]	MR[b]	MS[b]
+	–	2	0	5	0
–	+	0	1	0	15
+	+	5	0	3	0
Total		7	1	8	15
Grand total			8		23
%		87.5	12.5	34.7	65.3

[a] (+) agglutination   (–) no agglutination

[b] MR = mannose-resistant HA   MS = mannose-sensitive HA

5) After being cultured at 18°C, all *E. coli* strains which normally have MR- or MS–HA are unable to agglutinate RBCs. Under similar conditions, the adhesive property is clearly reduced in intensity or even becomes undetectable, particularly in *E. coli* devoid of HA under normal conditions (Table 3).

6) The effect produced by heating the bacterial suspension for one hour at different temperatures is much less clear. Globally, HA seems to be more heat-sensitive than the adhesive property, since at 65°C three out of five strains which were tested kept their ability to adhere whereas HA could no longer be detected or had greatly reduced activity. It must be emphasised that, in spite of heating at 80°C, one *E. coli* strain is still able to adhere to a cellular support (Table 3).

7) Only adherent strains were examined for fimbriae using an electron microscope. Only one of the bacterial strains which had HA activity did not present any fimbriae and, with only one exception, fimbriae were never found when HA was absent. On a simple EM image, it is not possible to differentiate MS–HA from MR–HA; the fimbriae are morphologically identical.

A few comments should be made on these first results. More than half of the adherent *E. coli* strains that we examined did not have

TABLE 3

Effect of Growth Temperature and Heating of Bacteria on Haemagglutination and
Adhesion Index of *E. coli* Strains Isolated from Urine

E. coli strains No	Pilia[a]	Erythrocytes[b] from		Haemagglutination[c]				Adhesion Index[d]			
				growth temperature		heating temperature		growth temperature		heating temperature	
		man	guinea-pig	18°C	37°C	65°C	80°C	18°C	37°C	65°C	80°C
1	+	+	−	−	+++	−	−	17	45	38	0
2	−	+	−	−	+	−	−	13	29	21	0
3	+	−	+	−	++	+	−	26	52	49	21
4	+	+	+	−	++	−	−	0	12	0	0
5	+	+	+	−	+++	+	−	1	81	1	0
6	−	−	−	−	−	−	−	0	81	0	0
7	−	−	−	−	−	−	−	0	33	1	0
8	+	−	−	−	−	−	−	0	64	55	0
9	−	−	−	−	−	−	−	0	11	1	0

[a] from electron microscopy

[b] (+) agglutination   (−) no agglutination

[c] agglutination: (+++) strong,   (++) mean,   (+) weak,   (−) no

[d] mean number of adherent bacteria per cell

any detectable surface HA. In addition, in some strains, the adhesive property existed without any fimbrial structures. Thus, this first study does not seem to indicate a fundamental difference between the MS−HA and MR−HA encountered in adherent or non adherent *E. coli*; but complementary studies should be conducted to confirm or refute this particular point.

When the adhesive property and a HA are both present, the HA is usually MR and occasionally MS. We were able to study an adherent strain with a MR−HA in more detail; adhesion was also D−mannose resistant in this particular case. This observation contradicts other recently published results which suggest that type I fimbriae or pili, i.e. a MS−HA, could also be responsible for adhesion in *E. coli* isolated from urine. If this is the case, D−mannose has an inhibitory effect not only on HA, but also on adhesion itself. On this point, I would like to mention that some enteropathogenic *E. coli* have a special K antigen which is a MR−HA bestowing the adhesive property.

Experiments on bacterial strains cultured at 18°C do not afford the expected arguments for understanding the process of adhesion. Even though the adhesive property and the K88 antigen, in piglet strains for example, are no longer detectable at this temperature, a study carried out long ago showed that other components of the bacterial surface, for example *Salmonella typhi* Vi antigen, are not synthesized under these culture conditions. The effect of the lower culture temperature is therefore too global and is not selectively limited to a single compound of the bacterial surface.

Some distinction might have been made between polysaccharide and protein compounds and their respective roles in adhesion by heating the strains. Here again, the effect obtained seems too global and is not very distinct.

The presence of a HA is not necessarily linked with the presence of fimbriae. This fact was reported by Duguid (1979) and is confirmed by our study.

When I presented the adhesion test which we currently use, I specified that one of the reasons for our choice was the fact that we found it very worthwhile to work with a cellular support in which vitality is ensured. Thus the *in situ* relationship between the adhering bacteria and the cellular support during the adhesion process can in fact be better revealed. For this study, we chose two adherent strains of *E. coli*, one of which has a MR—HA and fimbriae, the other has neither. The EM study was guided by the desire to discover if adherent *E. coli* devoid of HA had a surface structure which could be the molecular support for adhesion. Several observations were made:

1) A section prepared at the end of the adhesion test, then stained with uranyl acetate and lead citrate, shows the different constituents of the eucaryotic cell: the nucleus and a nucleolus, both surrounded by a thin layer of cytoplasm. The surface of the cell is irregular and slightly convex with bacteria adhering to the cytoplasmic membrane. At a higher magnification, the bacteria are seen to be adhering to the cell surface either directly or by means of cytoplasmic prolongations. This type of image is obtained with both strains of adherent *E. coli* whether or not they possess HA.

2) Specific staining of acid polysaccharides with ruthenium red reveals a very clear difference between the two strains. The one which has HA has a rough surface but the general appearance is that very frequently encountered in Gram-negative bacteria of the same family (Fig. 3). However, in the strain which is devoid of HA, a compound with an architectural structure and staining affinity resembling those of a glycocalyx is seen around the borders of the bacteria. The disposition can be seen more clearly at a higher magnification (Fig. 4).

3) A scanning microscope study further emphasises the relationships between the bacteria and the surface of the cellular support. In culture, the surface of the cell is normally spotted with small

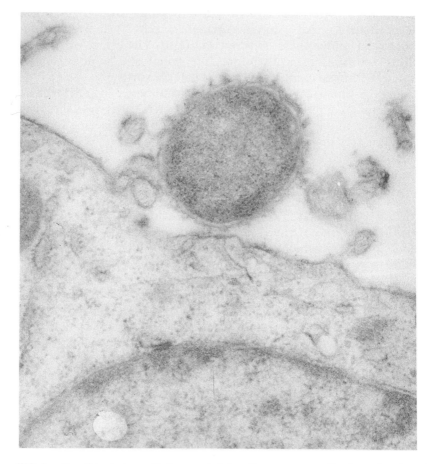

FIG. 3   *E. coli* bacterium with haemagglutinin adherent to one cell, after coloration of acid polysaccharide compounds by ruthenium red (x 68,200).

protrusions but when bacteria adhere, veritable microvilli emerge and attach them to the cell (Fig. 5).

Adhesion and Clinical Expression of Infection

The third and last part of this paper is devoted to the study of the role of *E. coli* adhesion in the clinical expression of urinary tract infection (UTI). In other words, what danger does a subject with UTI face through adherent bacteria?

The study covered 212 *E. coli* specimens isolated from the urine of two groups of patients: 17 subjects had acute or chronic pyelonephritis, and the other 195 subjects presented the usual clinical signs of uncomplicated acute cystitis.

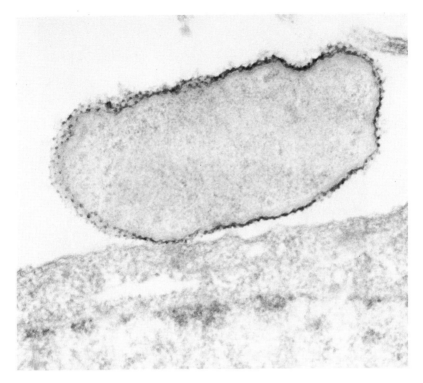

FIG. 4   *E. coli* bacterium without heamagglutinin adherent to one cell, after coloration by ruthenium red (x 68,200).

Three factors were considered in assessing the role of adhesion in the expression of UTI. Initially, the percentages of adherent and non adherent strains of *E. coli* isolated in acute cystitis were determined: only 19 strains (9.7%) had the property. Secondly, we sought for a relationship between bacterial adhesion and the clinical expression of cystitis when an adherent strain is isolated from urine: adhesion does not appear to influence either dysuria (either in frequency or intensity) or the frequency of miction or UTI relapse (when it occurs); however manifest haematuria is encountered more frequently during infection by adherent bacteria as shown in Table 4 where the observations on 19 already mentioned adherent strains are tabulated besides 19 other non-adherent strains. The difference is significant. Finally, a comparative study of number of adherent *E. coli* isolated in acute cystitis and pyelonephritis leads to the conclusion that adherent strains are encountered more frequently in acute pyelonephritis (respectively 9.7% and 29.4% of the isolated strains) (Chabanon *et al.*, 1979).

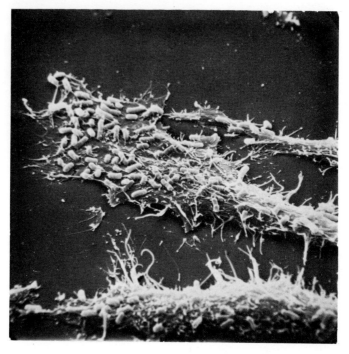

FIG. 5   Aspect under electron microscope of *E. coli* bacteria adherent to cells (x 2800).

TABLE 4

Repartition of *E. coli* Strains in Acute Cystitis in Relation to Haematuria

Haematuria in acute cystitis[a]	Number of *E. coli* strains		Total
	Adherent	Non-adherent	
+	8	2	10
0	11	17	28
Total	19	19	

[a] haematuria (+) present or (0) absent.

Conclusion

I would like to emphasise two points which, I feel, are essential. The first is that it has now been conclusively demonstrated that the adhesive property is an indisputable factor of virulence in strains which possess it. This observation again reinforces the "theory of specific pathogenicity" which is often evoked in the genesis of urinary tract infection. However adhesion alone can certainly not be responsible for the pathogenicity of urinary tract infection.

The second point concerns the future. Can we hope to interfere with this property in order to reduce the implantation and persistence of these bacteria, in short, the colonisation of the urinary tract? With our current knowledge, it is not easy to reply to this question. Several types of different structures are quite probably involved in adhesion; this implies a corresponding diversity in the possible inhibitory molecules. It can also be thought that the process of *E. coli* adhesion is composed of many steps which involve just as many different intermediaries, as it has been described for some streptococci. It was recently shown that various antibiotics can play such an inhibitory role (Svanborg-Eden *et al.*, 1978; Vosbeck *et al.*, 1979). Is this just a hope? It is still too early to know.

References

Chabanon, G., Hartley, C.L. and Richmond, M.H. (1979). *J. Clin. Microbiol.* **10**, 563–566.

Duguid, J.P., Glegg, S. and Wilson, M.I. (1979). *J. Med. Microbiol.* **12**, 213–227.

Duguid, J.P., Smith, I.W., Dempster, G. and Edmunds, P.N. (1955). *J. Path. Bacteriol.* **70**, 335–348.

Fowler, J.E., Jr. and Stamey, A. (1977). *J. Urol.* **117**, 472–476.

Hartley, L., Robbins, C.M. and Richmond, M.H. (1978). *J. Appl. Bacteriol.* **45**, 91–97.

Mardh, P.A. and Weström, L. (1976). *Infect. Immun.* **13**, 661–666.

Mardh, P.A., Colleen, S. and Hovelius, B. (1979). *Invest. Urol.* **16**, 322–326.

Svanborg-Eden, C., Hanson, L.A., Jodal, U., Lindberg, U. and Sohl-Akerlund, A. (1976). *Lancet* **II**, 490–492.

Svanborg-Eden, C., Sanberg, T., Stenquist, K. and Ahlstedt, S. (1978). *Infection* **6**, (Suppl. 1), 121–124.

Vosbeck, K., Handschin, H., Menge, E.B. and Zak, O. (1979). *Rev. Infect. Dis.* **1**, 845–851.

Discussion

Dr. Salem: I was fascinated by Dr. Chabanon's presentation. In our laboratories we have been working on a similar system, generated in order to study some new compounds with regard to their properties of inhibiting bacterial adherence. It is an *in vitro* system in which the cells used are human bladder carcinoma cells, and the organism is an *Escherichia coli* from a human urinary tract infection. With this system we have found that the adherence is not antagonised by mannose. Haemagglutination has not been investigated. We have confirmed the observation made by other people of inhibition by certain antimicrobial agents, notably ampicillin and nalidixic acid, in this system at concentrations below their m.i.c. against the particular strain being used. Further, of the large number of new compounds that we have screened, all except one of about 12 compounds which seemed to give interesting inhibition of bacterial adherence have antibacterial activity at higher concentration.

Can Dr. Chabanon comment on how far anti-adherence activity might contribute to the antibacterial efficacy of these compounds *in vivo*, by referring to known antibiotics, for example, ampicillin and nalidixic acid?

Secondly, does he believe that there is a role for compounds which purely inhibit bacterial adherence, in the treatment, for instance, of urinary tract infections?

Dr. Chabanon: The problem of adherence in the case of urinary tract infection is such that at the present time we should really know what we are faced with, as far as the molecular support of adherence is concerned. This is the essential point. Our first work seems to show that there are several possible behaviours of the bacteria which lead to the same effect, in other words adherence, so there are several possibilities. We can have mannose-resistant bacteria which can be adherent and in other cases we have a sensitive haemagglutination which works together with adherence. So we have to try and find out what is the responsibility of adherence, what is the responsibility of HA because there are some non HA bacteria which do adhere. Now, regarding the activity of a small dose of antibiotics, one of the most spectacular effects is due to tetracyclines, but they are not used for urinary tract infections. Ampicillin and nalidixic acid are probably more important. At the present time, I have not much of a personal opinion on this, because I have not worked on it long enough to give you general ideas about the interest of these products. However, if we do not want to go further into the analysis of the molecular structure responsible for adherence, we will have to take the problem from the other side. In other words, we will have to try and find out whether these products, whether these antibiotics, have an overall inhibitory effect on adherence in all strains, or on a lot of strains responsible for urinary tract infections. When you tested this, you probably used one strain and one product. But it seems that in fact there are several molecular types which are responsible for adherence. So if we do not want to go any further in the study of the molecular support, we will have to study more strains.

Professor Waldvogel: I would like to know whether, in your system, you tried to test the kinetics of adherence by adding up increasing concentrations of immunoglobulins against *E. coli* or against the pili. Second question: in order to validate the model as a biological model, did you try to modify your medium, as far as ion strength, pH and urea concentration are concerned, in order to approximately reconstitute the different conditions of normal urine.

Dr. Chabanon: As far as immunoglobulins are concerned, I think that everything that has been mentioned until now does not seem to be very strict to me. The antibodies usually used are agglutinating antibodies and if you agglutinate bacteria, you certainly interfere with adherence. Now, if you want to make tests with immunoglobulins, you need immunoglobulins that have been modified somehow beforehand, for example which have been partially cleaved in order to prevent them from agglutinating. This point is essential.

Now, about the pH and urea variations and others, there are in fact some discussions going on between various laboratories in Europe. It has been said that glucose had an inhibitory effect on the expression of bacterial adherence.

From the very beginning, I have always used a 1% glucose medium and bacteria do adhere. So I do not think that this constituent interferes as much as is being said. Concerning the pH, if you lower its value to about 4, then adherence does disappear. But in other tests at this pH, the cell monolayer disintegrates, so you cannot really carry out the test except with cell suspensions. The principle of our test is to have a solid support, as a cell layer, so it is prohibited to wash it thoroughly to assess the adherence. For this reason, we used PBS, pH 7.2. As to urea effect, I have not tested it myself.

Professor Tomasz: Did you test specificity in these interesting adhesion experiments; and was there any specificity with respect to the type of epithelial cell used?

Dr. Chabanon: As far as specificity of adherence is concerned, the tests we carried out could be questionable because we only used one reference strain which is just the first one we isolated from pyelonephritis. However, we see that there are two kinds of specificity. The first one is an histological or cellular specificity. In other words, when we take the cells from the same donor, for example from one animal or from one man, then we come across a problem. We find that there is a very good bacterial adherence on epithelial cells but the adherence on fibroblastic cells is practically zero. Now, when we test the adherence on the same type of cells, for instance epithelial cells coming from man or various animals, results are slightly different according to the source. Due to our visual method, it is not really possible to say whether the difference is significant or not. Apparently, the adherence is less intense with pig cells than with human cells. The same conclusion is true with other cell lines.

As Dr. Salem did, we also used a cell line coming from a bladder tumour, but we rapidly gave it up because it grew poorly in culture and, as a transformed cell, it was very different from a normal cell.

Professor Tomasz: Together with Drs. Frank Lawey and Neal Steigbigel of the Montefiore Medical Center in New York, we did some experiments using the rabbit heart model described by Professor Sande. The rabbits, which had traumatised heart valves, were injected with one to one mixtures of two *Streptococcus sanguis* cultures which were genetically marked. One of the component cultures was also pretreated with penicillin *in vitro*. As I mentioned this morning these bacteria are very difficult to kill by penicillin treatment *in vitro*. The treatment we applied was sufficient to cause the release of about 85% of the acylated lipoteichoic acids and about 40% of the lipids of the cells but the bacteria remained viable. After the mixture of cells were injected into the rabbits the animals were sacrificed; the heart valves were removed and the number of the adhering bacteria from the two genetically marked populations were determined. There was a very large difference in the titres, as if the penicillin pretreatment prevented the cells from effectively adhering to the heart valves.

Professor Sabath: First, I saw electron micrographs by Costerton showing enormous glycocalyx secreted by microorganisms grown in the bladders of animals, and also grown artificially. Did Dr. Chabanon take organisms directly from animals before measuring the adherence, to see whether there might be a greater degree of adherence when they are grown in an animal than when they come out of artificial media?

Secondly, concerning the specificity or the individual variation of the cell source to which there is adherence, as Dr. Chabanon probably knows, there is one school of thought which believes that, in patients with recurrent urinary tract infections, there is a greater adherence of faecal organisms to the vaginal vestibular cells than in individuals who do not have recurrent infection. This obviously raises a question about whether receptors are different in different human beings. Could Dr. Chabanon comment on differences in propensity for adherence in the host cell?

Dr. Chabanon: I shall answer first the second question. Some work has shown that women who had recurrent urinary tract infections, had vaginal cells that in fact fixed bacteria better. At the present time, the problem is that in adherence, the cell is not passive. The scanning microscopy pictures have shown it. There is in fact a cellular factor and a bacterial one, which must be studied altogether.

Second point: the *in vivo* culture of the bacteria to be tested; I did not study that precisely, but I looked at urinary strains from pigs to find whether there was any adherence on human cells; there was some. Nevertheless, I do not maintain that the strains are different in pigs and in humans.

Professor Acar: I shall just follow on what has just been asked by Dr. Sabath. I would like to know how you maintain your strains and if you checked the reproducibility of the adherence tests. A number of contradictory results are actually due to the fact that some people worked with strains coming from urinary infections, but without the same number of subcultures from the time of isolation. I would like to know whether you homogenised your group of urinary tract infections and whether you have any idea about the stability of the adherence property.

Dr. Chabanon: Very briefly, I would say that when we started this work, we were looking systematically for adherence of bacteria harvested on the urine test plates and just transferred on an agar slant medium. Later on, in most cases, we used bacteria after 5 or 6 subcultures. We did not find any major difference, but, for 2 strains out of our stock, there was a middle adherence property that disappeared. In fact, this raises the question of a possible plasmidic support, but limited tests we carried out with Professor Richmond on one strain demonstrated no plasmid.

Immunomodulating Activities of Antibiotics

P.H. LAGRANGE

Unité d'Immunophysiologie Cellulaire
Institut Pasteur, Paris, France

Introduction

In vitro antibiotics inhibit the growth of microorganisms or kill them: usually their activity is expressed by the minimal inhibitory concentration (m.i.c.). *In vivo* the main effect of antibiotics is also an antibacterial one. They reduce thereby the extent of changes induced by bacteria in the infected tissues and therefore may facilitate the natural mechanisms of defence and recovery which are more or less impaired by the infection. Thus, in many cases, the antibacterial activities measured *in vitro* and estimated in animals during experimental infection are in good agreement. However many reports in the literature indicate some discrepancies between *in vitro* potencies and responses observed in humans after antibiotherapy. Thus, for the last several years, the importance of natural resistance factors in the host has been emphasised as a primary determinant of antibiotherapy efficiency (Weinstein and Dalton, 1968). Hence several questions arise with respect to the activity of antibiotics on the immune response of an infected host. This response must be looked upon as a whole, including the specific and non specific mechanisms of antimicrobial protection.

Is the antibiotic treatment taking part in the healing mechanisms, and if so, is it synergistic, additive, antagonistic, or indifferent? Is there any interference between the antibiotic treatment and the induction of acquired resistance? Or is there any impairment of specific protecting functions normally induced during an infection? Finally, does antibiotherapy modify the natural outcome of infection, especially at the level of post-infectious immunopathologic phenomena?

Answers to these various questions were already partially given. But some uncertainties remain, which perhaps proceed from the different methodologies used by the authors dealing with these subjects.

As a matter of fact, several approaches may be selected when measuring the impact of antibiotics on the immune system, as indicated in Fig. 1. The evolution of a microbial infection depends

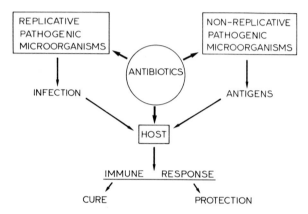

FIG. 1   Various impacts of antibiotics in the host-bacteria conflict.

on the capacity of bacteria to penetrate, grow, elaborate different metabolites – and on the power of host defence mechanisms. Then, the study of the mode of action of antibiotics must consider either the host's immune response or the infectious agent.

Effect of Antibiotics on the Immune Response

This effect may be analysed either in an infected individual or in a normal one.

The first attitude is a global approach *in vivo*, where it is often difficult to pinpoint the mechanism of action of antibiotics and to obtain other than indirect proofs. However some direct and indirect relationships between antimicrobial efficacy of an antibiotic and the immune response may be inferred. Here too, several experimental schemes have been considered.

With respect to the time of infection the treatment may be either simultaneous or delayed, either continuous or discontinuous. The infection rate may be estimated by counting either the number of survivors among the treated animals following infection with a lethal inoculum or the viable bacterial population in the target-organs. The models using infected normal animals usually give an estimate of the

antimicrobial therapy efficacy and of the experimental pharmacokinetics. In this way, the *in vivo* effect of antibiotics is estimated
from their direct antibacterial activity, which reduces the pathological effects of infection. For many antibiotics, particularly the
bactericidal ones the efficacy *in vitro* and *in vivo* are in good agreement. But such studies on antibiotics only take into account their
in vivo efficacy and not at all their indirect effect on the immune
defence mechanisms.

This last effect may be estimated by treating normal animals with
bacteriostatic antibiotics, or with bactericidal ones at subinhibitory
levels. Moreover particular animals deprived of one particular defence
system may be used. In this respect the study of Eagle *et al.* (1953)
on the optimal conditions for penicillin efficacy showed the relationships between the bactericidal and bacteriostatic properties and the
host defence. A single large dose was able to inhibit the growth of a
pneumococcus inoculum in mice as efficiently as *in vitro.* However
ultimately the surviving bacteria were able to kill the treated animals.
On the contrary, they survived when they had been previously
immunised. This led to the notion of potentialisation by an antibiotic of defence mechanisms which are ineffective during the first
step of bacterial disappearance. Such a synergism between bacteriostatic antimicrobials and antibodies was demonstrated several years
ago, particularly for sulfonamides (Fleming, 1938).

The studies on dependence of the antibiotic activity upon the
host's defence mechanisms have been experimentally performed with
immuno-deprived and infected animals. For instance in rabbits
exhibiting granulocytopenia induced by benzene injection, penicillin
cures the cutaneous wounds created by a pneumococcus injection
without any surrounding leucocytosis reaction (Gowans, 1953).
However, such an independence is not always as complete. In this
manner during a study on the survival of animals irradiated before
a systemic infection, the antibiotherapy, on an equal basis, is less
effective for these animals than for the normal ones (Marcus *et al.*,
1955). A bone marrow graft may restore the antibiotic effectiveness
(Byron *et al.*, 1964).

The same lack of *in vivo* efficacy of antibiotics, even with normally
active doses, has been observed in man in the course of immunosuppressive therapy, either in cancer patients or in patients receiving
transplants (Acar *et al.*, 1973). Moreover, regarding some intracellularly growing bacteria, like *Mycobacterium tuberculosis* or
Brucella melitensis, the *in vivo* antibiotic inefficacy, in comparison
with the *in vitro* activity may be related to the difficulty of
penetration into the infected cells. For instance the streptomycin

concentration inhibiting growth of the tubercle bacillus within macrophages is 200 times higher than the normal one *in vitro* (Mackaness and Smith, 1953). However this seems not to be true any longer when the macrophage is activated by an immune thymodependent reaction: in this situation, there is an extensive accumulation of antibiotics inside the secondary lysosomes (d'Arcy-Hart, 1974). The difference observed between *in vitro* and *in vivo* could be related to the pathogenic effect peculiar to mycobacteria which hinders the phagosome–lysosome fusion. This does not restrict the antibiotic accumulation within the normal macrophages, but inhibits its discharge into phagocyte vacuoles. In preimmunised mice a synergism with antibiotics may appear, since the fusion within the macrophage activated by an immune response is no longer inhibited.

Another type of synergism between antibiotics and immune reactions has been observed particularly when antibiotics acting on some bacteria *in vivo* prevent the formation of virulence factors. Thus, the accumulation of phagocytes inside infectious sites is higher in treated infected animals than in untreated ones (Kollath and Raabe, 1943). This could be explained by a reduction in the formation of phagocytosis-inhibiting factors. Still these effects seem simultaneous and unspecific. In other cases some relationship could exist between the appearance of pathogenicity factors and the sensitivity to antibiotics. Without emphasising the antibiotic effect on the natural flora, which are ecosystems actively inhibiting the potentially pathogenic bacteria (Sanders *et al.*, 1976), the existence of a BCG strain, selected for its streptomycin resistance, must be recalled. This mutant is able to grow *in vitro* in the presence or not of streptomycin, but is unable to multiply *in vivo* in mice. However mice infected with this mutant do not present any acquired immunity, as shown by a challenge test, nor do they exhibit any delayed hypersensitivity reaction (Mackaness *et al.*, 1973). Such an example shows how necessary is *in vivo* growth for evoking cell-mediated immunity against bacteria which grow intracellularly.

This fact has been confirmed in another way by using anti-tuberculous chemotherapy (rifampicin, isoniazide) as soon as the mycobacteria are inoculated into the mice. This efficient treatment inhibits the initial bacterial growth and thereby prevents the occurrence of specific defensive mechanisms (Mackaness *et al.*, 1973). Such inhibitions are observed only when antibiotics are given during the early period when the specific immunity sets in. When immunity is established, antibiotics act synergistically and apparently do not reduce the effectiveness of acquired resistance mechanisms. In some cases, they might even favour a return to normal of specific and unspecific immunological parameters impaired by infection (Goldstein *et al.*, 1976).

The specific immune responses and particularly antibody formation are usually reduced by infection in animals treated by antibiotics. As a result of antibiotic treatment, the antigenic stimulus normally triggered by the infectious agent is weakened by the rapid inhibition of bacterial growth. According to the antibiotic family and the administration time with regard to infection, antibody production may be totally, partially or not at all suppressed. Thus, as foreseen and usually stated in the clinic, the use of antibiotics when the illness is apparent does not alter the immune responses. However, one of the benefits of antibiotherapy on evolution of infectious diseases is the limitation of post-infectious immunopathological effects. Examples are plentiful and well known and do not deserve further consideration.

In its strict meaning, this "anti-allergic" activity may be double. As shown by the influence of efficient antibiotic treatments on the level of circulating immune complexes during septicaemia and endocarditis, there is an effect on the permanence of antigenic stimulus (Bacon *et al.*, 1974), (Hurwitz *et al.*, 1975). But antibiotic may also have its own immunosuppressive activity.

The direct immunomodulating activity of antibiotics have been estimated by treating non-infected normal animals with different kinds of products. By this way, a great number of antibiotics were tested for their immunosuppressive effects. Few of them were found active *in vivo* and *in vitro* and often, the suppressive activity when detected, appeared only at supranormal and toxic doses. Considering the nonspecific immune response, it was shown that several antibiotics, such as tetracyclines (Munoz and Geister, 1950), chloramphenicol (Hemmer *et al.*, 1953), amphotericin B (Björksten *et al.*, 1976) and gentamicin (Kahn *et al.*, 1976) impair granulocyte functions by acting either on the chemotactism or on the intracellular bactericidal effect. Anyway such effects observed *in vitro* are perhaps of no significance *in vivo*.

The immunomodulating effect of antibiotics on the specific immune response has been demonstrated *in vitro* and *in vivo*. Two major antibiotics, chloramphenicol and rifampicin and also actinomycin D seem to have an immunodepressive effect at therapeutic doses.

Actinomycin D inhibits and delays specific immune response *in vitro* (Wust, 1964) and *in vivo* in several animal species (Uhr, 1963). These phenomena seem related to a rapid and total inhibition of the RNA synthesis particularly affecting the DNA-dependent RNA polymerases. Such an activity concerns both cell-mediated immune reactions, as the *in vitro* lymphokine production, and antibody formation. However paradoxical effects were observed. For instance, the production of some immunoglobulin classes is stimulated when antibiotic is given one or two days before inoculation (Dobss *et al.*, 1968). It was inferred that antibiotic interferes with mechanisms regulating antibody formation.

Chloramphenicol as an inhibitor of protein synthesis, seems to stop antibody formation *in vitro* and *in vivo* as well as the blastogenic response of lymphocytes to mitogen stimulation (Weisberger *et al.*, 1969). However, the interest for this antibiotic, as an immuno-suppressive agent was limited by its age-dependent medullar toxicity. On the contrary, thiamphenicol, its less haematotoxic sulfonyl derivative, exhibits a better immunosuppressive activity at smaller doses. The effect of this derivative on antibody synthesis seems located not on the protein synthesis itself but on the growth of the morphological precursors of antibody forming cells. Thiamphenicol activity is effective only during 48 h after inoculation and disappears as soon as the treatment is interrupted. Then the activity is solely related to an inhibition of dividing cells (Petrescu, 1974).

Rifampicin beside its already mentioned direct antimicrobial activity shows a slight immunosuppressive effect, both on *in vivo* antibody formation and on *in vitro* cell-mediated responses. This effect appears *in vivo* only with large and toxic doses (Bassi *et al.*, 1973). The phagocytosis by macrophages is the main target for this antibiotic. But it does not apparently take part in the presentation to immunocompetent cells of the antigen when entrapped in macrophages. Since phagocytosis is very important, as a preliminary step in the thymodependent or independent specific immunological reactions, rifampicin could be an efficient tool to dissociate the various stages of immune response, especially those related to phago-cytosis and antigen presentation by macrophages.

Quite recently, it was shown that bestatin, a natural enzyme inhibitor isolated by Umezawa *et al.* (1976), was simultaneously an antitumour and immunostimulating agent acting both on humoral and cellular response. The effects observed in young mice are a macrophage activation, estimated by a rise of intracellular enzymes, an enhancement of humoral responses against thymo-dependent or -independent antigens and an increase of the antibody-mediated cytotoxic activity of splenic cells (Florentin *et al.*, 1978). In older animals, multiple injections, each one of 100 μg of bestatin, during 6 months partially restored immune responses made deficient by age and in parallel reduced the number of spontaneous tumours in comparison with controls (Bruley-Rosset *et al.*, 1979). Since this well defined immunorestoring compound is without any chronic toxicity in man and animals, new immunostimulating agents could be designed by chemical or biochemical modification of products only known as antibacterial.

Impact of Antibiotics on Infectious Bacteria

In addition to the studies on direct or indirect effects of antibiotics on the immune response of normal or infected host, some researches have been recently directed to their activity against the pathogenic bacteria themselves. At this point, the antibiotic actions are not considered any further on the multiplication mechanisms but rather on the modification of bacterial metabolism and on their ultimate influences upon the host's antiinfectious mechanisms. Have the antibiotic treated and not treated bacteria an identical immunological behaviour? In the past years the observations on the effects of subinhibitory concentrations on bacteria *in vitro*, were gathered and showed bacterial modification of cellular morphology, serological properties, sensitivity both to antibiotics and bactericidal factors of normal serum. In the same way, some bacteria grown in the presence of subinhibitory doses of antibiotic, for instance *Staphylococcus aureus* with nafcillin, are phagocytized more readily by polymorphonuclear leucocytes (Friedman and Warren, 1974). Such effects have been studied *in vitro* and *in vivo* with several kinds of antibiotics. Antibiotics inhibiting cell-wall biosynthesis are the most effective in potentiating the bactericidal agents present either in serum or inside the phagocyte lysosomes (Lorian and Atkinson, 1979), (Nishida *et al.*, 1976).

These authors investigated *in vitro* the bactericidal and phagocytic activity of rabbit leucocytes on *Pseudomonas aeruginosa* in the presence or not of different antibiotics at several concentrations in a medium containing no serum. Only inhibitors of cell wall biosynthesis at subinhibitory concentrations could enhance phagocytosis and polymorphonuclear bactericidal activity: probably the bacteria become weaker and more sensitive to the leucocyte bactericidal systems. At the same time, several studies *in vivo* demonstrated the potentialisation of defensive mechanisms by subinhibitory doses of antibiotic (Lorian *et al.*, 1978). Such doses may have complementary activities on bacteria beside a curing effect, like a decrease in the formation of pathogenicity or virulence factors and a modification of immunogenic determinants.

It seems that adherence of bacteria to cells contributes to their pathogenicity. According to several authors, bacteria grown in the presence of an antibiotic at subinhibitory level lost their property of adherence on the surface of epithelial cells *in vitro* (Sugarman and Donta, 1979) as well as *in vivo* (Davis and Savage, 1976). The antibiotic effect on the immunogenicity expression, i.e. the ability to elicit an immune response, was noted from several models.

Thus there are:

— a change in agglutination of *Salmonella*, when treated by an antibiotic and brought in contact with anti—0—serum (Lorian *et al.*, 1976);

— an increase of specific humoral responses when *E. coli* is grown in presence of cyclacillin and injected into animals (Friedman and Warren, 1977);

— a rise in anti–H and anti–0 antibody levels, in rabbits immunised with killed *Salmonella wien* then injected with the live bacteria grown in presence of fosfomycin at a subinhibitory level (Viano *et al.*, 1979).

Likewise, in our laboratory, some preliminary tests showed that subinhibitory concentrations (from 1/4 to 1/16 of m.i.c.) of carbenicillin, ticarcillin or amoxicillin make *P. aeruginosa* better able to bind their specific antibodies. In the same way there was a significant increase of specific antibody level in mice when injected with antibiotic-treated and heat-killed bacteria by comparison with only heat-killed microorganisms (Fig. 2) in identical amount. It must be emphasised that such an increase was obtained only with large doses. At first sight, it may be inferred that treating bacteria with subinhibitory doses, which alter their morphology (lack of segmentation), also modifies their antigenic determinants. This change was demonstrated *in vitro*, since the treated bacteria can bind a large amount of specific antibody on their surface. Likewise, *in vivo* an equivalent amount of bacteria (as evaluated by optical density) induces a higher humoral immune response when the bacteria are treated by an antibiotic and inactivated by heat than when they are heat-inactivated without previous antibiotic treatment.

However, from preliminary experiments concerning the evolution of immunity induced by different doses of bacteria injected after they had been treated or not with subinhibitory amounts of antibiotic, the responses, when evaluated from resistance against a new challenge by bacteria, are identical. However, there is some relationship between the number of bacteria in liver and the level of antibodies. Some experiments using adoptive transfers of specific cellular or humoral compartments are now in progress in order to determine whether the observations are related or not to the defensive specific mechanisms.

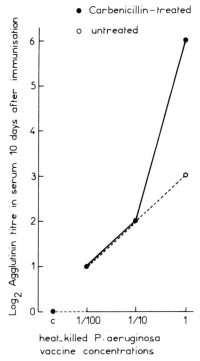

FIG. 2   Effect of *in vitro* antibiotic treatment on immunogenicity of *Pseudomonas aeruginosa* (serum pools from 5 mice).

Conclusion

The main effect of antibiotic *in vivo* seems to be a direct antibacterial activity which in some occasions is associated with the host's natural defence mechanisms to cure the infection and to prevent certain postinfectious immunopathological disorders. When some antibiotics elicit a transient immunosuppression in normal animals, it is a minor phenomenon with regard to the beneficial antibacterial effect of the treatment. On the contrary, the discovery of antibiotics endowed with immunostimulating properties and in particular able to restore the immune functions altered by age, seems to be an interesting goal. This indicates a need for developing immunopharmacological investigations on antibiotics. Likewise, the studies on changes in pathogenic and antigenic components of bacterial cell walls, occurring as an effect of antibiotics, should bring about a better knowledge of mechanisms leading to the cure of an infection and then give rise to a more logical use of antibiotics in human and animal infectious pathology.

334   P.H. Lagrange

References

Acar, J.F., Lagrange, P.H., Bedrossian, J., Huraux, J.M., Bricout, F. and Idatte, J.M. (1973). *In* "Cours International de Transplantation", pp. 289–301. SIMEP Editions (Villeurbanne).

d'Arcy-Hart, P. (1974). *In* "Activation of macrophages". (W.H. Wagner and H. Hahn, eds), pp. 131–137. Excerpta Medica, Amsterdam.

Bacon, P.A., Davidson, C. and Smith, B. (1974). *Quart. J. Med.* **43**, 537.

Bassi, L., Di Berardino, L., Arioli, V., Silvestri, L.G. and Cherie Ligniere, E.L. (1973). *J. Infect. Dis.* **128**, 736–744.

Björksten, B., Ray, C. and Quie, P.G. (1976). *Infect. Immun.* **14**, 315–317.

Bruley-Rosset, M., Florentin, I., Kiger, N., Schulz, J. and Mathé, G. (1979). *Immunology* **38**, 75–83.

Byron, J.W., Haigh, M.V. and Lajtha, L.G. (1964). *Nature* (London) **202**, 977–979.

Davis, C.P. and Savage, D.C. (1976). *Infect. Immun.* **13**, 180–188.

Dobbs, J., Rivero, I., Sabb, F. and Lee, S.L. (1968). *Immunology* **14**, 213–224.

Eagle, H., Fleischman, R. and Levy, M. (1953). *J. Lab. Clin. Med.* **41**, 122–132.

Fleming, A. (1938). *Lancet* **II**, 564–567.

Florentin, I., Kiger, N., Bruley-Rosset, M., Schulz, J. and Mathé, G. (1978). *In* "Human Lymphocyte Differenciation" (B. Serrou and C. Rosenfeld, eds), p. 299. North Holland Biomedical Press.

Friedman, H. and Warren, G.H. (1974). *Proc. Soc. Exp. Biol. Med.* **146**, 707–711.

Friedman, H. and Warren, G.H. (1977). *Chemotherapy* **23**, 324–336.

Goldstein, R.A., Hun Ang, U., Foellmer, J.W. and Janicki, B.W. (1976). *Am. Rev. Respir. Dis.* **113**, 197–202.

Gowans, J.L. (1953). *Brit. J. Exp. Path.* **34**, 35–43.

Hemmer, M.L., Novak, M.V. and Taylor, W.I. (1953). *Antibiot. Chemother.* **3**, 773–777.

Hurwitz, D.A., Quismorio, F.P. and Friou, G.J. (1975). *Clin. Exp. Immunol.* **19**, 131–141.

Kahn, A.J., Evans, H.E., Glan, L., Kahn, P. and Chang, C.T. (1976). 16th ICAAC, Chicago, Abstract N⁰ 108.

Kollath, W. and Raabe, F. (1943). *Zbl. Bakt. Par. Inf. Hyg.* **149**, 434–440.

Lorian, V. and Atkinson, B.A. (1979). *Rev. Infect. Dis.* **1**, 797–806.

Lorian, V., Atkinson, B. and Ewing, W.H. (1976). *Am. J. Clin. Path.* **66**, 1004–1011.

Lorian, V., Koike, M., Zak, O., Zanon, V., Sabath, L.D., Grassi, C.G. and Stille, W. (1978). *In* "Current Chemotherapy", Vol. 1. (W. Siegenthaler and R. Lüthy, eds), p. 72. ASM. Washington.

Mackaness, G.B. and Smith, N. (1953). *Am. Rev. Tuberc.* **67**, 322–340.

Mackaness, G.B., Auclair, D.J. and Lagrange, P.H. (1973). *J. Nat. Cancer Inst.* **51**, 1655–1667.

Marcus, S., Donaldson, D.M. and Esplin, D.W. (1955). *J. Immunol.* **74**, 494–497.

Munoz, J. and Geister, R. (1950). *Proc. Soc. Exp. Biol. Med.* **75**, 367–370.

Nishida, M., Mine, Y., Monoyama, S. and Yokota, Y. (1976). *Chemotherapy* **22**, 203–210.

Petrescu, D. (1974). *Postgrad. Med. J.* **50** (Suppl. 5), 97–104.

Sanders, C.C., Sanders, W.E. and Harrowe, D.J. (1976). *Infect. Immun.* **13**, 808–812.

Sugarman, B. and Donta, S.M. (1979). *J. Infect. Dis.* **140**, 622–625.

Uhr, J.W. (1963). *Science* **142**, 1476–1477.

Umezawa, H., Aoyagi, T., Suda, H., Hamada, M. and Takeuchi, T. (1976). *J. Antibiot.* **29**, 97–99.

Viano, I., Martinetto, P., Valtz, A., Santiano, M. and Barbaros, S. (1979). *Rev. Infect. Dis.* **I**, 858–861.

Weinstein, L. and Dalton, A.C. (1968). *N. Engl. J. Med.* **279**, 467–473; *ibid.*, 524–531; *ibid.*, 580–588.

Weisberger, A.S., Wessler, S. and Avioli, L.V. (1969). *J. Am. Med. Assoc.* **209**, 97–103.

Wust, C.J. (1964). Bacteriol. Proc., 64th A.S.M. Annual Meeting. Abstract M 107, p. 64.

Intracellular Penetration and Distribution of Antibiotics: The Basis for an Improved Chemotherapy of Intracellular Infections

A. TROUET and P. TULKENS

International Institute of Cellular and Molecular Pathology, I.C.P. and Université Catholique de Louvain, Brussels, Belgium

Introduction

Clinical experience gained during treatment of leukaemia and solid tumours illustrates very well the fact that host defences against bacterial infections rely primarily on white blood cells, and that the most potent antibiotics are of little help in the fight against infections if these cells are absent or present in very small number.

The processes by which these cells, i.e. polymorphonuclears and monocytes, kill bacteria will not be reviewed here in detail and it is sufficient to point out that bacteria must be phagocytised and are then killed inside lysosomes or phagolysosomes by various mechanisms involving lysosomal enzymes, bactericidal proteins, production of peroxide and halogenation (Fig. 1).

Several bacterial species are, however, able to escape this bactericidal effect either by evading phagocytosis, by killing the cells or by resistance to the intracellular killing mechanisms.

Amongst the bacteria resisting intracellular killing one distinguishes the facultative and obligatory intracellular parasites. The former are bacteria which multiply mainly outside cells but which may survive and sometimes proliferate inside the host cells, mainly the macrophages. Amongst these bacteria one finds: *Mycobacterium tuberculosis, Salmonella, Brucella, Listeria, Pasteurella.* The obligatory intracellular parasites like *Mycobacterium leprae, Toxoplasma*, not only survive inside cells but require the intracellular medium for growth and multiplication.

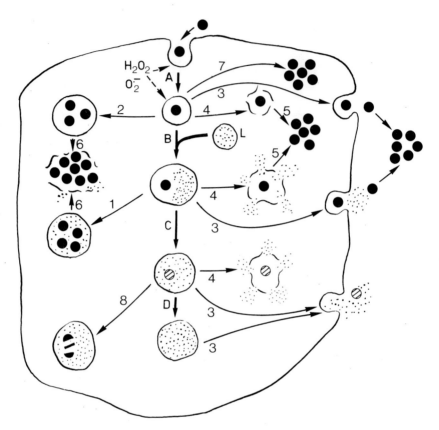

FIG. 1   Pathogeny of cellular infection (modified from de Duve and Trouet, 1973). The central part illustrates the normal pathway of microorganism destruction by phagocytes: (A) phagocytosis, accompanied by production of H_2O_2 and O_2^-; (B) fusion of the phagosome with lysosome (L). These two processes lead to killing (C) and then on to digestion (D). Pathogenic events may result from a failure of killing, causing intracellular survival or proliferation, either (1) in secondary lysosomes (for instance *M. leprae*) or (2) in phagosomes (for instance *M. tuberculosis, Toxoplasma*). The latter phenomenon results from inhibition of fusion of the phagosome with the lysosomes.

Other pathogenic mechanisms may depend on production of toxins released from live or killed microorganisms; and causing (3) exocytosis; (4) rupture of phagosomal or lysosomal membranes. Intracytoplasmic proliferation may be observed after toxic (5) or mechanical (6) rupture of the lysosomal or phagosomal membrane, or because the microorganism is able to pass across the phagosomal membrane (7) (example: *Trypanosoma cruzei*) under trypomastigote and transition forms. Finally, persistence of undigested residues (8) has been found causative in inflammatory processes or cell overloading.

Most of the intracellular bacteria reside in the lysosomal vacuoles while a few seem to escape the intracellular killing processes by inhibiting the fusion of phagosomes with lysosomes. These latter phagosomal parasites are mainly *Mycobacterium tuberculosis* (Armstrong and d'Arcy Hart, 1971), *Toxoplasma gondii* (Jones and

Hirsch, 1972) and *Chlamydia psittaci* (Friis, 1972). There is no evidence available at this time in favour of survival or multiplication of bacteria in the cytoplasm or in other cell compartments than the lysosomes and phagosomes.

Intracellular bacteria seem to be protected from the action of antibiotics (Shaffer *et al.*, 1953; Shepard, 1957; Mackaness, 1960; Ekzemplyarov, 1965; Holmes *et al.*, 1966; Alexander and Good, 1968; Solbert, 1972). This protective effect may explain the difficulties in treating infections caused by obligatory intracellular parasites and also stress the great pathological importance of the intracellular "reservoir of bacteria" that may exist in infections caused by facultative intracellular parasites. They can, indeed, defeat the curing effects of antibiotics by escaping from the cells as soon as the extracellular concentration of the drugs have fallen below active levels.

The relative inefficiency of antibiotics in dealing with intracellular bacteria may be due either to their inability to penetrate cells or to the fact that after penetration in cells they are excluded from the cellular compartments which like lysosomes harbour bacteria. Conflicting results have been reported in the literature with regard to the intracellular penetration of penicillin and streptomycin. Penetration of penicillin was claimed by Eagle and Saz (1955) but could not be observed by Mandell (1973). Ekzemplyarov (1965) failed to demonstrate the accumulation of streptomycin in macrophages while Bonventre and Imhoff (1970) reported the accumulation of ^{3}H in cells incubated in the presence of [^{3}H] dihydrostreptomycin. Rifampicin was reported to accumulate about two fold in leucocytes (Mandell, 1973).

For that reason we have been led to study the uptake and subcellular localisation of aminoglycosides, like streptomycin, amikacin, gentamicin and kanamycin, and also of phenoxymethylpenicillin and rifampicin, in cultured rat fibroblasts, using microbiological assay and cell fractionation techniques (Tulkens *et al.*, 1974; Tulkens *et al.*, 1980).

Cellular Pharmacology of Aminoglycosides

When incubated for 4 days in the presence of streptomycin, gentamicin, amikacin or kanamycin at a concentration of 0.5 mg/ml, fibroblasts accumulate the antibiotic from 5 μg/mg of cell protein for streptomycin up to 13 μg/mg of cell protein for gentamicin. There is a linear relationship between drug concentration and uptake at least up to 1 μg/mg. Since the fibroblast cell volume corresponding to 1 μg of protein was found close to 5 μl, the intracellular concentration of the antibiotic varies from 1 mg/ml for streptomycin up to 2.6 mg/ml for gentamicin. The uptake of aminoglycosides proceeds at a slow rate, more than 4 days being required for a stable intracellular content to be reached.

Cytoplasmic extracts obtained from fibroblasts incubated for 4 days in the presence of streptomycin (350 μg/ml) were fractionated by isopycnic centrifugation. The distribution of streptomycin, protein, RNA, catalase and of marker enzymes for mitochondria (cytochrome oxidase), plasma membrane (5′–nucleotidase), endoplasmic reticulum (NADH: cytochrome c reductase) and lysosomes (N–acetyl–β–glucosaminidase and cathepsin) were determined and are given in Fig. 2.

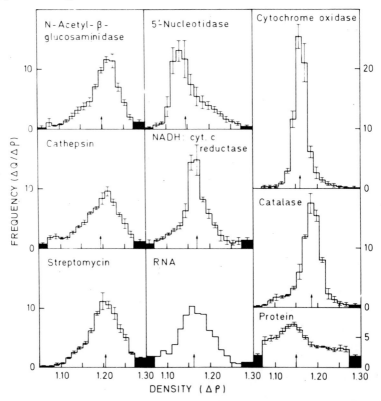

FIG. 2   Fractionation of cytoplasmic extracts of fibroblasts by density equilibration in linear sucrose gradients. The graphs show the mean results (± standard deviation) of 5 independent experiments. These results are presented as normalised histograms of density distribution of constituents or activities (Leighton *et al.*, 1968). The abscissa is the density span of the gradients divided in 15 sections of equal density increment; the ordinate is the frequency of constituents or activities in each section.

Similar experiments were performed with fibroblasts incubated during 4 days in the presence of 200 μg/ml of dihydrostreptomycin,

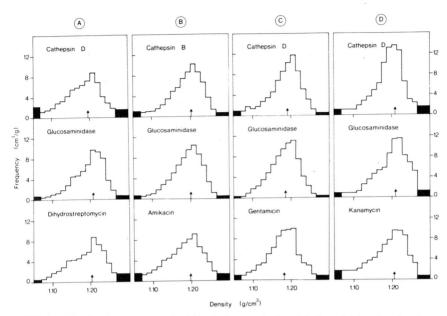

FIG. 3   Distribution patterns of acid hydrolases and of antibiotic activities after fractionation of cytoplasmic extracts of fibroblasts by density equilibration. Results are presented
as in Fig. 2.

amikacin, gentamicin or kanamycin. In Fig. 3 we present the
distribution patterns of these antibiotics in comparison with those of
the lysosomal enzymes N–acetyl–β–glucosaminidase and cathepsin
D or B.

We observed a constant association and similarity between the
antibiotic distribution and those of lysosomal hydrolases. Moreover,
the distribution of streptomycin is clearly distinct from that of the
marker enzymes of the other cell constituents. This association does
not result from an absorption on the organelles during homogenisa-
tion and fractionation and it is not a consequence of the destruction
or loss of activity of the antibiotics in the other cell compartments.
These results indicate strongly that the aminoglycosides are mostly
localised in the lysosomes. Since lysosomes of rat embryo fibroblasts
occupy about 3% of the cell volume (Tulkens *et al.*, 1975), one can
estimate that the concentration ratio between the lysosomal content
and the culture medium varies between 60 and 150.

The exact mechanism by which aminoglycosides enter cells is still
not known with certainty. Most probably they permeate through the
cell membranes and are concentrated exclusively as basic compounds
in the acid compartment of the lysosomes. This process of lysosomal
accumulation described in detail by de Duve *et al.* (1974) rests on the

assumption that the uncharged and sufficiently lipophilic molecules cross more rapidly biological membranes whereas the protonated forms of the drug permeate only very slowly if at all. The steady state level depends mainly on the difference between the pH of the extracellular medium and that of lysosomes which has been estimated to vary between 4.5 and 5 (Ohkuma and Poole, 1978).

The kinetics of accumulation of aminoglycosides are compatible with such a mechanism. It is, however, surprising that streptomycin with two strongly basic guanidinium groups (pKa ± 12) and kanamycin or gentamicin having ionisable groups with a maximum pKa of 10 enter cells at the same slow rate. It is not possible at this stage to exclude completely the possibility that aminoglycosides enter cells by endocytosis.

The major point to stress here is that whatever the mechanism of entry, aminoglycosides are concentrated in lysosomes and that the ratio of their protonated versus unprotonated form must vary between 10^7 for streptomycin and 10^5 for kanamycin and gentamicin.

If these results are extended to other cells like macrophages or polymorphonuclear leukocytes, they may explain the relative inefficiency of aminoglycosides against intracellular bacteria. These antibiotics are concentrated in the lysosomal compartment of cells but will be inactive on these bacteria which are localised in the phagosomes and on those residing in the lysosomes since the activity of aminoglycosides is strongly pH dependent and extremely low at a pH around 4 and 5. This pH effect is such that the efficiency of streptomycin will be similar at pH 5 and at pH 7, even if it is 30 to 40 times more concentrated at the former value. This inefficiency of aminoglycosides at low pH may easily be explained by the fact that they are almost exclusively protonated and are not able as such to cross the membranes of either cells or bacteria.

Cellular Pharmacology of Phenoxymethylpenicillin and of Rifampicin

Penicillins and ansamycins are organic weak acids or zwitterions and they behave differently from aminosides regarding their intracellular distribution.

Phenoxymethylpenicillin

Penicillin is much less active on intracellularly growing *Staphylococcus aureus* (Solberg, 1972) and is active in moderately acid media (pH 6–6.5). We have first investigated the uptake of phenoxymethylpenicillin by fibroblasts and determined its subcellular localisation by cell fractionation techniques in cultivated fibroblasts. Phenoxy-methylpenicillin was chosen because of its much greater stability in acid media making it thus possible to detect its eventual localisation in lysosomes.

When incubated in the presence of phenoxymethylpenicillin (360 μg/ml) fibroblasts take up the antibiotic in increasing amounts over the first 24 h but the intracellular steady state level reached was about 35% of that of the extracellular concentration. The subcellular localisation of the antibiotics was then investigated by isopycnic centrifugation of cytoplasmic extract obtained from cells incubated with phenoxymethylpenicillin (600 μg/ml) for 48 h. As shown in Fig. 4, all the penicillin activity remains on the top of the gradient

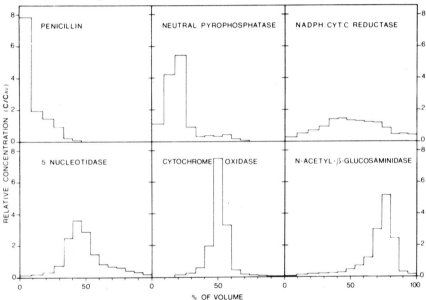

FIG. 4   Isopycnic centrifugation of a cytoplasmic extract of fibroblasts incubated for 48 h in the presence of phenoxymethylpenicillin (600 μg/ml). Results are presented in the form of histograms of relative concentration distributions as a function of the volume.

suggesting the presence of the antibiotic in the cytosol. It has been checked that phenoxymethylpenicillin is not inactivated when incubated for several hours at pH 5 in presence of lysosomal enzymes.

The low intracellular levels of phenoxymethylpenicillin and the exclusion of this antibiotic from the lysosomes can be explained on the assumption that the acid drug permeates freely through the membrane under its non-ionised form. The concentration of this latter form will, however, be higher in the acid medium of lysosomes than in the other cell compartments and extracellular space and as a consequence, the drug will be unable to accumulate inside the lysosomes.

Preliminary studies with penicillin G and with the zwitterionic ampicillin seem to give similar indications in fibroblasts and macrophages.

Ansamycins

Rifampicin and rifamycin SV are stable in acid media down to pH 3 and are optimally active around pH 6–6.5. These ansamycins are accumulated about 3 to 5 times by fibroblasts, a steady state level being obtained after 20 h. After fractionation of fibroblasts incubated with rifampicin or rifamycin SV, the distribution of the antibiotics is similar to that of the cytosolic marker enzyme neutral pyrophosphatase.

The behaviour of zwitterionic drugs like the ansamycins is more complex and more difficult to interpret on the basis of the hypothesis formulated for phenoxymethylpenicillin. Our results may explain why penicillins are ineffective against intralysosomal bacteria since these drugs do not accumulate inside cells and are excluded from lysosomes. But, the 3 to 5 fold intracellular concentration of rifampicin inside the cell is compatible with its activity intracellular *Mycobacterium tuberculosis* which resides in the phagosomes. The content of these vesicles, which we are unable to identify by cell fractionation, is probably in equilibrium with the cytosol.

Prospects for Drug Development

The relative inefficiency of antibiotics against intracellular bacteria can be related to the following facts:

1) Bacteria residing in the acid lysosomal content are not actively duplicating or only at a very low rate. In this dormant state, they are very much resistant to the action of most antibiotics.
2) Basic drugs like aminoglycosides which are most active at a basic or neutral pH accumulate inside lysosomes but are inactive at the acid lysosomal pH.
3) Acid or zwitterionic drugs active at an acid pH, like penicillins or ansamycins, accumulate very little in the cells and in lysosomes.

If one excepts the case of leprosy, the major therapeutic problem caused by the presence of bacteria inside the lysosomes is that they constitute a reservoir of infection agents which are shielded against the activity of antibiotics.

We think that it would be possible to circumvent this problem by introducing, into the infected lysosomes, acid antibiotics at the required concentration to penetrate inside the intralysosomal bacteria and to be retained in the more neutral bacterial cytoplasm. The drugs could then interfere with the bacterial metabolism either immediately or after release of the bacteria from the cells.

Such a lysosomotropism of acid antibiotics could be obtained by two processes, either by linking to endocytosable macromolecules or by a reversible masking of their acidic groups.

Linking to Endocytosable Carrier Molecules

The acid drug should be linked to the carrier via a bond which remains stable in the blood stream but which will be split by lysosomal enzymes and release the drug in its active acid form. The carrier should be a molecule which is recognized and endocytised selectively by macrophages. Glycoproteins with terminal mannosyl residues would be very good candidates for such carriers (Sly and Stahl, 1978). The main limitation of this approach will be the increased risk of antibody production and anaphylactic reactions with drugs such as penicillin.

Reversible Masking of Acid Functions of the Drug

In order to promote the intralysosomal accumulation of acid drugs, the acid function of these latter should be masked by another group displaying a basic function. This added chemical moiety should, however, be sensitive to the acid medium or enzymes of the lysosomes and its removal should release the acid drug which would then leave the lysosomes to permeate and accumulate inside the intralysosomal bacteria.

The chemotherapy of intraphagosomal bacterial infections seems to be less problematic. Although the characteristics of phagosomes are much less known than those of lysosomes, the phagosomal environment is less hostile to bacteria and more compatible with bacterial multiplication. The susceptibility to antibiotics of the phagosomal bacteria will thus be greater than those of the intralysosomal ones. On the other hand, the pH of the phagosomal content is probably very close to that of the cytoplasm and as a consequence antibiotics which permeate into cells and which distribute through most of the non acid compartments of the cell should be suitable to cope with phagosomal infections provided the bacteria are sensitive to the given antibiotic.

References

Alexander, J.W. and Good, R.A. (1968). *J. Lab. Clin. Med.* **71**, 971–983.

Armstrong, J.A. and d'Arcy Hart, P. (1971). *J. Exp. Med.* **134**, 713–740.

Bonventre, P.F. and Imhoff, J.G. (1970). *Infect. Immun.* **2**, 89–95.

de Duve, C. and Trouet, A. (1973). *In* "Non-specific factors influencing host resistance". (W. Brown and J. Ungar, eds), pp. 153–170. Karger, Bern.

de Duve, C., de Barsy, T., Poole, B., Trouet, A., Tulkens, P. and Van Hoof, F. (1974). *Biochem. Pharmacol.* **23**, 2495–2531.

Eagle, H. and Saz, A.K. (1955). *Annu. Rev. Microbiol.* **9**, 173–226.

Ekzemplyarov, O.N. (1965). *Antibiotiki* **10**, 420–424.

Friis, R.R. (1972). *J. Bacteriol.* **110**, 706–721.

Holmes, B., Quie, P.G., Windhorst, D.B., Pollara, B. and Good, R.A. (1966). *Nature* (London) **210**, 1131–1132.

Jones, T.C. and Hirsch, J.G. (1972). *J. Exp. Med.* **136**, 1173–1194.

Leighton, F., Poole, B., Beaufay, H., Baudhuin, P., Coffey, J.W., Fowler, S. and de Duve, C. (1968). *J. Cell. Biol.* **37**, 482–513.

Mackaness, G.B. (1960). *J. Exp. Med.* **112**, 35–53.

Mandell, G.L. (1973). *J. Clin. Invest.* **52**, 1673–1679.

Ohkuma, S. and Poole, B. (1978). *Proc. Nat. Acad. Sci. U.S.A.* **75**, 3327–3331.

Shaffer, J.M., Kucera, C.J. and Spink, W.W. (1953). *J. Exp. Med.* **97**, 77–89.

Shepard, C.C. (1957). *J. Bacteriol.* **73**, 494–498.

Sly, W.S. and Stahl, P. (1978). *In* "Transport of Macromolecules in Cellular Systems". (S. Silverstein, ed.), pp. 229–244. Dahlem Konferenzen, Berlin.

Solberg, C.O. (1972). *Acta Med. Scand.* **191**, 383–387.

Tulkens, P., Beaufay, H. and Trouet, A. (1974). *J. Cell. Biol.* **63**, 383–401.

Tulkens, P., Van Hoof, F. and Trouet, A. (1975). *Arch. Int. Physiol. Biochim.* **83**, 1004–1006.

Tulkens, P., Schneider, Y.-J. and Trouet, A. (1980). *In* "Mononuclear Phagocytes: Functional Aspects". (R. Van Furth, ed.), pp. 613–647. N. Nijhoff Pub., The Hague.

Discussion

Professor Sande: I am slightly confused by Professor Trouet's data indicating that rifampicin concentrates in the cytoplasm. If, for example, chronic granulomatous disease polymorphs, or even normal polymorphs take up staphylococci, it can be shown both in the abnormal and the normal cells that there is a fairly significant proportion of viable bacteria remaining within the cells, and supposedly therefore within the phagosomes. If the cells are treated with rifampicin, contrary to almost any other drugs including the aminoglycosides, vancomycin, or the penicillins, the intracellular organisms are killed very effectively. This suggests, at least functionally, that rifampicin is reaching the location of the bacteria.

Professor Trouet: I omitted to mention that one limitation of our fractionation technique is that it is impossible to identify phagosomes, because these behave like 5'–nucleotidase. With regard to the bacteria which are inside the phagosomes, the problems are much less difficult than with those inside the lysosomes, because the pH of the phagosomes is probably much closer to 7 than is the pH of the lysosomes.

Professor Sande: We are fairly certain, though, that we cannot kill the intracellular organisms with aminoglycosides. We have gone as far as wrapping the aminoglycosides in lipid membranes, making liposomes, thus getting high concentrations of aminoglycosides into the phagosomes — the liposomes can be seen within the phagosomes — but it is still impossible to kill the bacteria. This suggests, that, perhaps, degranulation of lysosomes has occurred and that the pH within the phagosomes is probably quite low.

Professor Trouet: Are you sure that these are phagosomes?

Professor Sande: Not absolutely sure, no.

Professor Trouet: It is very difficult to distinguish between lysosomes and phagosomes, even with electron microscopy.

Professor Sande: It is possible to see the liposome in the same granule in which there is the microorganism.

Professor Trouet: But you certainly agree they could be lysosomes. In this case, the aminoglycosides will be inactive because of the low pH.

Professor Vilde: Concerning penetration of vancomycin and penicillin into the cells of chronic granulomatosis, we carried out tests with vancomycin and penicillin G on a strain of *Staphylococcus* sensitive to both antibiotics and it did not change the score, in other words the bacteria remained viable in a perfectly identical manner compared to the control. The question I wish to ask you concerns the possible utility, this is somewhat futuristic, of an antibiotic, like vancomycin, that would bind on the bacteria and penetrate inside cells with them. In other words, could not bacteria penetrate into the phagocytic cell and the vacuole with antibiotics that would continue to exert an action on the bacteria *in situ*?

Professor Trouet: Yes, that could be. Once you have got an antibiotic bound to bacteria, it will probably exert its action unless it dissociates insides the lysosomes. Penicillin G for instance, which we have studied, is excluded from the lysosomes because of its acid property. The situation is more complicated for drugs that have acid and basic moieties, hence the interest of introducing antibiotics into lysosomes since they have a certain chance to inhibit the bacteria present there. But that is a prospective point of view.

Professor Fillastre: A few questions and comments. First of all, I would like to say that you have explained a fact which appeared curious to clinicians. In the past, when we noted the extremely high concentration of aminoglycosides in the kidney, we thought that we could treat infectious renal diseases by making injections at extremely long intervals; this was done by Pr. Fabre, who gave an injection at 8-day intervals. We know that it did not work and you gave us the explanation by proving precisely that there was an inactivation due to pH conditions. The other question I wish to ask is how do you account for the fact that, in spite of penetration that you have demonstrated for streptomycin and for kanamycin, there is a difference in the renal toxicity between these two antibiotics and the other aminoglycosides, for instance gentamicin. Do you have arguments pertaining to the modification of the latent lysosomal structure or on the modifications of the behaviour of certain hydrolases or other enzymes within the lysosome, accounting for this difference in nephrotoxicity? This point is important for us, because if we can now understand a common mechanism of penetration, we still do not understand the mechanism of nephrotoxicity. Finally I wish to evoke a problem and suggest an answer. I think that we can possibly eliminate a process of active resorption which you have evoked in certain cells and in tubular renal cells because studies by Whelton have shown that penetration into the kidney was entirely independent first of all from the volume of diuresis, but also from the reabsorption of glucose, organic bases and organic acids. The only point that remains to be elucidated is the competition with certain amino-acids. So my question is: do you have arguments to account for nephrotoxicity?

Professor Trouet: Dr. Tulkens and his wife made such a study on nephrotoxicity. They observed inhibitions of lysosomal enzymes but we cannot at present say whether these are truly the cause of the toxic phenomena observed. We found no correlations between the effects on lysosomes and the differences that you have mentioned between the various antibiotics. So the situation is not quite clear.

Professor Fillastre: There is another important point. We are sure that gentamicin provokes an extremely marked and persistent reduction of sphingomyelinase. So we have here the experimental model which provides a comparison between what we know in human pathology in the case of phospholipidoses and what we see experimentally with gentamicin. It seems that with other aminoglycosides you do not find this action on sphingomyelinase whilst you find it on other enzymes. Perhaps it is the way to better understand nephrotoxicity.

Professor Waldvogel: As Professor Trouet, we have performed similar experiments using a model with polymorphonuclear neutrophils and radioactive gentamicin. Our results, published in the December issue of "Antimicrobial Agents and Chemotherapy" are in keeping with yours concerning the uptake of the antibiotic. We also tried to stimulate the metabolism of polymorphonuclear leucocytes by giving complement coated bacteria or particles, and asked the question whether the uptake could be increased. It was not. Prolonged incubations of leucocytes with gentamicin however showed surprisingly that the uptake varied from one experiment to the other. When we tested the viability of the polymorphonuclears with trypan blue after 12 h of incubation with bacteria or antibiotics, we discovered that part of them were lysed. Addition of the same amount of lysate to intact cells now reproduced the binding in a reliable manner. In your experiments, 4 day incubations were performed, which is very long. Could you exclude in your experiments the possibility of an uptake of aminoglycosides due to increased permeability of the cells by a slow degradation process?

Professor Trouet: It is the reason for which we used fibroblasts and macrophages because it is possible to maintain these cells, even in the presence of reasonable concentrations of aminoglycosides, in a good condition in terms of morphology and biochemistry (protein synthesis, etc.). There is no toxic effect. However, it is not surprising that, after 12 h, polymorphonuclears are altered.

May I add that I was very interested in what Professor Tomasz has told us today. One of the possible interactions between antibiotics and enzymes could occur intracellularly, inside the lysosomes and not only extracellularly. Has he tested other possible lysosomal enzymes which could co-operate with the antibiotic effect in this way?

Professor Tomasz: No, I did not.

Portage Transport

C. GILVARG

Princeton University, Princeton, N.J., U.S.A.

Introduction

The lipid elements of the cell membrane serve to minimise the loss of metabolic intermediates and to restrict access of external molecules to the cell's interior. This barrier is then selectively breached by transport systems whose specificity dictates which components of the environment may enter the cell. In general, this specificity is sufficiently stringent so that slight modification of a substrate eliminates its uptake by the cell.

It was, therefore, initially at any rate, somewhat of a surprise to discover that the system that was responsible for the admission of oligopeptides to *E. coli* was remarkably tolerant with respect to the nature of the side chains of the amino acids comprising the peptide. Attention was first drawn to this point by the observation that while acetylation of the amino terminus of a peptide virtually eliminated its ability to be taken up, acetylation of the ϵ-amino groups of lysine residues, though it destroyed the nutritional effectiveness of those particular residues, did not interfere with the transport of the peptide nor with the utilisation of the unsubstituted amino acids (Gilvarg and Katchalski, 1965; Losick and Gilvarg, 1966). Further evidence for side chain tolerance became apparent with the recognition that a single transport system was responsible for the uptake of peptides containing the full gamut of acidic, basic, neutral, aromatic, hydrophobic and hydroxy amino acids (Barak and Gilvarg, 1975).

In view of the fact that employing the twenty amino acids that commonly occur in protein, one can construct 400 dipeptides, 8000 tripeptides, or 160,000 tetrapeptides, it should not have occasioned any surprise that *E. coli* was not going to match that kind of substrate diversity with an equal number of exacting transport systems. Apparently, given the commitment to utilise oligopeptides (Gilvarg, 1972), *E. coli* has evolved a system that emphasises those elements common to all peptides and largely ignores the diversity based on the variety of side chains.

"Portage Transport" of Substances Required for Bacterial Growth

It is a logical extension of this notion to imagine that virtually any substance, including those that would ordinarily be impermeable to *E. coli*, could be brought into the cell by incorporating it into a peptide. In fact, by using a molecule that could not enter *E. coli* as a model, one would simultaneously have the most severe test of the proposal as well as the most convincing experimental demonstration of the principle since alternative entry portals would not exist.

Homoserine phosphate was chosen as the substance to be examined for the transport. It was selected since, in common with almost all phosphorylated compounds, it was anticipated that it could not pass through the cell membrane. Moreover, the detection of such a passage would be easily determined in a threonine auxotroph, in terms of a simple growth response, since the compound is an intermediate in the pathway of biosynthesis of threonine. Finally, the incorporation of homoserine phosphate into a peptide structure is straightforward since the compound is an amino acid.

It was shown that dilysylhomoserine phosphate could indeed support the growth of a threonine auxotroph that was unable to use homoserinephosphate to meet its threonine requirement (Fickel and Gilvarg, 1973). A substrain of that auxotroph, selected for its inability to transport oligopeptides, would not utilise the dilysylhomoserine phosphate proving that the oligopeptide transport system had been the entry portal. A concern that the peptide might conceivably have been dephosphorylated in the periplasm by alkaline phosphatase and that only the transport of homoserine had been demonstrated, was eliminated by repeating the experiment with a threonine auxotroph lacking homoserine kinase. In this strain only homoserine phosphate can act as a threonine replacement (see Fig. 1). An analogous experiment involving histidinolphosphate and diglycylhistidinolphosphate was carried out with *S. typhimurium* by Ames *et al.* (1973).

These experiments demonstrate the validity of the principle that if one covalently links a compound to a peptide in such a way as not to interfere with recognition of the substrate the compound can be brought into the cell. Moreover, the fact that the compound itself

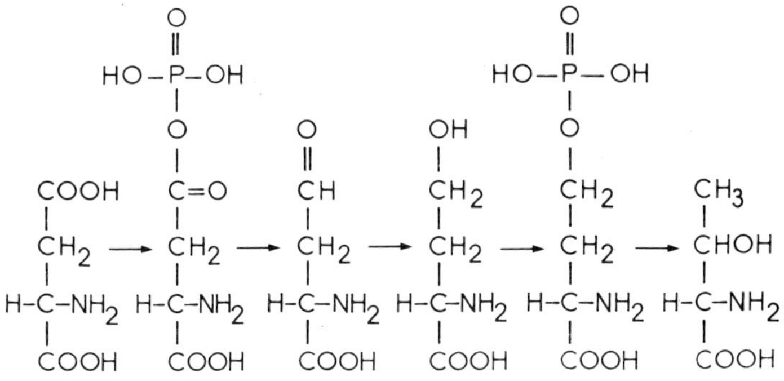

FIG. 1   Threonine biosynthesis.

may be impermeant to the cell does not preclude its transport. Operationally this is a peptide assisted transport. It has been referred to as "illicit transport" (Ames *et al.*, 1973) or "smuggling" (Payne, 1977). However, these terms, apart from their needlessly pejorative quality, do not convey any aspect of the mechanism. The term "portage transport" meets this requirement.

Natural Examples of "Portage Transport"

It is an astonishing coincidence that at the time the above experiments were being carried out, two peptides were isolated from *Streptomyces* fermentation broths whose structures strongly suggested that they represented natural examples of portage transport (Bayer *et al.*, 1972; Pruess *et al.*, 1973). In one instance, 2–amino–4–(methyl-phosphino)–butanoate (phosphinothricin) is linked to L–alanyl–L–alanine (Fig. 2); in the other, L–(N^5–phosphono)–S–sulphoximinyl-methionine is the N–terminal amino acid joined to dialanine (Fig. 3).

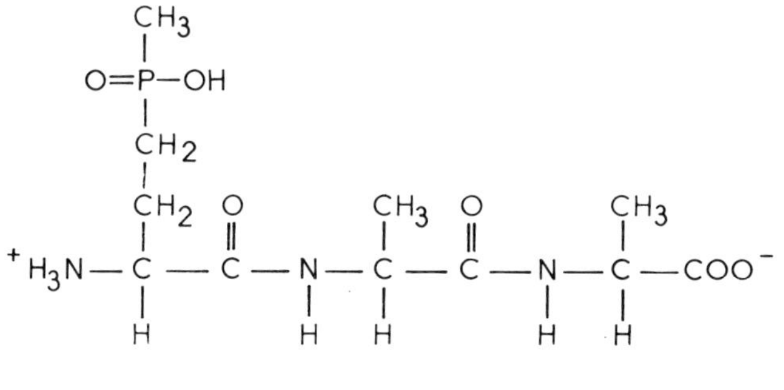

FIG. 2   Structure of L–phosphinothricyl–L–alanyl–L–alanine.

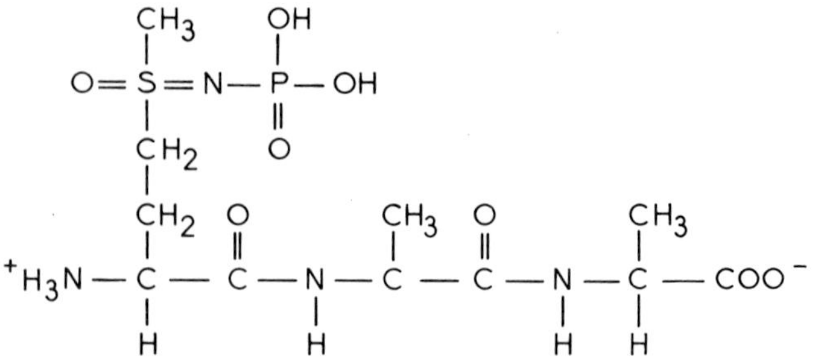

FIG. 3   Structure of L–(N^5–phosphono)–S–sulphoximinyl–methionyl–L–alanyl–L–alanine.

In both cases the unusual amino acid has little antibacterial activity in the free form though both as free amino acids are effective antagonists of glutamine synthetase. However, the peptides themselves do not inhibit the enzyme. Since the *in vivo* antibacterial activity of the peptides can be reversed by glutamine, it is clear that these tripeptides participate in the portage transport of the amino acids.

Moreover it was demonstrated that oligopeptide transport deficient mutants of *E. coli* were resistant to the action of either tripeptide proving that the oligopeptide transport system is indeed the vehicle for bringing these materials into the cell (Diddens and Zähner, 1976).

In reexamining the earlier reports of the isolation from fermentation broths of di- and tripeptides that contained unusual amino acids it is clear that these were not recognised as examples of portage transport. Possibly this was because it was not so obvious, as in the examples cited above, that the free amino acids might be impermiant to the organisms against which the peptides were screened.

The recent characterisation of the structure of plumbemycin (Fig. 4) provides yet another clear cut natural example of portage transport (Park *et al.*, 1977). Moreover the discovery that it contained 2–amino–5–phosphono–3– cis–pentenoic acid, an obvious analogue of homoserine phosphate, provides a reinforcement of one of the laboratory examples. It should also be noted that it meets the criterion of failing to inhibit an oligopeptide transport deficient strain of *E. coli* (Diddens *et al.*, 1979).

It is interesting to contrast the laboratory and natural examples of portage transport. In both of the former cases peptides were constructed that facilitated the entrance of substances that made it possible for cells to grow. Nature appears less beneficent. In all the instances of the biosynthetically elaborated peptides considerable metabolic effort appears to have been invested in transforming a

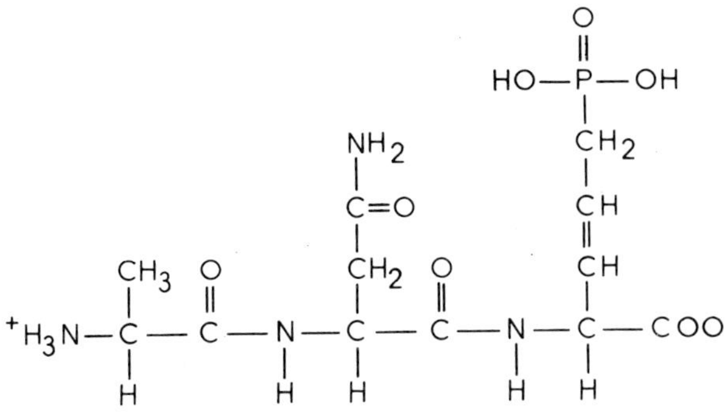

FIG. 4   Structure of plumbemycin.

benign amino acid into an antibacterial peptide. In the scales which weigh the proposition that some antibiotics are not merely secondary metabolites but are elaborated to eliminate competitors, these peptides would appear to add heavily to that view.

Recently another candidate for portage transport in nature has surfaced. The structure of the toxin elaborated by *Pseudomonas phaseolicola* (Fig. 5), the causative agent of halo bean blight disease

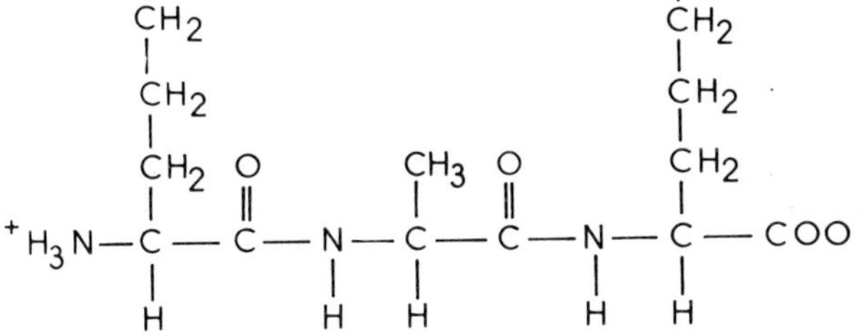

FIG. 5   Structure of phaseotoxin.

has been elucidated (Mitchell, 1976). In common with the other materials discussed above it is a tripeptide one of whose amino acids contains phosphorus. This sulfamyl phosphoryl derivative of ornithine is almost certainly an antagonist of ornithine carbamoyl transferase, a key enzyme at the start of the pathway leading to arginine bio-synthesis. Strikingly, the tripeptide also contains homoarginine, a likely antagonist of arginine itself. The design of this peptide, and one is strongly tempted to use that anthropomorphic term, is most instructive. Given the proposition that one were going to place two antimetabolites within a single peptide the question would immediately arise as to whether it would be better to have each anti-metabolite directed against different pathways or whether the two antagonists should be directed against the same pathway. Throttling down two parallel pathways, each by 90%, could not lead to a greater than 90% effect on the organism. However if one were to inhibit two steps in a single pathway, a synergistic response is certainly to be expected. It is difficult to accept the idea that the inclusion of two substances antagonistic to the same pathway within the structure of a peptide could have arisen purely adventitiously. Contrariwise one would have to conclude that the structure of phaseotoxin is a forceful argument for the deliberate production of an antibiotic by an organism. The term "antibiotic" is used in its broadest sense since it is not clear in what physiological context *Pseudomonas phaseolicola* operates, i.e. whether it is advantageous for the microorganism to destroy its host, the bean plant, or possible competitors at its table. At any rate the message conveyed by the structure of phaseotoxin should not be lost on those interested in the design of antibiotics.

Design of Synthetic Transport Peptides

Most recently even laboratory products related to portage transport are following nature's lead in converting innocuous amino acids into noxious peptides. A synthetic attempt at a transition state analogue of ornithine carbamoyltransferase $N-\delta-$(phosphonoacetyl)$-L-$ornithine, was found to be a very potent inhibitor of the enzyme with a K_i of 0.77 μM. However, it was without effect on *E. coli* until two glycine residues were added to its $\alpha-$amino group (Fig. 6) (Penninckx and Gigot, 1979). The tripeptide was bacteriostatic and as expected the peptide itself was quite inert with respect to the ornithine carbamoyl transferase.

An example of a portage transport substrate, different in several respects from most of the compounds discussed above, is alaphosphin (Fig. 7). The compound is a dipeptide analogue of alanylalanine in which the C$-$terminal carboxyl group has been replaced by phos-phonic acid. It represents a departure from an exact adherence to a peptide backbone as did diglycylhistidinol phosphate. In the guise of a dipeptide it can presumably enter *E. coli* both by way of the

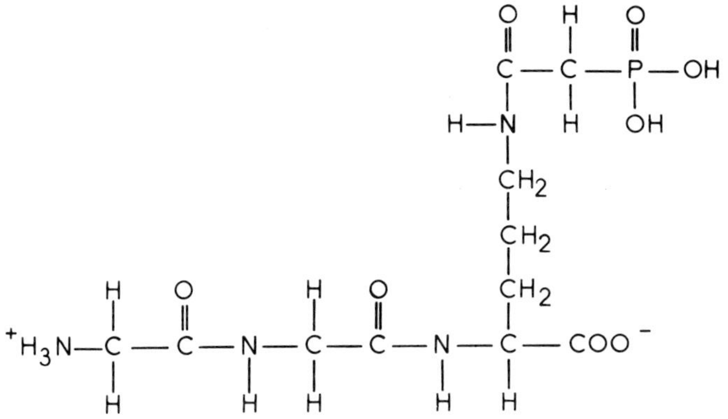

FIG. 6   Structure of diglycyl–δ–N–(phosphonoacetyl)–L–ornithine.

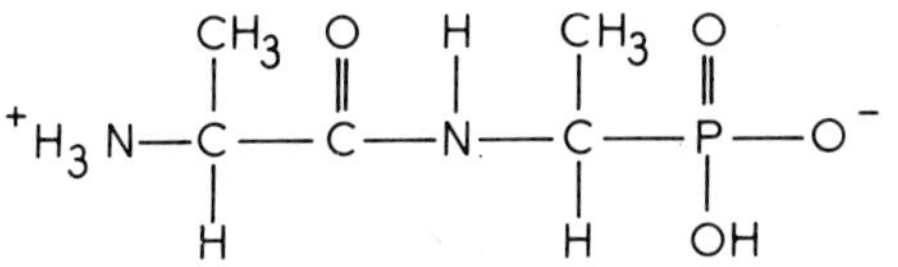

FIG. 7   Structure of alaphosphin.

dipeptide transport and the oligopeptide transport systems. The compound was synthesised as part of a series aimed at antagonising the D–alanyl–D–alanine that is an essential part of the disaccharide pentapeptide precursor of the peptidoglycan component of the bacterial cell wall (Allen *et al.*, 1978). Interestingly, the D,D enantiomer of alaphosphin is inactive and only the L,L stereoisomer which permits portage transport, is effective and allows the potency of the L–amino ethyl phosphonic acid to be displayed (Atherton *et al.*, 1979b). The activity of the dipeptide was sufficiently great to warrant an extensive programme to test the range and basis of its antibacterial activity as well as the synthesis of a large number of homologues (Allen *et al.*, 1979; Atherton *et al.*, 1979a).

The most detailed information on oligopeptide transport exists for *E. coli* though it is clear from sporadic reports in the literature that this capability exists in many other bacterial species as well (Barak and Gilvarg, 1975). However the extensive testing of alaphosphin and in particular its higher homologues has provided convincing evidence that the oligopeptide as well as the dipeptide system is widespread in both Gram-positive and Gram-negative organisms.

Conclusions

A priori there is no reason to expect that the information gleaned from the studies with *E. coli* will be capable of exact transliteration to other bacterial species. Indeed the size of peptide that will be accepted by the transport system appears to be species specific (Atherton *et al.*, 1979b). This is not unanticipated since the porosity of the bacterial cell envelope varies greatly and this barrier must be surmounted first, before a substance can gain access to the permeases of the cytoplasmic membrane. This is a limitation on the range of possible substances that can be considered for portage transport that must be taken into account. The discrimination against a substance that is too large for the pores of the cell envelope is a very sharp one (Gilvarg and Katchalski, 1965). In this connection it might also be mentioned that molecular weight is not a good guide to serve as a basis for establishing limits on the size of possible candidates for portage transport. The more relevant parameter is the hydrodynamic volume that the peptide sweeps out in solution and this can be assessed more meaningfully by determining its elution volume on a molecular sieve column rather than by reference to its molecular weight (Payne and Gilvarg, 1968).

Clearly, from a practical point of view, the ease with which resistant strains can arise will also be an important consideration in the assessment of portage transport applications. Here too, one would expect considerable species variability. However it should be pointed out that for those species that possess both dipeptide and oligopeptide transport systems there is every reason to use mixtures of di- and tripeptides containing the antimetabolite in order to exploit the enormous advantage to be gained in forcing a cell to mutate simultaneously at two independent loci to achieve resistance. Of course in those instances in which the antimetabolite has its own transport portal there is no reason not to employ it in free as well as in peptide form.

In a consideration of how the peptide carrier structure can be modified to accomodate its role as a participant in portage transport, all of the instances discussed above are examples of direct incorporation of an amino acid or close analogue into the peptide backbone. There would appear to be no limit to the tolerance for the kind of side chain employed. This suggests that, in principle, one could attach any antimetabolite to an appropriate side chain residue and expect it to be ferried into the cell. Naturally, the kind of linkage to the side chain would then determine whether the antimetabolite would be released once the peptide were within the cell.

For *E. coli* the N–terminal amino acid would appear to be an unpromising site for acyl linkages. The C—terminal carboxyl group, though not essential for transport, contributes importantly to affinity and is not a reasonable focus for chemical substitutions, though obviously, the closely mimetic phosphonic group is easily tolerated. It is not yet clear to what extent these various structural features are applicable to other bacterial and fungal species. Some preliminary information exists for *Saccharomyces* and *Candida* suggesting that the amino terminus is not as critical a determinant in these fungi as is true in *E. coli* and this was used as a basis for deciding to attach 5—fluorocytosine to the amino terminus of a peptide through a succinyl linker. However the linkage was not sufficiently stable to provide a critical test of these kinds of peptide derivatives (Steinfeld *et al.*, 1979).

Despite all these strictures it is clear that one should not overlook the point that the parable of the Trojan horse has direct applicability to antibacterial warfare.

References

Allen, J.G., Atherton, F.R., Hall, M.J., Hassall, C.H., Holmes, S.W., Lambert, R.W., Nisbet, L.J. and Ringrose, P.S. (1978). *Nature* **272**, 56–58.

Allen, J.G., Atherton, F.R., Hall, M.J., Hassall, C.H., Holmes, S.W., Lambert, R.W., Nisbet, L.J. and Ringrose, P.S. (1979). *Antimicrob. Agents Chemotherapy* **15**, 684–695.

Ames, B.N., Ames, G.F., Young, J.D., Isuchiya, D. and Lecocq, J. (1973). *Proc. Nat. Acad. Sci. U.S.A.* **70**, 456–458.

Atherton, F.R., Hall, M.J., Hassall, C.H., Lambert, R.W., Lloyd, W.J. and Ringrose, P.S. (1979a). *Antimicrob. Agents Chemotherapy* **15**, 696–705.

Atherton, F.R., Hall, M.J., Hassall, C.H., Lambert, R.W. and Ringrose, P.S. (1979b). *Antimicrob. Agents Chemotherapy* **15**, 677–683.

Barak, Z. and Gilvarg, C. (1975). *Biomembranes* **7**, 167–218.

Bayer, E., Gugel, K.H., Hägele, K., Hagenmaier, H., Jessipow, S., König, W.A. and Zähner, H. (1972). *Helv. Chim. Acta* **55**, 224–239.

Diddens, H. and Zähner, H. (1976). *Eur. J. Biochem.* **66**, 11–23.

Diddens, H., Dorgerloh, M. and Zähner, H. (1979). *J. Antibiot.* **32**, 87–90.

Fickel, T.E. and Gilvarg, C. (1973). *Nature, New Biol.* **241**, 161–163.

Gilvarg, C. (1972). *In* "Peptide Transport in Bacteria and Mammalian Gut", Ciba Foundation Symposium, Elsevier, Excerpta Medica, North Holland. Associated Scientific Publishers, Amsterdam, London, New York.

Gilvarg, C. and Katchalski, E. (1965). *J. Biol. Chem.* **240**, 3093–3098.

Losick, R. and Gilvarg, C. (1966). *J. Biol. Chem.* **241**, 2340–2346.

Mitchell, R.E. (1976). *Phytochemistry* **15**, 1941–1947.

Park, B.K., Hirota, A. and Sakai, H. (1977). *Agric. Biol. Chem.* **41**, 573–579.

Payne, J.W. (1977). *In* "Transport and Hydrolysis of Peptides by Micro-organisms", Ciba Foundation Symposium, Elsevier, Excerpta Medica, North Holland. Associated Scientific Publishers, Amsterdam, London, New York.

Payne, J.W. and Gilvarg, C. (1968). *J. Biol. Chem.* **243**, 6291–6299.

Penninckx, M. and Gigot, D. (1979). *J. Biol. Chem.* **254**, 6392–6396.

Pruess, D.L., Scannell, J.P., Ax, H.A., Kellett, M., Weiss, F., Demny, T.C. and Stempel, A. (1973). *J. Antibiot.* **26**, 261–266.
Steinfeld, A., Naider, F. and Becker, J.M. (1979). *J. Med. Chem.* **22**, 1104–1109.

Discussion

Professor Davies: Did Professor Gilvarg say what the antibacterial spectrum of phaseotoxin was? Is the range of bacteria against which it is effective known?

Professor Gilvarg: A number of people have worked on this compound and Mitchell determined its structure. A paper will appear shortly indicating that phaseotoxin is picked up by *Escherichia coli*, and I believe that at extraordinarily low concentrations it is effective in killing *Escherichia coli*. I have no idea of what its host range is.

Dr. Bost: Does not Professor Gilvarg think that one of the limitations of the portage transport is due to the fact that these peptides might be very sensitive to extracellular protease?

Professor Gilvarg: It is possible that that problem was avoided by the ala-phosphin because of the phosphonic acid derivative which may have assisted the peptide to escape attack. I have no personal experience with serum peptidases but it is something which might have to be taken into account. Obviously, the examples at the moment are very limited. It is my hope that there will be many attempts at using this technique for introducing materials into the cell. There may be sufficient peptidases in the blood for the antimetabolite to be rapidly released, which would lead to difficulties. However it is my understanding that human serum is rather low in peptidase activity, as compared to the serum of, say, the mouse. We should not jump to conclusions from results in test animals in this regard, but should assess the stability of the compound with respect to the peptidase spectrum in human serum.

Professor Sabath: I very much enjoyed Professor Gilvarg's paper. Would he comment on the transport across the human gut as an aspect of absorption of oral antibiotics, and the way in which that may or may not correlate with getting these oligopeptides into bacteria?

Professor Gilvarg: As Professor Sabath may know, in recent years the tide has turned from the original concept that all our amino–nitrogen is taken in by breaking down peptides to the level of the free amino acids, transporting the free amino acid into the enterocyte and hence into the portal circulation. There is now fairly good evidence that about 50% of amino–nitrogen is brought into the enterocyte in the form of at least dipeptides. Experiments performed by Matthews have shown that even a tripeptide is capable of entering the enterocyte. However, as far as I know, peptide transport has not been generally demonstrated for other mammalian cell types. It would therefore be anticipated that these peptides could at least be ferried into the enterocyte. Again, possibly because of the phosphonic acid, the alaphosphin may have escaped the usual fate of dipeptides, which is to be broken down in the enterocyte to the amino acids.

Professor Braun: Do these ornithine derivatives interfere with arginine bio-synthesis?

Professor Gilvarg: That has been proven for the tripeptide that I showed. The Belgian workers demonstrated that the free amino acid but not the peptide affects ornithine transcarbamylase.

Professor Tomasz: How frequent are mutations in *Escherichia coli* leading to the loss of peptide transport?

Professor Gilvarg: With respect to the oligopeptide transport system which I have studied, these mutations arise with great frequency. However I would like to stress that dipeptides can be ferried in by transport systems specific for dipeptides and also by the oligopeptide transport system. There are thus two portals of entry for a dipeptide. This represents a double guarantee against having a permeability-type mutant.

Secondly, it is important not to immediately jump to the conclusion that a strain which is going to lose the oligopeptide transport system will be virulent. As I understand it, in Spain, phosphonomycin is used clinically. The compound was previously excluded on the basis of the ease with which resistant mutants arose. On more thorough and detailed study it appears that these resistant mutants are not very virulent.

Professor Richmond: Returning to the subject of peptides and resistance, the problem with alaphosphin is the very rapid emergence of resistance, despite what Professor Gilvarg says about there being two transport systems.

Professor Gilvarg: I do not know whether alaphosphin itself is taken up by both systems — that point was never studied. It seems to me that it would have been a very good idea to have employed higher homologues along with the alaphosphin. That might thereby have avoided the emergence of resistant strains. In fact, with *Escherichia coli*, some of the higher homologues are just as effective as the alaphosphin. The two should have been employed simultaneously.

Professor Tomasz: Is there any regulatory connection known between the transport of an amino acid in the free amino acid form versus transport of that amino acid in the peptide form, such that if a bacterium was presented with the alternatives...?

Professor Gilvarg: I have no information other than in the case of *Escherichia coli*. With *Escherichia coli* the peptide transport system is insensitive to the amino acid, both from the point of view of co-transport, in that it does not act as an inhibitor, and also of absence of any regulatory effect. The oligopeptide transport system is constitutive in *Escherichia coli*.

Increase in Drug Efficacy by Combination

R. LABIA and M. GUIONIE

CNRS – CERCOA, Thiais, France

Introduction

The concept of drug combination has been widely developed and has proved to be very useful, particularly in the field of antibacterial therapy. Very often, the use of antibacterial drugs or antibiotics encounters resistance problems. Mostly, this situation arises through two mechanisms: (1) natural or intrinsic resistance, which simply defines the activity limits of a given antibiotic molecule; (2) acquired resistance, an evolutionary phenomenon which describes the more or less rapid development of microbes towards lower sensitivity to antimicrobial agents. As an example, resistance to penicillin G appeared very early in *Staphylococcus* (1946–1948), while resistance to the same antibiotic appeared in *Streptococcus* or *Gonococcus* only during the last decade (1970–1977).

Thus, by appropriate combination of antibacterial drugs, one can try to obtain more effective therapy, which here implies that the m.i.c. value of the combination can be considerably lower than that of each compound taken alone. It is worth noting that sometimes one of the compounds of the combination shows very poor antibacterial activity by itself, as is the case, for example, with clavulanic acid (Reading and Cole, 1977) or the sulphone CP 45899 (English *et al.*, 1978).

Another purpose of combinations might be to prevent the more or less rapid development of microbes resistant to a given monotherapy. A very famous and historic example is given by antituberculous treatments (Kendig and Brummer, 1970). Meanwhile, in this special case, the increase of drug efficacy follows as a consequence of a statistical decrease in the risk of appearance of resistant bacteria. Nevertheless, this aspect is fundamental when one considers the efficiency of the therapy.

At this time, the field of application of drug combinations is very wide.

Characterisation of Synergy

From a qualitative point of view, synergy is quite easy to show by techniques related to antibiotic sensitivity determination (Bonifas, 1952). By these methods, synergy (Fig. 1) was very clearly distinguished from antagonism (Figs 2 and 3) or indifference (Fig. 4). In the present paper, we shall consider indifference and addition to be synonymous.

From a quantitative point of view, synergy (and also antagonism or indifference) depicted by the isobologram, can be used to determine the optimum proportions of the two components of the combination. Thus an interaction index can be determined as the sum of the two fractional inhibitory concentrations (f.i.c.): $a_1/a_2 + b_1/b_2$, where a_1 and b_1 are the concentrations of the two antibiotics in the m.i.c. of the combination, and a_2 and b_2 are the m.i.c. values of the antibiotics acting separately. An interaction index of < 1, 1 and > 1 indicates synergy, indifference or antagonism respectively. However, examination of the interaction index must take into account the usual accuracy of the m.i.c. measurements (Sanderson and Drabu, 1979).

Nevertheless, *in vivo*, it appears quite impossible to maintain the optimum ratio of the two compounds previously determined, since various factors must be taken into consideration:

1) each component of the combination possesses its own individual pharmacokinetic and pharmacodynamic characteristics,
2) one of the two constituents of the combination could generate more acute intolerance or toxicity problems,
3) there are some economic problems, related to the cost of each compound, which could also influence the ratio chosen finally.

When a given ratio is adopted, it is necessary to evaluate the true

FIG. 1 (opposite)   Synergic effect obtained with cefotaxime and cloxacillin. The bacterial strain is *Enterobacter cloacae* P 99 (constitutive cephalosporinase producer).
FIG. 2 (opposite)   Antagonism observed between cefoxitin and cefuroxime. The bacterial strain is *Enterobacter cloacae* R 12 (inducible cephalosporinase producer).
FIG. 3 (opposite)   Antagonism observed between cefoxitin and cefotaxime. The bacterial strain is the same as in Fig. 2.
FIG. 4 (opposite)   Indifference between cefoxitin and mecillinam. Same bacterial strain as in Fig. 2.

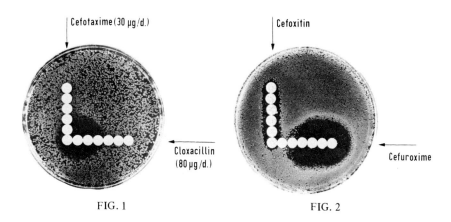

Cefotaxime (30 μg./d.)

Cloxacillin
(80 μg./d.)

FIG. 1

Cefoxitin

Cefuroxime

FIG. 2

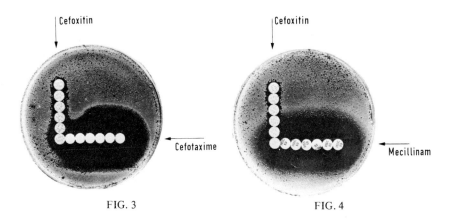

Cefoxitin

Cefotaxime

FIG. 3

Cefoxitin

Mecillinam

FIG. 4

synergic effect *in vivo*, by determination of the protective dose (PD_{50}) in experimental infections with laboratory animals.

Molecular Mechanisms usually Involved in Synergy

If the notion of indifference or addition between antibiotics might seem "natural" and self-explanatory, this is not the case for synergy or antagonism. Unfortunately, very often these last two phenomena can find only partial interpretation, if any. Thus we will only examine a few examples of synergic combinations for which a molecular mechanism is known or postulated. Mostly, we will examine recently proposed combinations, with special attention to those involving beta-lactams.

One very "didactic" synergistic combination is that of trimethoprim and sulphamethoxazole, substances which interfere with bacterial folic acid metabolism. Folic acid is a cofactor involved in the transport and activation of one carbon units, and also in their oxido—reduction. Sulphamethoxazole, like most antibacterial sulphonamides, inhibits dihydropteroate synthetase, by competition with p—aminobenzoate. This property had been demonstrated very early in the particular case of sulphanilamide (Woods, 1940; Lascelles and Woods, 1952). Thus sulphonamides inhibit and decrease folic acid synthesis.

The combination of sulphonamides with trimethoprim is usually synergic, since the latter substance inhibits dihydrofolate reductase, an enzyme involved in oxido—reduction of the cofactor. Thus the total decrease of active cofactor appears to be the product of the partial decrease effected by each compound. From the enzymatic point of view, the inhibition by these substances seems to be competitive and reversible.

Bacterial strains resistant to sulphonamides have been known for a very long time, and it has been shown by various authors that this resistance is related to alterations of the dihydropteroate synthetase. The "new" enzyme is then poorly inhibited by sulphonamides but has not lost its catalytic properties (see for example: Ortiz, 1970; Ho *et al.*, 1974).

More recently, bacterial strains resistant to trimethoprim have been isolated (O'Grady *et al.*, 1973). The resistance character may be chromosomally or R—factor mediated (Hamilton-Miller, 1979; Acar *et al.*, 1977). These strains produce an altered dihydrofolate reductase which is no longer inhibited by trimethoprim (Datta *et al.*, 1979).

Recently a new combination of this type has been proposed: tetroxoprim plus sulphadiazine (Bywater *et al.*, 1979).

A cycloserine (CS) and deuterofluoroalanine (DFA) combination has been proposed by the Merck company. In fact, in this combination,

CS was introduced in the form of "prodrug" derivative (PCS) in order to improve pharmacokinetic equivalence of the components of the combination (Kollonitsch and Barash, 1976). Cycloserine itself is an old product used previously in tuberculosis therapy. In the latter indication, the dosage of this substance was quite critical because of side-effects.Cycloserine inhibits bacterial alanine racemase by a competitive and progressively irreversible process characteristic of suicide substrates (Wang and Walsh, 1978). A similar mechanism may also be involved in DFA action (Soper *et al.*, 1976). If these last two statements are true, the reasons for this combination remain unclear. The true mode of action of these substances might well be more complex. They could also inhibit other enzymatic systems such as transaminases and ligases. Therefore much more needs to be known about these compounds.

Combinations which Involve Beta-Lactams

Synergy with Beta-Lactams and Aminoglycosides

The synergy obtained with these two families of antibiotics is well known. The reasons for the synergy are mostly speculative.

In one explanation the beta-lactam antibiotics, for which the cell wall is the target, might facilitate the penetration of aminoglycosides into the bacteria in order to reach the ribosome. The synergic effect is then related to the fact that beta-lactam antibiotics induce detectable alterations in the cell wall, even at concentrations considerably lower than the m.i.c. Conversely, a decrease in ribosomal protein biosynthesis induced by low concentrations of aminoglycosides will facilitate the action of beta-lactam antibiotics. The bacteria will thus not be able to restore the cell wall proteins bound by the beta-lactam antibiotics.

Synergy Involving Two Beta-Lactam Antibiotics

Mecillinam is an amidinopenicillin which binds selectively to a cell wall target termed PBP–2 (Penicillin Binding Protein) (Spratt, 1975, 1977). Mecillinam very often synergises with other beta-lactam antibiotics (penicillins or cephalosporins) which mostly bind other PBP's, such as 1 and 3 (Baltimore *et al.*, 1976; Chattopadhyay *et al.*, 1979; Tybring and Melchior, 1975). Mecillinam interacts with *E. coli* giving osmotically stable round forms, which may then be more easily lysed by the other beta-lactam compounds.

Recently, special attention has been paid to beta-lactamase inhibitors. This idea is rather old (Hamilton-Miller, 1977), and one of the first synergic combinations of this type was probably that of ampicillin and cloxacillin. Cloxacillin inhibits some beta-lactamases able to hydrolyse ampicillin at a moderate rate. Ampicillin is thus "protected" from degradation and retains its antibacterial activity. For various reasons this combination has not undergone further development.

We now know that cloxacillin mainly inhibits cephalosporinases, through a competitive and reversible process. Thus all beta-lactam antibiotics which are destroyed to any physiologically significant extent by these enzymes are liable to show synergy with cloxacillin. This was found previously with the first cephalosporins (Sykes and Matthew, 1976), but can be also demonstrated with the new cephalosporins (Labia and Guionie, 1979). For example, Fig. 1 shows the synergic effect of cefotaxime–cloxacillin that we obtained against *Enterobacter cloacae* P 99. This strain is a laboratory mutant which is a constitutive cephalosporinase hyperproducer (Sykes and Matthew, 1976). Hydrolysis of cefotaxime by P 99 cephalosporinase is difficult to demonstrate, since the maximum velocity of hydrolysis is low (Vmax = 0.2 compared to penicillin G = 100), but the affinity is very high (Km = 0.1 μM). Consequently, the parameter γ = Km/Vmax (Labia, 1974), which is related to the half-life of the beta-lactam at "low concentrations", is probably rather small. In fact, Fig. 1 shows clearly that cefotaxime hydrolysis by P 99 cephalosporinase has a physiological meaning: the strain is resistant to cefotaxime, but the antibiotic's activity increases in the presence of a beta-lactamase inhibitor.

This point is further substantiated by combinations of cefoxitin with other cephalosporins. Cefoxitin is a powerful inducer of cephalosporinases, and thus antagonises the activity of beta-lactams which are susceptible to hydrolysis by these enzymes. With another *Enterobacter cloacae* strain, R 12 (Dr. Pitton, Geneva), which produces an inducible cephalosporinase we have demonstrated powerful antagonism between cefoxitin and cefuroxime (Fig. 2), and a lesser effect with cefoxitin and cefotaxime (Fig. 3). This confirms that cefotaxime is hydrolysed by *Enterobacter cloacae* cephalosporinase, and also shows that cefuroxime is hydrolysed to a much greater extent.

Figure 4 shows a clear indifference between cefoxitin and mecillinam. Mecillinam is very resistant to hydrolysis by *Enterobacter cloacae* cephalosporinase: the enzyme has a low Vmax ($\simeq$ 1 compared to penicillin G = 100) and low affinity (Km $\geqslant$ 300 μM) for the substrate.

At present, examples of antagonism by cefoxitin and synergy with cloxacillin must be considered essentially as useful enzymatic tools. We have to take into account the fact that cloxacillin is itself destroyed by the R–factor mediated beta-lactamases (Labia *et al.,* 1979), which might suppress any synergic effect in such beta-lactamase producing strains.

A new class of R–factor mediated beta-lactamase (or more specifically penicillinase) inhibitors has been introduced, starting with clavulanic acid (Reading and Cole, 1977). Clavulanic acid and also the sulphone CP 45899 are suicide substrates (or suicide inhibitors) of the penicillinases. Suicide inhibition is characterised by a competitive and progressively irreversible process. This allows one to define and measure at least three important parameters: an affinity constant (Ki), an inactivation constant (k_{inact}) and a "turnover number", which characterises the number of inhibitor molecules necessary to give irreversible inhibition of one mole of enzyme (Labia *et al.*, 1980). Three R–factor mediated beta-lactamases (TEM–1, TEM–2 and Pitton's type 2) show similarly high affinities (Ki = 0.6 to 1.8 μM) for clavulanic acid and sulphone CP 45899, but in the time dependent inhibition phase, clavulanic acid appears somewhat more efficient (Labia *et al.*, 1980).

Conclusion

In the field of antimicrobial agents, drug combinations have given remarkable results which rival improvements made in monotherapy. These two fields of research are effectively complementary. Because a given substance gives good results in combinations, it does not follow that only compounds of the same chemical series will possess these same properties. Thus, at present, a variety of new beta-lactam antibiotics have emanated from research conducted specifically for this purpose. They include thienamycin, olivanic acid, PS 5 and, very recently, moxalactam.

References

Acar, J.F., Goldstein, F.W., Gerbaud, G.R. and Chabbert, Y.A. (1977). *Ann. Microbiol.* (Inst. Pasteur) 128 A, 41–47.

Baltimore, R.S., Klein, J.O., Wilcox, C. and Finland, M. (1976). *Antimicrob. Agents Chemother.* 9, 701–705.

Bonifas, V. (1952). *Experientia* 8, 234–239.

Bywater, M.J., Holt, H.A. and Reeves, D.S. (1979). *J. Antimicrob. Chemother.* (supp. B) 5, 51–60.

Chattopadhyay, B. and Hall, I. (1979). *J. Antimicrob. Chemother.* 5, 549–553.

Datta, N., Nugent, M., Amyes, S.G.B. and Mc Neilly, P. (1979). *J. Antimicrob. Chemother.* 5, 399–406.

English, A.R., Retsema, J.A., Girard, A.E., Lynch, J.E. and Barth, W.E. (1978). *Antimicrob. Agents Chemother.* **14**, 414–419.

Hamilton-Miller, J.M.T. (1977). *J. Antimicrob. Chemother.* **3**, 195–203.

Hamilton-Miller, J.M.T. (1979). *J. Antimicrob. Chemother.* (supp. B) **5**, 61–73.

Ho, R.I., Corman, L., Morse, S.A. and Artenstein, M.S. (1974). *Antimicrob. Agents Chemother.* **5**, 388–392.

Kendig, E.L. and Brummer, D.L. (1970). *In* "Antimicrobial Therapy". (B.M. Kagan, ed.), pp. 294–312. Saunders W.B. Co., London.

Kollonitsch, J. and Barash, L. (1976). *J. Am. Chem. Soc.* **98**, 5591–5593.

Labia, R. (1974). C.R. *Hebd. Séances Acad. Sci. Sér. D* **279**, 109–112.

Labia, R. and Guionie, M. (1979). *In* "Microbial Drug Resistance", Vol. II. (S. Mitsuhashi, ed.), pp. 301–308. Tokyo Univ. Press.

Labia, R., Lelièvre, V. and Peduzzi, J. (1980). *Biochim. Biophys. Acta* **611**, 351–357.

Lascelles, J. and Woods, D.D. (1952). *Brit. J. Exp. Path.* **33**, 288–301.

O'Grady, F., Kelsey-Fry, I., Mc Sherry, A. and Cattell, W.R. (1973). *J. Infect. Dis.* **128**, S652–S656.

Ortiz, P.J. (1970). *Biochemistry* **9**, 355–361.

Reading, C. and Cole, M. (1977). *Antimicrob. Agents Chemother.* **11**, 852–857.

Sanderson, P.J. and Drabu, Y.J. (1979). *J. Antimicrob. Chemother.* **5**, 728–730.

Soper, T.S., Jones, W.M., Lerner, B., Trop, M. and Manning, J.M. (1976). *J. Biol. Chem.* **252**, 3170–3175.

Spratt, B.G. (1975). *Proc. Nat. Acad. Sci.* (USA) **72**, 2999–3003.

Spratt, B.G. (1977). *Antimicrob. Agents Chemother.* **11**, 161–166.

Sykes, R.B. and Matthew, M. (1976). *J. Antimicrob. Chemother.* **2**, 115–157.

Tybring, L. and Melchior, N.H. (1975). *Antimicrob. Agents Chemother.* **8**, 271–276.

Wang, E. and Walsh, C. (1978). *Biochemistry* **17**, 1313–1321.

Woods, D.D. (1940). *Brit. J. Exp. Path.* **21**, 71–90.

Discussion

Professor Chabbert: The recent cephalosporins, as the oxa derivatives, cefotaxime, cefoperazone analogues and even cefotiam, all these products are obviously resistant to cephalosporinases secreted by enterobacteria, but some of these enzymes are known as being inducible, specially by cefoxitin. There is something that seems serious to me concerning their future, since it is relatively easy to obtain mutants or variants. I do not really know what these mutants are, and which are high producers of enzymes. Anyway, it would be desirable to avoid the mutant selection because the mutation rates for some enterobacteria are very high and you end up with hyperproductive strains. So, to try and avoid this mutation process, what would be the best solution?

Dr. Labia: It is obvious that a substance can more or less induce beta-lactamases; cefoxitin, in this respect, is very bad because it is the best inducer known. Now, to find antibiotics which would not give rise to mutants is a different problem.

Professor Chabbert: What about thienamycin? Do you think that it could not induce mutants and even allow to avoid their selection?

Dr. Labia: This is quite possible. It seems that this substance is very refractory to hydrolysis since it does not have any affinity for the enzymes. Nothing can happen, at least between them. But there might be other interactions.

Professor Chabbert: There is another question: why does cefoxitin induce more β–lactamase than the other cephalosporins?

Dr. Labia: In the laboratory, we carried out comparative measurements of the inducing capacity of cefamandole, cefoxitin and a few others. Cefoxitin induces 100 to 1000 times more than the others. Why? I do not know. It might be due to a sort of much more irreversible interaction of cefoxitin with the repressor gene, the acylation reaction of which for instance would become irreversible.

Professor Richmond: In connection with a question asked by Professor Chabbert about the emergence of resistance to thienamycin, it is interesting to know that, as Spratt has shown, thienamycin binds primarily to penicillin-binding protein 2. That is a behaviour which is also characteristic of mecillinam. I have taken a number of mecillinam resistant mutants and a number of so-called *vodY* mutants (where there is a mutation in the penicillin-binding protein 2, which has the effect of decreasing the affinity of that binding site for mecillinam) and these mutants are substantially less sensitive to thienamycin: the m.i.c. is increased about 10 or 15 fold.

Dr. Labia: It seems that bacterial resistance to mecillinam might involve few other mechanisms in addition with PBP–2 alterations, or mutations.

Part 3

*Suggestions on Methods for
Obtention of New
Antibiotics*

Screening for New Antibiotic Producers: The Selection of Wild Strains

H. A. LECHEVALIER

Waksman Institute of Microbiology, Rutgers –
The State University, New Jersey, U.S.A.

Introduction

According to the usually accepted definition, antibiotics are substances, produced by microorganisms, small amounts of which
inhibit the growth of microorganisms. Thus our interest is limited
to microorganisms and to substances active in trace amounts.

As far as the concentrations necessary for activity are concerned,
an antibiotic should be active against some microorganisms at least at
the concentration of 10 to 50 $\mu g/ml$. Most antibiotics are active in
the 1 $\mu g/ml$ range and many are active at the 0.1 to 0.01 $\mu g/ml$ range.

Now what are microorganisms? It is generally accepted that microorganisms include viruses, bacteria, fungi, algae and protozoa. Also
associations among organisms of these groups, such as lichens, are
considered to be microbes (Korzybski *et al.*, 1978).

My aim is to discuss the selection of wild strains of microorganisms
capable of producing antibiotics which have a chance of being novel.

Short Survey of Antibiotic Producers

We all take for granted that everything which is obvious and comparatively easy to do in the selection of potential antibiotic producers
has been done. Thus, for the isolation of novel antibiotics from wild
strains we can either keep doing what is easy and obvious in the hope
that eventually a rare type of microbe will show up, or alternatively,
grow easily isolated microorganisms in a novel fashion in the hope
that novel metabolites will thus be formed. A third approach would
be to try to use isolation methods which will permit us to grow the

organisms of nature which have not been grown as yet using our conventional procedures and hope that novel organisms produce novel metabolites.

Viruses are organisms that contain only one type of nucleic acid and which can reproduce only by growing within the cells of organisms that have both DNA and RNA. The culture of viruses involves the destruction of cells of higher forms of life, and although during that process antibiotics might be formed, I am not aware of any screening programme geared to their detection.

Protozoa, algae and lichens can produce antibiotics. Bérdy in 1974 counted 23 antibiotics produced by algae, 56 by lichens and 8 by protozoa.

The rate of growth of lichens is proverbially slow, and they cannot readily be cultivated; thus, antibiotics from lichens can only be extracted from specimens having grown in nature. In addition, we are told that due to the overall pollution of the world, the lichens are a disappearing breed. Lichen products may thus become fossil chemicals.

Some algae can be grown in the laboratory, though at a comparatively slow pace; others can be found in nature in large enough quantities to be used as a source of natural products. Our lack of experience with algae and protozoa will induce us to drop them from consideration and we will mainly turn our attention to bacteria and fungi as sources of antibiotics.

Bérdy (1974) counted about 2500 antibiotics produced by bacteria and about 800 by fungi. These are the organisms that we know how to handle in the laboratory most easily. Production of large biomasses of these organisms is possible with comparative ease, making the production of a useful antibiotic on a commercial scale a profitable venture. Among the bacteria, the actinomycetes have been the most prolific producers of antibiotics, accounting for about 2100 antibiotics or 84% of Bérdy's bacterial antibiotics.

In order to find novel antibiotics, one could argue with equal conviction that one should not screen actinomycetes and concentrate on other groups of microorganisms because actinomycetes have been over-exploited as sources of new antibiotics, or inversely that a screening programme should concentrate on actinomycetes because they have been the most prolific source of antibiotics. Thus the isolation of novel actinomycetes would be an attractive source of potentially new antibiotics.

Thirty-two years ago, I was told that it was not worth looking for a new antibiotic since the chances of seeing one's discovery reach the market was so low as to be non-existent. Such pessimism is certainly more appropriate now than it was a third of a century ago. As Conover has shown in 1971, we have passed from a period of rapid expansion in the field of discovery of new useful antibiotics to one where modifications of already known substances has yielded compounds of therapeutic value. In that field also, success did not come easily and it takes the preparation of about 1000 derivatives of penicillin to see one accepted for clinical practice.

Prospects for Anaerobes

If one looks at Bérdy's compilation of 1974, one notes that the two most prolific genera of bacteria, as far as antibiotic production is concerned, are *Streptomyces* and *Bacillus*. Also, one is struck by the paucity of antibiotics produced by anaerobic bacteria.

There are two possible explanations for the lack of reports on the production of antibiotics by anaerobes: one is that the anaerobic type of metabolism does not lead to the formation of secondary metabolites; the second possibility is that anaerobes have not been screened vigorously for the production of these metabolites.

Concerning the first possibility, it is probably taken for granted by most microbiologists that the products of life without air are not extremely varied. However, not all anaerobic microorganisms have the same type of metabolism. One can differentiate at least the large groups of the photosynthetic bacteria, the fermenters that produce methane, organic solvents and acids, and the organisms capable of anaerobic respiration in presence of nitrates. As reported by Evans (1977), the products of degradation of aromatic compounds under anaerobic conditions are varied, thus suggesting that from this diversity, antibiotics might emerge.

This takes us to the second question: Is it possible that anaerobes have escaped the scrutiny of those screening for antibiotics?

In 1974, I asked this very question to two well known specialists of anaerobes. Dr. R.E. Hungate could not recall that any systematic search had been made for the detection of antibiotics by anaerobes. On the other hand, Dr. Louis D.S. Smith remembered that such screening programmes had been run in the 1950's but that nothing of value had been found.

We never published the results of our own screening programme using anaerobes as a potential source of antibiotics. I shall summarise it here.

In one screen, one hundred and sixty-five cultures of bacteria were isolated by plating out anaerobically various substrates on a few media, the most commonly used one containing beef extract, peptone, glycerol and yeast extract (NYG–2). The anaerobes were streaked on NYG–2 agar plates and incubated anaerobically before cross-streaking with *Escherichia coli, Staphylococcus aureus, Pseudomonas aeruginosa* and *Candida albicans.* Twenty-five of the isolates gave wide (15 mm or more) zones of inhibition against the bacteria at least. The pH of the agar in the zones of inhibition was measured and the widths of the zones of inhibition were not always proportional to the acidity. Each of the active strains was grown anaerobically in four different liquid media. Testing for activity of the liquid cultures by dilution assay revealed little activity and, what there was, disappeared upon neutralisation of the filtrates.

We concluded from this first screen that the inhibition was due to the production of acids of various types but that various acids do not all have the same range of biological activity.

A second screen consisted in the testing of cultures of anaerobic bacteria directly in liquid media. Samples of soil, such as mud, suspected of having rather low redox potentials were plated out on water agar fortified with 0.05 g/l of L–cysteine. After one month of anaerobic incubation at 28°C, a selection of the anaerobes was transferred directly to liquid media and was again incubated anaerobically. After one and two weeks of incubation the cultures that grew (about 50% did not grow) were tested by streak-dilution against the four test organisms that I mentioned previously. Of the 286 cultures that grew under these conditions, 43 had some activity against one of the test organisms. We decided that to be of interest to us, an active substance would have to be produced only anaerobically and be filterable, through a bacteriological filter. None of the active strains produced such a compound. The most common type of activity was when the cells of the anaerobe were placed in direct contact with those of the test organisms.

Our neighbours at E.R. Squibb and Sons, have also experimented with the screening of anaerobes. They found some active strains and in every case the active compound was a fatty acid (Richard Sykes, pers. comm.).

Perhaps, an anaerobe will be found one day that will produce a wonder drug, but the prospect does not look very bright to me on the basis of what we have done and what has been published so far.

Prospects for Actinomycetes

Now, I would like to turn my attention to the actinomycetes since they have been the main subject of my attention during my professional life.

In 1948, when I joined the staff of Dr. Selman A. Waksman, he considered that soil actinomycetes were composed only of strains of

Streptomyces, Micromonospora, and *Nocardia.* It is with suspicion that he witnessed the explosion of the new genera of actinomycetes which started with John N. Couch's rediscovery of sporangia-bearing actinomycetes (Lechevalier, 1968) in 1950.

In Table 1 are listed some of the genera of aerobic soil actinomycetes which can be considered potential sources of antibiotics. Some

TABLE 1

Selected List of Genera of Soil Actinomycetes to be Considered for Antibiotic Production

Nonsporate	Polysporate
Agromyces	*Actinomadura*
Intrasporangium	*Actinosynnema*
Mycoplana	*Chainia*
Nocardia	*Micropolyspora*
Nocardioides	*Nocardiopsis*
Oerskovia	*Pseudonocardia*
Promicromonospora	*Saccharomonospora*
Rhodococcus	*Saccharopolyspora*
	Streptomyces
Monosporate	*Streptoverticillium*
Micromonospora	
Thermoactinomyces	Sporangiate
Thermomonospora	
	Actinoplanes
	Amorphosporangium
Bisporate	*Ampullariella*
	Dactylosporangium
Microbispora	*Microellobosporia*
	Planomonospora
Muriform	*Spirillospora*
	Streptosporangium
Geodermatophilus	

of these forms, such as *Microbispora*, and all the sporangiate actinomycetes were unknown during the first half of this century. Others such as *Actinomadura, Nocardiopsis* and *Nocardioides* could have been classified into the system of Waksman before the advent of chemotaxonomic criteria (Lechevalier and Lechevalier, 1965).

Rare Genera as Potential Producers

We attempted in 1964 to gauge the frequency with which members of the so-called rare genera of actinomycetes were isolated. We observed about 5000 colonies of actinomycetes obtained by plating out 16 soil samples (Lechevalier, 1964). No attempt was made to isolate what appeared to be streptomycetes and the related streptoverticillia, nor was any effort made to isolate morphologically uninteresting actinomycetes which could have been nocardiae. The results of our survey is shown in Table 2, together with an estimate

TABLE 2

Occurrence of "Rare" Forms of Actinomycetes in 16 Soil Samples.
About 5000 colonies of actinomycetes were examined.

Genus	No. of strains	Antibiotics[a]
Micromonospora	70	41
Micropolyspora	28	2
Actinoplanes	10	23
Microbispora	9	4
Thermoactinomyces	8	9
Streptosporangium	5	10
Microellobosporia	2	3

[a] Estimate of the number of antibiotics known to be produced by the genus.

of the number of antibiotics known to be produced by members of these various genera. One will note that in general, the estimate of the number of antibiotics known to be produced by strains of a given genus is proportional to the ease with which members of the various genera can be isolated. Thus the conclusion can be reached that as more "rare" actinomycetes will be isolated and screened, the more antibiotics there will be found to produce (Nara *et al.*, 1977).

Originality and Potentiality of Antibiotics from Rare Genera

The next question is: How novel are the antibiotics which are produced by the rare forms of actinomycetes?

Let us select the genus *Actinoplanes* since our task has been made easy by a recent review by Parenti and Coronelli (1979). As you can see from an examination of Table 3, some of the antibiotics produced by strains of *Actinoplanes* belong to families of antibiotics produced by streptomycetes. These include mixtures of macrocyclic lactones and depsipeptides of the virginiamycin-type, antifungal polyenic macrolides, peptides, and naphthoquinones. In one case at least, the same sulfur-containing polypeptide has been isolated from actinoplanetes and from streptomycetes.

In contrast, there is also some chemical novelty, for example, chuangxinmycin is composed of a unique bicyclic system formed of an indole nucleus fused to a thiopyran residue (Fig. 1). Some of the antibiotics of *Actinoplanes* characterised so far represent classes of compounds unknown as products of actinomycetes. Such is the case of Antibiotic A/15104Y (Fig. 2) which represents the first example of a halogenated pyrrole from an actinomycete. Such compounds had been found previously only as products of sponges and pseudomonads (Parenti and Coronelli, 1979).

TABLE 3

Antibiotics Produced by Strains of *Actinoplanes*

Name	Chemical nature	Type of activity	Producing *Actinoplanes*	Year of discovery
Taitomycin	S-containing poly-peptide	Gram + including anaerobes	*taitomyceticus* also streptomycetes	1969
A/672	acid	Gram +	*brasiliensis*	1969
A/4696	base	Gram + fungi	*sp.*	1972
A/477	Cl-containing base	Gram +	*sp.*	1972
A/287	cyclic peptides	Gram +	*utahensis*	1974
Purpuromycin	naphthoquinone	Gram + Gram − fungi	*ianthinogenes*	1974
Lipiarmycin	Cl-containing base	Gram +	*deccanensis*	1975
A/2315 Plauracins	virginiamycin-group	Gram + Gram − fungi	*philippinensis auranticolor*	1975
SE73 SE73−B	macrolides (?)	Gram + Gram −	*sp.*	1975
Gardimycin	S-containing poly-peptide	Gram +	*garbadinensis liguriae*	1976
A/7413	S-containing poly-peptides	Gram +	*sp.*	1977
	naphtoquinone dimer	Gram +	*cyaneus*	1977
Chuangxinmycin	acid with fused indole and thiopyran nuclei	Gram + Gram −	*tsinanensis*	1977
67−121 Sch−16656	heptaenes	fungi	*caeruleus azureus sp.*	1977
41.012	acidic polypeptide	Gram +	*nipponensis*	1977
Teichomycin A$_1$	phosphoglycolipid	Gram + Gram −	*teichomyceticus*	1978
A$_2$	Cl-containing glyco-peptide	Gram +	,,	
A/15104	chlorophenols	Gram + Gram − fungi	*sp.*	1978
5−aza−cytidine		Gram − tumors	*missouriensis*	1978
A/17002	virginiamycin group	Gram + Gram −	*sp.*	1979
A−10947	S-containing peptide	Gram + mycoplasmas	*sp.*	1979

From Parenti and Coronelli, 1979; Yaginuma *et al.*, 1979.

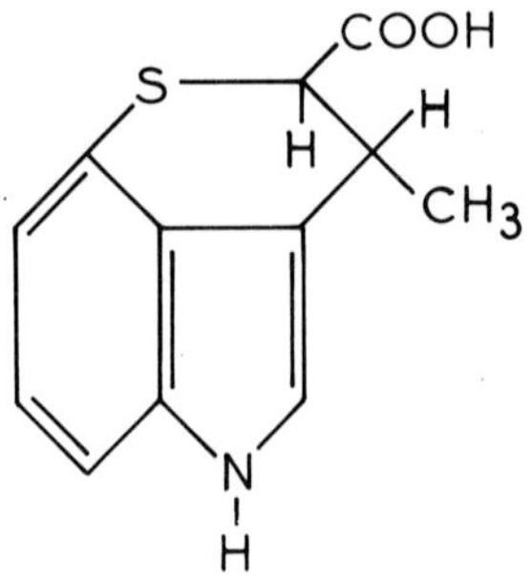

FIG. 1   Structure of chuangximycin.

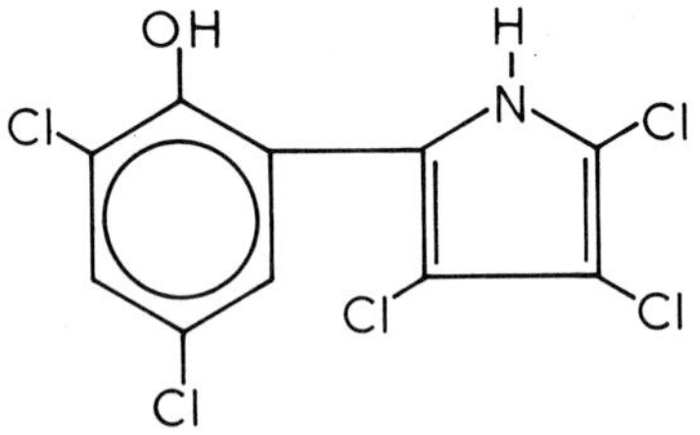

FIG. 2   Structure of antibiotic A/15104 Y.

One could add, in an optimistic note, that many of the antibiotics listed in Table 3 are rather non-toxic. When tested intraperitoneally in mice, 12 of them had LD_{50}'s of more than 200 mg/kg and 8 of these were 1000 mg/kg or more.

We can thus conclude from this survey of the antibiotics known to be produced by *Actinoplanes* that, when investigated, a group of "rare" actinomycetes was found to produce a number of new antibiotics most of which belonged to families of compounds previously known as metabolites of other groups of actinomycetes but that new types of structures had been spotted.

We cannot always recognise the novelty of the actinomycetes which are described as producers of new antibiotics from the literature. I could give as an example the case of the genus *Actinosynnema*.

Toru Hasegawa, while working in our laboratory, isolated from a grass blade which was floating in river water an actinomycete which formed synnemata bearing chains of flagellated spores (Fig. 3) (Hasegawa *et al.*, 1978). The organism had a Type III cell wall and a sugar pattern of Type C. We proposed the genus *Actinosynnema* to accommodate such organisms. We became aware that ATCC 21806, described by Aoki *et al.* in 1976 and named by them *Nocardia*

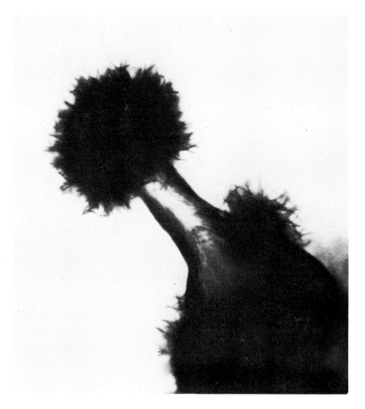

FIG. 3   Synnema of *Actinosynnema mirum*. Bright field microscopy. x 625.

uniformis subsp. *tsuyamanensis* had these properties, although we would not have been able to guess it from their description. This organism produces β–lactam antibiotics called nocardicins. We also became aware that the so-called *"Nocardia"* producing the anti-tumour compound, ansamitocin, was also an *Actinosynnema* (Higashide *et al.*, 1977).

The nocardicins are very non-toxic antibacterial antibiotics and the antitumour ansamitocins are of interest since they are the first maytansinoids which can be produced by fermentation, the others previously known being products of tropical plants (Fig. 4). We thus see that a small group of rare actinomycetes which can easily be characterised morphologically and chemically, has been found to produce compounds of potential therapeutic importance.

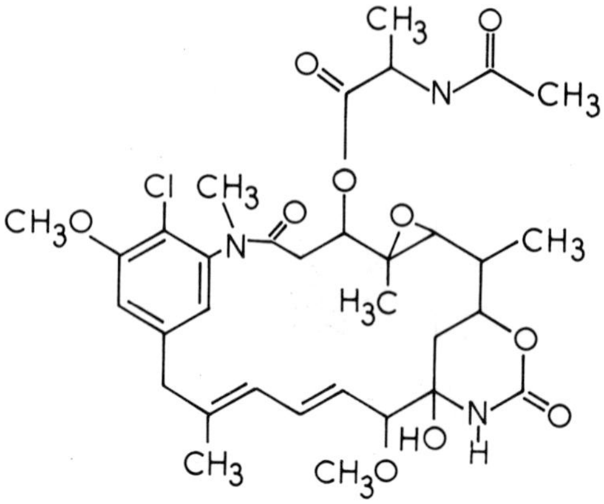

FIG. 4   Structure of maytansine from *Maytenus ovatus* (Celastraceae).

Unusual Culture Conditions and Relationships with Strain Morphology and Antibiotic Production

I would like now to discuss briefly the production of antibiotics by strains which are not grown under the usual set of conditions and see if this might lead to the detection of novel types of metabolites. The most common way of obtaining an antibiotic from actinomycetes is to isolate streptomycetes and to grow them in aerated liquid media. But there are indications that antibiotics are also formed under different conditions.

For example, it has been known for almost as long as antibiotics have been studied, that it was possible to get large zones of inhibition on solid media but that the cultures producing this type of inhibition were not always the producers of antibiotics when grown on liquid media or that the antibiotics produced under the two sets of circumstances seemed to be different since they did not have the same antibiotic spectra (Routien and Finlay, 1952; Hsu and Lockwood, 1969; Hamill, 1977). Another possibility, which is but a variation on the previous theme, is that different mixtures of antibiotics are formed under both sets of circumstances.

This problem has recently interested Shomura and co-workers (1979) who, having found 1300 strains of actinomycetes which were active on a solid glycerol—peptone—meat extract medium, against at least one of 7 test organisms (bacteria and yeasts), grew them in five liquid media. They found 25 strains that were active only on the solid medium. One of these was selected for further study. It was identified as *Streptomyces halstedii* and it was noted that the mycelium remained intact on the solid medium but fragmented in liquid media, where no antibiotic production took place. It was also found that if the liquid media were made more dilute, the mycelium retained its integrity and the antibiotic, which was characterised as N—carbamoyl—D—glucosamine (Omoto *et al.*, 1979) was produced.

This very non-toxic antibiotic, which is mainly active against Gram-negative bacteria, is produced not only on dilute media where the mycelium does not fragment but also by non-fragmenting mutants of *S. halstedii* indicating a connection between cellular morphology and antibiotic production. Links between morphology and antibiotic production have long been suspected. For example, the very fact that members of the genera *Bacillus* and *Streptomyces* are producers of spores, though of a different type, and are prolific antibiotic producers, has suggested some relationship between the production of antibiotics and the ability to sporulate.

In a recent study, McCann and Pogell (1979) reported on the production of a highly saturated alicyclic compound by a strain of *Streptomyces alboniger* which had activity against Gram-positive bacteria and *Neurospora* and which was also a stimulator of the production of aerial mycelium by the producing organism. The antibiotic was isolated from cultures of the actinomycete grown on solid media.

These studies point to the fact that actinomycetes may produce metabolites which are more easily detected when the organisms are grown on solid rather than in liquid media. In addition, they suggest various approaches to be prospected in the search for new antibiotics. For example one could isolate fragmenting actinomycetes and obtain from them nonfragmenting mutants which might be screened for the production of unusual antibiotics, or screening programmes could be set up for the detection of stimulators of sporulation in the hope that these will turn out to be also antibiotics of unusual virtue.

Indirectly, the stimulation of sporulation might also lead to the production of various metabolites. It has been noted that the loss of the ability to form aerial mycelium was accompanied with the simultaneous loss of several functions such as the ability to produce metabolites of the geosmin-type, loss of the ability to produce pigments and the loss of the ability to synthesise arginine (Redshaw *et al.*, 1979).

It is only logical to conclude that some of the bald actinomycetes found in soil are derived from aerial mycelium-forming parents. Such strains could be subjected to the action of sporulation stimulators and an effort could be made to see if antibiotic production was also generated. The studies of Redshaw *et al.* (1979) however would indicate that the aerial mycelium-deficient form of streptomycetes, which would be the synthetically less-gifted form, would also be the most stable morphologically, though the most vulnerable physiologically, since they would require preformed amino acids such as arginine. If such is the case, one could argue that it is not so much the capability to produce antibiotics which favours the survival of the antibiotic producers in nature but the fact that they do not require preformed amino acids.

Recently, in our laboratory, Thomas Umbreit compared by thin layer chromatography, the production of pigments by a strain of *Streptomyces viridochromogenes* grown under a variety of cultural conditions. He noted that a certain green pigment, probably a quinone, was produced on solid rice cultures but not in 9 liquid media which included rice extract. The pigment was, however, produced in thick slurries of a number of cereals. This observation lends support to the concept that certain metabolites are not formed when actinomycetes are grown in our conventional aerated liquid media. There is thus still room for experimentation not only in the selection of the wild strains to be screened for antibiotic production but also in the conditions under which we grow them.

Conclusion

I would conclude that the screening for new metabolites from cultures of comparatively rare microorganisms is a valid approach. I would add that an effort should be made not only to isolate a diversity of rare forms to feed into the screens but that the conditions of growth of the organisms should be varied. I would add that this approach to the search of new metabolites should not be the only one used but that it is the most likely approach to yield completely new types of molecules. Other approaches, such as mutasynthesis, recombination, bioconversions, are more likely to yield variations on known chemical themes.

Acknowledgments

I wish to thank M.P. Lechevalier for Figure 3 and the support of the Charles and Johanna Busch Fund for the experimental work reported.

References

Aoki, H., Sakai, H.-I., Kohsaka, M., Konomi, T., Hosoda, J., Kubochi, Y., Iguchi, E. and Imanaka, H. (1976). *J. Antibiot.* **29**, 492—500.
Bérdy, J. (1974). *Adv. Appl. Microbiol.* **18**, 309—406.
Conover, L.H. (1971). *In* "Advances in Chemistry, Series No. 108, Drug Discovery", pp. 33—80. American Chemical Society.

Evans, W.C. (1977). *Nature* **270**, 17–22.

Hamill, R.L. (1977). *Jap. J. Antibiot.* **30**, S164–S173.

Hasegawa, T., Lechevalier, M.P. and Lechevalier, H.A. (1978). *Inter. J. Syst. Bacteriol.* **28**, 304–310.

Higashide, E., Asai, M., Ootsu, K., Tanida, S., Kozai, Y., Hasegawa, T., Kishi, T., Sugino, Y., and Yoneda, M. (1977). *Nature* **270**, 721–722.

Hsu, S.C. and Lockwood, J.L. (1969). *J. Gen. Microbiol.* **57**, 149–158.

Korzybski, T., Kowszyk-Gindifer, Z. and Kurylowicz, W. (1978). "Antibiotics. Origin, Nature and Properties". American Society for Microbiology, Washington, D.C.

Lechevalier, H.A. (1964). *In* "Principles and Applications in Aquatic Microbiology". (H. Heukelekian and N.C. Dondero, eds), pp. 230–253. John Wiley, New York.

Lechevalier, H.A. (1968). *Inter. J. Syst. Bacteriol.* **18**, 203–206.

Lechevalier, H.A. and Lechevalier, M.P. (1965). *Ann. Inst. Pasteur* **108**, 662–673.

McCann, P.A. and Pogell, B.M. (1979). *J. Antibiot.* **32**, 673–678.

Nara, I., Kawamoto, I., Okachi, R. and Oka, T. (1977). *Jap. J. Antibiotics* **30**, S174–S189.

Omoto, S., Shomura, T., Suzuki, H. and Inouye, S. (1979). *J. Antibiot.* **32**, 436–441.

Parenti, F. and Coronelli, C. (1979). *Annu. Rev. Microbiol.* **33**, 389–411.

Redshaw, P.A., McCann, P.A., Pentella, M.A. and Pogell, B.M. (1979). *J. Bacteriol.* **137**, 891–899.

Routien, J.B. and Finlay, A.C. (1952). *Bacteriol. Rev.* **16**, 51–67.

Shomura, T., Yoshida, J., Amano, S., Kojima, M., Inouye, S. and Niida, T. (1979). *J. Antibiot.* **32**, 427–435.

Yaginuma, S., Muto, N. and Otani, M. (1979). *J. Antibiot.* **32**, 967–969.

Discussion

Professor Rinehart: The question of maytansine production by *Maytenus ovatus* is still open. It is not really clear whether it is produced by a plant. There has been considerable speculation that it might be microorganisms simply working on the plant. Many of us were very happy to see that it was produced by *Nocardia* – or, at least, something related to it.

Professor Lechevalier: It is not produced by *Nocardia*, but by *Actinosynnema*.

Dr. Gero: In this respect, is the maytansine identical with Takeda's and Kupchian's product, or is it a different maytansine structurally?

Professor Lechevalier: It is not identical, but different. The microbial product has different substitution, and I gave only the formula of the parent compound. The structures are known and there are slight differences, but not many.

Professor Demain: I have always been interested in the fact that the yeasts were such poor producers of antibiotics, and now Professor Lechevalier has told us about the clostridia. Would he agree that there certainly seems to be some type of ecological relationship between antibiotic production and a particular niche? It seems to me that organisms which have ability to live in restricted environments do well without antibiotic production, whereas organisms in the soil that have to compete with many other species produce many antibiotics. Could Professor Lechevalier comment on this idea?

Professor Lechevalier: I cannot really comment. It is a rather difficult question to answer. It seems to imply some sort of function for the production of secondary metabolites. The main difference between aerobes and anaerobes is that the anaerobic pathways do not lead to the formation of such diverse secondary metabolites — that is the basic difference. I do not know whether life without air is a difficult and restrictive environment for a microorganism. After all, it was the first environment that there was on earth before the presence of photosynthetic organisms. I do not know whether such an environment is specifically taxing. On the contrary, it may well be a rather non-taxing way of life because it is both primitive and easy.

Screening of Specific Inhibitors of Cell Wall Peptidoglycan Synthesis: An Approach to Early Identification of New Antibiotics

S. ŌMURA

Kitasato University and The Kitasato Institute,
Minato-ku, Tokyo, Japan

Introduction

Many kinds of attempts to isolate new antibiotics have been made and a large number of antibiotics have been discovered in the past four decades; many infectious diseases have been conquered by using antibiotics as chemotherapeutics. However, additional useful antibiotics are needed for the treatment of disease caused by drug resistant microbes, of super infections and of opportunistic infections.

Unfortunately, finding a new antibiotic has become more and more difficult. In these circumstances, to put a relatively narrow target among many kinds of antibiotics seems useful for early identification of antibiotics and reaching an effective success for the new antibiotics. Among the various types of antibiotics which have various modes of action, specific inhibitors of cell wall peptidoglycan synthesis are characterised in general by their low toxicities. Consequently, we attempted to establish a new screening method for such an inhibitor (Ōmura *et al.*, 1979a).

Figure 1 shows the biosynthetic pathway of cell wall peptidoglycan in bacteria and inhibition sites of its inhibitors. It seems possible to find new inhibitors having different targets in this pathway. Our screening method for cell wall synthesis inhibitors is based on the inactivity of cell wall inhibitors against mycoplasmas, which lack a cell wall, and on the inhibition of incorporation of radioactive precursors into macromolecules in *Bacillus* sp.

In this screening programme, we could find a new cell wall synthesis inhibitor, azureomycin, and also new antibiotics other than cell wall synthesis inhibitors, nanaomycins, frenolicin B, asukamycin, setomimycin and vineomycin (OS–4742).

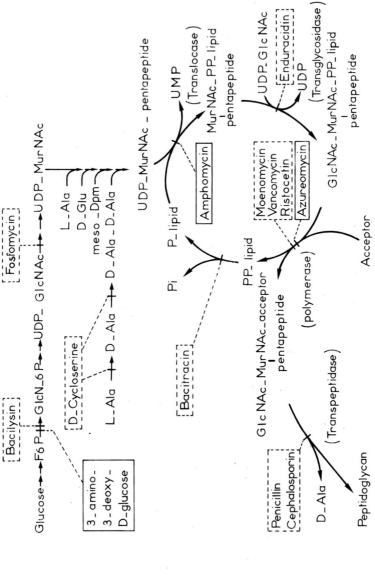

FIG. 1 Biosynthetic pathway of cell wall peptidoglycan and its inhibitors. Azureomycin, amphomycin and 3-amino-3-deoxy-D-glucose were located in the figure by the present work.

The present paper deals with the screening method and the new antibiotics found in this screening work, and the mechanism of action of azureomycin, amphomycin and 3–amino–3–deoxy–D–glucose (3–AG).

Screening Methods

Primary Screening Method: Antimycoplasmal Activity of Antibiotics

As mycoplasmas have no cell wall, cell wall synthesis inhibitors have no activity against mycoplasmas. Among strains of mycoplasmas, *Mycoplasma gallisepticum* KP–13 and *Acholeplasma laidlawii* PG8 were used as test organisms for paper disk method. Antimycoplasmal and antibacterial activities of various antibiotics were compared to determine whether comparative activity can be useful as the primary test for screening for specific inhibitors of the synthesis of bacterial cell wall peptidoglycan.

Table 1 shows the comparison of the activities of various antibiotics against *M. gallisepticum, A. laidlawii, Bacillus subtilis* and *Escherichia coli.* Inhibitors of protein biosynthesis or nucleic acid synthesis, such as tetracyclines, macrolides, actinomycin D, iyomycin, daunorubicin, streptonigrin, mitomycin C and hedamycin, were active against both mycoplasmas and bacteria. Penicillin G, D–cycloserine, vancomycin, ristocetin and cephaloridine, inhibitors of bacterial cell wall synthesis, were active against *B. subtilis* but did not affect the growth of both *Mycoplasma* and *Acholeplasma. M. gallisepticum* KP–13 was not sensitive to aminoglycoside antibiotics (100 µg/ml) such as streptomycin, kanamycin and so on, but these antibiotics that are inhibitors of protein synthesis were active against *A. laidlawii* PG8. Some antibiotics such as lividomycin, viomycin and colistin were found to be inactive against the mycoplasmas at the concentrations tested.

From these results, it was ascertained that cell wall inhibitors could be selected in the primary screen by picking out antibacterial substances that were inactive against mycoplasmas.

Secondary Screening Method: Influence of Antibiotics on Incorporation of [³H] Diaminopimelic Acid and [¹⁴C] Leucine into Acid-Insoluble Fraction of Bacterial Cells

As described above, there are some antibiotics which are not cell wall synthesis inhibitors and have no activity against mycoplasma. These antibiotics other than the cell wall synthesis inhibitors could be

TABLE 1

Antimicrobial Activities of Various Antibiotics against *M. gallisepticum*, *A. laidlawii*, *B. subtilis* and *E. coli*

Antibiotic (100 μg/ml)	Mode of Action*	Antimicrobial activity**			
		M. gal.	*A. lai.*	*B. sub.*	*E. coli*
Tetracycline	P	+	+++	+	+
Oxytetracycline	P	++	++	+	−
Leucomycin	P	++	++	+	±
Amaromycin	P	++	+	+	−
Streptomycin	P	−	++	+	++
Dihydrostreptomycin	P	−	++	++	+
Kanamycin	P	−	+	+	++
Kanendomycin	P	−	+	+	++
Lividomycin	P	−	−	+	+
Bluensomycin	P	−	+	+	+
Viomycin	P	−	−	+	+
Colistin	M	−	−	−	+
Actinomycin D	N	+++	+++	++	−
Iyomycin	N	+	+	+	−
Daunorubicin	N	+	+	+	−
Streptonigrin	N	+	++	+	+++
Mitomycin C	N	++	+++	++	+++
Hedamycin	N	++	+	+	+
Kinamycin D		+	+	+	+
Cerulenin	L	+	−	++	++
Azalomycin		−	+	+	−
Xanthomycin		+	+	+	−
Penicillin G	W	−	−	+	−
D−Cycloserine	W	−	−	+	−
Vancomycin	W	−	−	+	−
Ristocetin	W	−	−	+	−
Cephaloridine	W	−	−	++	+

* P: Inhibition of protein synthesis
   N: Inhibition of nucleic acid synthesis
   M: Interference with cytoplasmic membrane
   L: Inhibition of lipid synthesis
   W: Inhibition of cell wall synthesis
** −: negative,   +: 10−20 mm,   ++: 10−30 mm, +++: 30−40 mm of diameter of inhibitory zone
.(reprinted with permission of The Japan Antibiotics Research Association)

eliminated by the estimation of the inhibition of selective incorporation of precursor of cell wall synthesis. For this purpose, effects of various antibiotics on incorporation of radioactive precursors into macromolecules were examined. *Bacillus* sp. KB152 (Dpm⁻) was used as the test organism. The organism contains *meso*−diaminopimelic acid (Dpm) in cell wall peptidoglycan. Dpm is an amino acid which is not incorporated into macromolecules other than peptidoglycan, while leucine (Leu) is an amino acid which is not incorporated into peptidoglycan. The cold L—lysine was added to the medium to prevent the formation of labelled L—lysine from [³H] Dpm. In early stage of this work we used prototrophic *Bacillus subtilis* PCI 219. However, Dpm was little incorporated into peptidoglycan, and good incorporation of [³H] Dpm was accomplished by using the Dpm-requiring mutant. Table 2 shows the estimation method of inhibition

TABLE 2

Estimation Method of the Inhibition of Incorporation of [³H] Diaminopimelic Acid and [¹⁴C] Leucine into Macromolecular Fraction

---

Fresh slant culture of *Bacillus* sp. KB—152 (Dpm⁻)
   ↓   suspend in 5 ml of a medium (0.5% peptone, 0.5% meat ext., 10 μg/ml Dpm,
        200 μg/ml L—Lys, pH 7.0)
Cell suspension
   | inoculate into 10 ml of the medium to make OD_{660}: 0.05
   ↓   incubate at 37°C until OD_{660} reaches 0.2
Culture for the incorporation of isotopes

      Incorporation mixture
      ⎧ Culture   0.8 ml
      ⎨ [³H] Dpm   0.1 μCi ⎫
         L—[¹⁴C] Leu 0.5 μCi ⎬ 0.1 ml
      ⎩ Sample   0.1 ml

      Reaction: at 37°C for 10 min
      Assay: radioactivity of TCA-insoluble fraction was counted by liquid scintillation
          counter.

---

of incorporation of [³H] Dpm and [¹⁴C] Leu into macromolecular fraction. To the exponentially growing culture of *Bacillus* sp. KB152 (Dpm⁻) were added the isotopes and an antibiotic and then the culture was incubated at 37°C for 10 min. The radioactivity of TCA-insoluble fraction was counted by liquid scintillation counter.

In order to examine whether the method is useful for selecting cell wall synthesis inhibitors, known antibiotics with various modes of action were tested at various concentrations. As shown in Table 3, all antibiotics known to be cell wall synthesis inhibitors inhibited the incorporation of [³H] Dpm, while they did not prevent that of [¹⁴C] Leu.

Among the cell wall synthesis inhibitors, the inhibition of [³H] Dpm by moenomycin-group antibiotics was limited. The inhibition by β—lactam antibiotics, such as penicillin G and cephaloridine seems also to be limited. This may be explained by the site of action of these antibiotics: they inhibit cross-linking reaction of nascent peptidoglycan chain, but do not inhibit formation of single chain of peptidoglycan.

On the other hand, as shown in Table 4, protein synthesis

TABLE 3

Influence of Cell Wall Synthesis Inhibitors on the Incorporation of [^{3}H] Dpm and [^{14}C] Leu
into Acid-Insoluble Fraction in *Bacillus* sp. KB−152 (Dpm⁻)

Antibiotic	Concentration (μg/ml)	Incorporation (%)	
		[^{3}H] Dpm	[^{14}C] Leu
Bacillin	5	45	103
(Tetaine)	50	10	119
	500	9	99
D−Cycloserine	2	97	100
	20	32	103
	200	9	102
Enduracidin	0.1	35	99
	1	9	96
	10	9	93
Ristocetin	10	8	108
	100	8	90
Vancomycin	10	9	95
	100	4	98
Moenomycin	100	98	105
	1000	59	103
Macarbomycin	10	85	97
	100	52	98
Bacitracin	10	21	92
	100	7	95
Penicillin G	10	36	103
	100	32	104
Cephaloridine	10	44	101
	100	41	100
A−16886 A	10	74	103
	100	51	99

(reprinted with permission of The Japan Antibiotics Research Association)

inhibitors such as kanamycin and gentamicin did not affect the incorporation of [^{3}H] Dpm, while streptomycin, leucomycin and tetracycline prevented it somewhat. In contrast, incorporation of [^{14}C] Leu was inhibited more strongly than that of [^{3}H] Dpm. Colistin and polymyxin B inhibited the incorporation of both [^{3}H] Dpm and [^{14}C] Leu. Inhibitors of DNA synthesis did not affect the incorporation of both [^{3}H] Dpm and [^{14}C] Leu. Rifampicin, an inhibitor of RNA synthesis, and cerulenin, an inhibitor of fatty acid synthesis, inhibited the incorporation of [^{3}H] Dpm by lesser extent than that of [^{14}C] Leu.

From these results, it was shown that the cell wall synthesis inhibitors were the only antibiotics that inhibited [^{3}H] Dpm incorporation but did not inhibit [^{14}C] Leu incorporation even when the antibiotics were used at relatively high concentrations. Thus, it

TABLE 4

Influence of Antibiotics other than Cell Wall Synthesis Inhibitors on the Incorporation of [³H] Dpm and [¹⁴C] Leu into the Acid-Insoluble Fraction in *Bacillus* sp. KB-152 (Dpm⁻)

Antibiotic	Concentration (μg/ml)	Incorporation (%) [³H] Dpm	[¹⁴C] Leu
Streptomycin	1	109	93
	10	70	25
Kanamycin	10	100	18
	100	99	7
Gentamicin	10	94	14
	100	83	5
Leucomycin	10	40	10
	100	37	4
Tetracycline	10	72	9
	100	2	7
Colistin	1	93	95
	10	4	20
	100	1	3
Polymyxin B	1	69	127
	10	5	31
Mitomycin C	1	110	105
	10	100	94
Novobiocin	1	102	105
	10	100	81
	100	91	70
Bleomycin	100	109	111
Rifampicin	100	91	45
Cerulenin	100	71	49

(reprinted with permission of The Japan Antibiotics Research Association)

seemed reasonable to eliminate antibiotics having a mode of action other than inhibition of cell wall synthesis by this procedure.

Elimination of Antibiotics of High Molecular Weight: Molecular Weight and Passing Ratios of Antibiotics through Diaflo UM–2 Membrane Filter

Elimination of antibiotics of high molecular weight was attempted at an early stage of the screening system, because in general they are often useless in medical field. Identification of antibiotics of molecular weight under 1000 was tried with a membrane filter. Table 5 shows passing ratios of various antibiotics through Diaflo UM–2 membrane filter. The passing ratio of colistin (molecular weight: 967) was 7.0%. Vancomycin and ristocetin having molecular weights of over 1000 also passed by several per cent. Thus, the criterion for

TABLE 5

Passing Ratios of Various Antibiotics through Diaflo UM−2 Membrane Filter

Antibiotic	Molecular weight	Passing ratio (%)
D−Cycloserine	90	72.5
Penicillin G	356	22.0
Cephalosporin C	415	17.5
Streptomycin	581	32.0
Colistin	967	7.0
Vancomycin	1600	5.4
Ristocetin B	>1000	6.0

(reprinted with permission of The Japan Antibiotics Research Association)

eliminating an antibiotic having a molecular weight of larger than 1000 was set about 7−8%.

From the above-mentioned results, the following procedure was established for the screening of specific inhibitors of cell wall peptidoglycan synthesis. In the primary test, culture broths were selected that showed activity against *B. subtilis* but lacked activity against *A. laidlawii.* In the secondary test, the broths were further selected by retaining those which inhibited only the incorporation of [^{3}H] Dpm into the acid-insoluble fraction of *Bacillus* sp. KB152 (Dpm$^-$). Finally, antibiotics having molecular weights under 1000 were retained.

Results of this Screening Programme

Azureomycin Discovery

Broth filtrates of about ten-thousand strains including bacterial, fungal and actinomycetal soil isolates were submitted to this screening programme (Table 6). One new antibiotic, azureomycin, (Ōmura *et al.,* 1979b), was found, and several known antibiotics such as amphomycin, 3−amino−3−deoxy−D−glucose, D−cycloserine and penicillin G were identified in this programme. Among these known antibiotics, the mechanism of action of amphomycin and 3−amino−3−deoxy−D−glucose have not been known.

The new antibiotic, azureomycin, is a complex. Major components A and B were isolated from the culture filtrate of a soil isolate named as *Pseudonocardia azurea* nov. sp. They are water-soluble, basic substances containing sugar, amino acid and phenolic chromophore (Table 7), and are active against Gram-positive bacteria including penicillin resistant staphylococci, mycobacteria and clostridia at a range from 0.1 to 12.5 μg/ml (Table 8). When azureomycin B was administered intraperitoneally in mice at 500 mg/kg, it had no influence as to acute toxicity.

TABLE 6

Steps in Screening for Inhibitors of Cell Wall Synthesis in Bacteria (CSI: Cell Wall Synthesis Inhibitor)

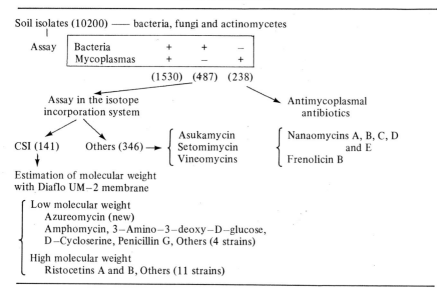

TABLE 7

Physico-Chemical Properties of Azureomycins A and B (HCl Salts)

	Azureomycin A	Azureomycin B
Anal. Found %	C: 43.5 H: 4.46 N: 4.97	C: 47.6 H: 5.27 N: 4.74
MP	231°C (decomp.)	220°C (decomp.)
$[\alpha]_D^{22}$	−124° (c 0.5, water)	−116° (c 2, water)
Mol. wt.	850 ± 40	870 ± 20
Formula	$C_{30-34}H_{36-44}N_3O_{21-24}\cdot HCl$	$C_{35-36}H_{46-48}N_3O_{19-21}\cdot HCl$
UV λ_{max} ($E_{1\ cm}^{1\%}$)		
in 0.05 N HCl	282 (54)	279 (50)
in 0.05N NaOH	301 (81)	286 sh. (77)
Nature	basic, colorless, water-soluble	
Color reaction	—	
positive to	Rydon-Smith, Anisaldehyde−H_2SO_4, $KMnO_4$	
negative to	Elson-Morgan, Ehrlich, TTC, Sakaguchi	

(reprinted with permission of The Japan Antibiotics Research Association)

As by-products of this screening, we obtained several new antibiotics as described later.

TABLE 8

Antimicrobial Spectra of Azureomycins A and B

Microorganism	m.i.c. (μg/ml)*	
	A	B
Staphylococcus aureus FDA 209P	6.25	12.5
S. aureus FS 1277 (penicillin resistant)	6.25	12.5
Bacillus subtilis PCI 219	1.56	1.56
B. cereus T	6.25	6.25
B. megaterium KM	0.39	0.10
Sarcina lutea PCI 1001	0.78	0.78
Mycobacterium smegmatis ATCC 607	12.5	12.5
Nocardia asteroides KB 54	3.13	3.13
Streptococcus pneumoniae III	3.13	1.56
S. pyogenes C203	3.13	1.56
Clostridium perfringens PB6KN5	3.13	6.25
C. perfringens MB 2237	1.56	6.25
C. botulinum IFO 3733	1.56	0.39
C. kainantoi IFO 3353	–	0.39
C. sporogenes IFO 3987	–	0.39
Escherichia coli NIHJ	>100	>100
Salmonella typhimurium KB 20	>100	>100
Pseudomonas aeruginosa P3	>100	>100

* Heart infusion agar, 20 h at 37°C.
  Clostridium strains were incubated for 48 h at 37°C in Gifu Anaerobic Medium (Nissui).
  (reprinted with permission of The Japan Antibiotics Research Association)

Mechanism of Action of Azureomycin, Amphomycin and 3–Amino–3–deoxy–D–glucose

To evaluate this screening method for cell wall synthesis inhibitors, we studied the detailed mechanism of action of azureomycin, amphomycin and 3–amino–3–deoxy–D–glucose. Azureomycin B induced lysis of the growing cells of *B. cereus* T, and caused accumulation of a precursor of cell wall peptidoglycan synthesis, UDP–MurNAc–pentapeptide, in the azureomycin-treated cells (Spiri-Nakagawa et al., 1979). As shown in Fig. 2, azureomycin B inhibited the peptidoglycan synthesis from labelled UDP–MurNAc–pentapeptide by a particulate fraction of *B. megaterium* KM, while it caused a little accumulation of lipid intermediates. The inhibition of peptidoglycan synthesis by azureomycin was reversed by the addition of cell wall preparation isolated from the same organism (Spiri-Nakagawa et al., 1980).

From these results, we speculated that azureomycin inhibits polymerase by binding probably to nascent peptidoglycan, which is one of the substrates of the polymerization reaction (Fig. 1). It can be said that the inhibition of polymerase by azureomycin B causes lysis of bacterial cells.

120
100
80
60
40
20
0
Relative activity (%)
Lipid intermediates
Peptidoglycan
0
5
10
20
50
Azureomycin B (µg/ml)

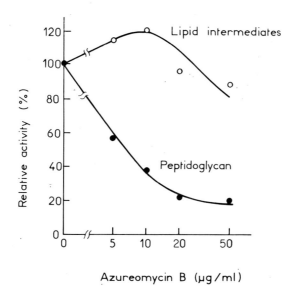

FIG. 2 Effect of azureomycin B on lipid intermediate accumulation and peptidoglycan synthesis by a particulate fraction of *B. megaterium*. [Reaction mixture (30 μl): 3.3 x 10^{-4} M UDP–MurNAc–pentapeptide ([^{3}H] Dpm-labelled); 3.3 x 10^{-4} M UDP–GlcNAc; 2.5 x 10^{-2} M $MgCl_2$; 1.0 x 10^{-3} M dithiothreitol; 0.25 M Tris–HCl (pH 8.5); particulate fraction (10 μl). Incubation: 25°C, 2 hours. Determination of lipid intermediates (in *n*–BuOH extract) and of peptidoglycan (in acid-insoluble fraction of water layer) by LSC (liquid scintillation counter).]

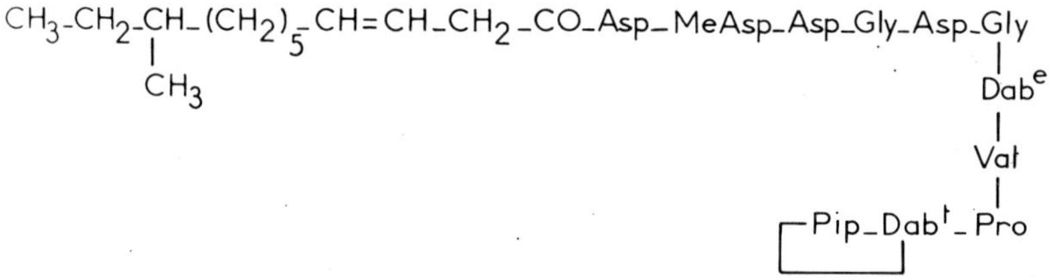

CH3-CH2-CH-(CH2)5-CH=CH-CH2-CO-Asp-MeAsp-Asp-Gly-Asp-Gly
CH3
Dab^e
Val
Pip-Dab^t-Pro

Dab^e: D-*erythro*-α,β-diaminobutyric acid

Dab^t: L-*threo*-α,β-diaminobutyric acid

Pip: D-pipecolic acid

FIG. 3 Structure of amphomycin.

Amphomycin (Fig. 3) is an antibiotic discovered by Heinemann *et al.* in 1953, but the mode of action was not known (Heinemann *et al.*, 1953; Bodanszky *et al.*, 1973). During the work on the screening for cell wall synthesis inhibitors, we found that amphomycin is a specific inhibitor of cell wall peptidoglycan synthesis (Ōmura *et al.*, 1975; Tanaka *et al.*, 1977). As shown in Fig. 4, amphomycin inhibited

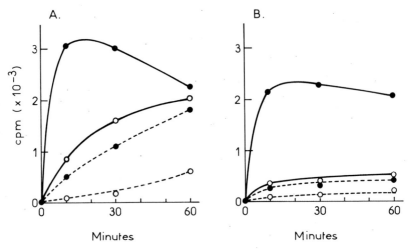

FIG. 4   Effect of amphomycin on lipid intermediates accumulation and peptidoglycan synthesis by a particulate enzyme of *B. megaterium.* – ● –, lipid intermediates; – ○ –, peptidoglycan; ——, no antibiotic; – – –, amphomycin (100 μg/ml). Reaction mixture as for Fig. 2: (A) complete or (B) without UDP–GlcNAc.

lipid intermediates accumulation and peptidoglycan synthesis by a particulate enzyme of *B. megaterium* KM, but did not inhibit transglycosylation and polymerisation. Thus, it was concluded that the primary site of action is phospho–MurNAc–pentapeptide translocase, the first step in the lipid cycle of peptidoglycan synthesis (Tanaka *et al.*, 1979a). Recently, amphomycin has been reported by Kang *et al.* (1978) to inhibit the incorporation of mannose and N–acetylglucosamine (GlcNAc) into lipid-linked saccharides by pig aorta extract. It will be of interest to know whether amphomycin interferes with syntheses of various lipid-linked saccharides in prokaryotes and eucaryotes.

3–Amino–3–deoxy–D–glucose, one · of the constituents of kanamycin, was isolated in this screening programme and was found to be a specific inhibitor of cell wall synthesis (Iwai *et al.*, 1977). In contrast, kanamycin is well known to be a protein synthesis inhibitor. 3–Amino–3–deoxy–D–glucose was produced by *B. cereus* var. SA–1127 in our laboratory, but it had previously been isolated from

B. aminoglucosidicus (Umezawa *et al.*, 1967). The inhibition of the growth of *Staphylococcus aureus* by the antibiotic was reversed by GlcNAc, and it inhibited the incorporation of [^{14}C] fructose into cell wall fraction of the organism (Table 9) (Tanaka *et al.*, 1979b). From

TABLE 9

Effect of 3–amino–3–deoxy–D–glucose (3–AG) on the Incorporation of [^{14}C] Fructose into the Cell Wall Fraction in *S. aureus*. (The Organism was Incubated in the Presence of D–[^{14}C] Fructose and Chloramphenicol, and then Nucleic Acids and Lipids were Removed from the Acid-Insoluble Fraction. The Radioactivity of the Residual Acid-Insoluble Material (Cell Wall Fraction) was Counted)

Addenda (μg/ml)	Incorporation cpm (%)
None	43,068 (100)
3–AG (20)	22,348 (52)
3–AG (100)	12,046 (28)
3–AG (200)	10,050 (23)
Penicillin G (100)	3,464 (8)

this, the primary site of action was speculated to be the formation of glucosamine–6–phosphate from fructose–6–phosphate, a reaction catalysed by glucosamine synthetase.

By-Products of this Screening

Fortunately, in this screening work we could find several new anti-biotics other than cell wall synthesis inhibitors.

Nanaomycins (Ōmura *et al.*, 1974 and 1976b; Tanaka *et al.*, 1975a, b,c; Kasai *et al.*, 1979) and frenolicin B (Iwai *et al.*, 1978) (Fig. 5) are active against mycoplasmas in the primary test in contrast with cell wall synthesis inhibitors. Nanaomycins are also very active against *Trichophyton*, the pathogen of ring worm, especially of cattle.

In the secondary test of the inhibition of incorporation of radio-active precursors into macromolecules in *Bacillus* sp. KB152 (Dpm⁻), some antibiotics produced by soil isolates inhibited the incorporation of [^{3}H] Dpm alone at a relatively low concentration, but inhibited also that of both [^{3}H] Dpm and [^{14}C] Leu at a high concentration. This pattern of the inhibition was not observed in the known anti-biotics tested except polymyxin B (Table 3). Thus, it was expected that these antibiotics had high possibility to be new. In fact, we could find several new antibiotics among these antibiotics.

Asukamycin (Fig. 6) (Ōmura *et al.*, 1976a; Kakinuma *et al.*, 1979) was isolated from the culture broth of *Streptomyces nodosus* subsp. *asukaensis*. It is active against Gram-positive bacteria and effective in reducing mortality of chicks infected with *Eimeria tenella*.

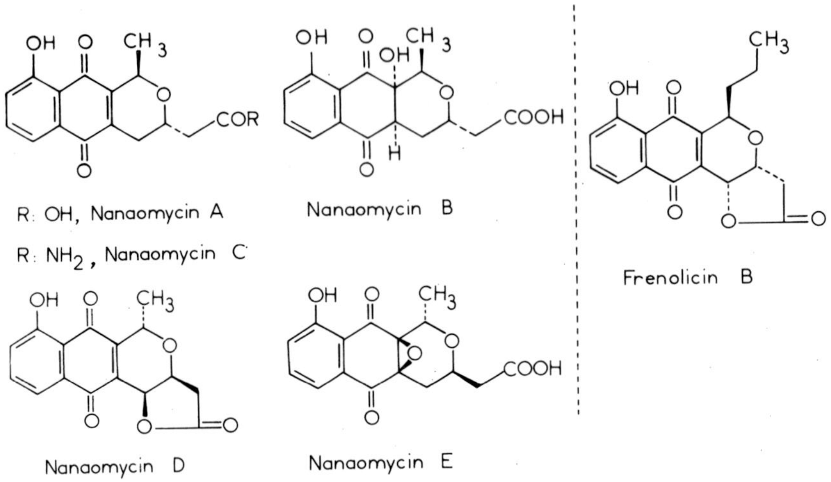

FIG. 5 New antibiotics discovered as antimycoplasma antibiotics. Nanaomycin A, B, C, D, E from *Streptomyces rosa* var. *notoensis*. Frenolicin B from *S. roseofulvus* strain AM—3867.

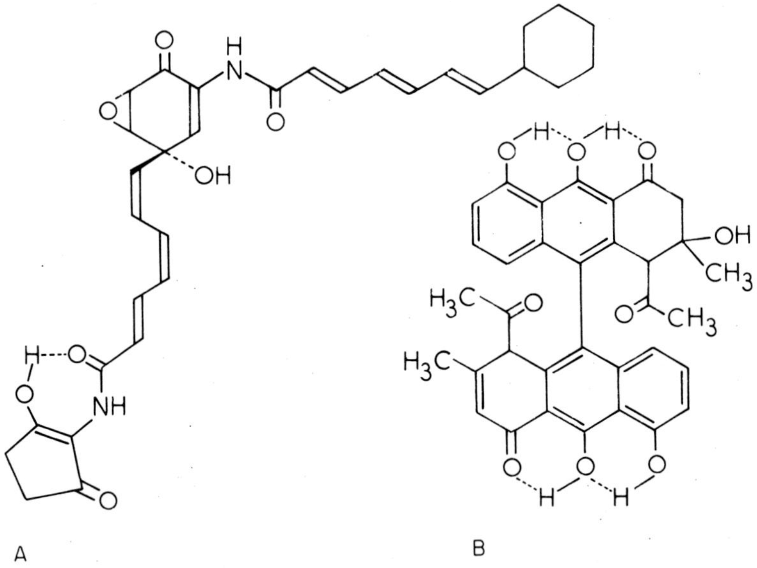

FIG. 6 Structures of (A) asukamycin and (B) setomimycin.

Setomimycin (Ōmura *et al.*, 1978; Kakinuma *et al.*, 1980) was isolated from *Streptomyces pseudovenezuelae*. It is active against Gram-positive bacteria and has antitumour activity against Sarcoma—180 solid tumour in mice.

Vineomycins (OS–4742–A_1, A_2, B_1 and B_2) (Ōmura *et al.*, 1977) are new neutral anthracycline antibiotics (Table 10) isolated from *Streptomyces matensis* subsp. *vineus*. They possess antibacterial

TABLE 10

Physico-Chemical Properties of Vineomycins A_1, A_2, B_1 and B_2

	A_1	A_2	B_1	B_2
Nature	Neutral Orange needles	Neutral Orange powder	Neutral Yellow powder	Neutral Yellow powder
MP (°C)	162–163	173–176	132–135	128–131
$[\alpha]_D^{26}$ (in $CHCl_3$)	+ 92° (c, 0.5)	+ 3° (c, 0.4)	+ 76.°8 (c, 0.5)	+ 30.°8 (c, 0.5)
Anal. Found C	62.51	61.60	59.53	62.37
% H	6.23	6.44	5.93	6.21
N	0	0	0	0
Formula	C_{47-50} H_{58-60} O_{16-18}		C_{39-44} H_{46-52} O_{17-19}	C_{42-48} H_{50-58} O_{16-18}
Mol. wt.	880–950		786–872	810–922
UVλ_{max} ($E_{1\,cm}^{1\%}$) in MeOH	218 (441) 318 (59) 438 (61)	216 (364) 315 sh. (107) 425 (50)	230 (325) 258 (185) 295 (60) 427 (89) 440 (87)	230 (421) 258 (226) 294 (76) 427 (107) 440 (107)

(reprinted with permission of The Japan Antibiotics Research Association)

activities against Gram-positive bacteria and antitumour activities against Sarcoma–180 solid tumour in mice.

Conclusion

In summarising up, we established a new, simple screening method for specific inhibitors of cell wall peptidoglycan synthesis. In this screening programme, we found a new cell wall synthesis inhibitor, azureomycin, and proposed the mode of action of azureomycin, amphomycin and 3–amino–3–deoxy–D–glucose. The sites of action of these antibiotics are shown in Fig. 1.

Also we could find several new antibiotics other than cell wall synthesis inhibitors as by-products of this screening work.

Acknowledgements

Present study was supported in part by Grant for Scientific Research from The Ministry of Education, Science and Culture of Japan. The author thanks Dr. H. Tanaka for valuable discussion and preparation of this paper.

References

Bodanszky, M., Sigler, G.F. and Bodanszky, A. (1973). *J. Am. Chem. Soc.* **95**, 2352–2357.

Heinemann, B., Kaplan, M.A., Muir, R.D. and Hooper, I.R. (1953). *Antibiot. Chemother.* **3**, 1239–1242.

Iwai, Y., Kōra, A., Takahashi, Y., Hayashi, T., Awaya, J., Masuma, R., Ōiwa, R. and Ōmura, S. (1978). *J. Antibiot.* **31**, 959–965.

Iwai, Y., Tanaka, H., Ōiwa, R., Shimizu, S. and Ōmura, S. (1977). *Biochim. Biophys. Acta* **498**, 223–228.

Kakinuma, K., Ikekawa, N., Nakagawa, A. and Ōmura, S. (1979). *J. Am. Chem. Soc.* **101**, 3402–3404.

Kakinuma, K., Imamura, N., Ikekawa, N., Minami, S., Tanaka, H. and Ōmura, S. (1980). *J. Am. Chem. Soc.* **102**, 7493–7498.

Kang, M.S., Spencer, J.P. and Elbein, A.D. (1978). *J. Biol. Chem.* **253**, 8860–8866.

Kasai, M., Shirahata, K., Ishii, S., Mineura, K., Marumo, H., Tanaka, H. and Ōmura, S. (1979). *J. Antibiot.* **32**, 442–445.

Ōmura, S., Kitao, C., Tanaka, H., Ōiwa, R., Takahashi, Y., Nakagawa, A., Shimada, M. and Iwai, Y. (1976a). *J. Antibiot.* **29**, 876–881.

Ōmura, S., Tanaka, H., Iwai, Y., Nishigaki, K., Awaya, J., Takahashi, Y. and Masuma, R. (1978). *J. Antibiot.* **31**, 1091–1098.

Ōmura, S., Tanaka, H., Koyama, Y., Ōiwa, R., Katagiri, M., Awaya, J., Nagai, T. and Hata, T. (1974). *J. Antibiot.* **27**, 363–365.

Ōmura, S., Tanaka, H., Ōiwa, R., Awaya, J., Masuma, R. and Tanaka, K. (1977). *J. Antibiot.* **30**, 908–916.

Ōmura, S., Tanaka, H., Ōiwa, R., Nagai, T., Koyama, Y. and Takahashi, Y. (1979a). *J. Antibiot.* **32**, 978–984.

Ōmura, S., Tanaka, H., Okada, Y. and Marumo, H. (1976b). *J. Chem. Soc., Chem. Commun.* 320–321.

Ōmura, S., Tanaka, H., Shinohara, M., Ōiwa, R. and Hata, T. (1975). *Chemotherapy* (Proc. 9th Int. Cong. Chemoth.) **5**, 365–369.

Ōmura, S., Tanaka, H., Tanaka, Y., Spiri-Nakagawa, P., Ōiwa, R., Takahashi, Y., Matsuyama, K. and Iwai, Y. (1979b). *J. Antibiot.* **32**, 985–994.

Spiri-Nakagawa, P., Tanaka, Y., Ōiwa, R., Tanaka, H. and Ōmura, S. (1979). *J. Antibiot.* **32**, 995–1001.

Spiri-Nakagawa, P., Ōiwa, R., Tanaka, Y., Tanaka, H. and Ōmura, S. (1980). *J. Biochem.* **88**, 565–570.

Tanaka, H., Iwai, Y., Ōiwa, R., Shinohara, S., Shimizu, S., Oka, T. and Ōmura, S. (1977). *Biochim. Biophys. Acta* **497**, 633–640.

Tanaka, H., Koyama, Y., Awaya, J., Marumo, H., Ōiwa, R., Katagiri, M., Nagai, T. and Ōmura, S. (1975a). *J. Antibiot.* **28**, 860–867.

Tanaka, H., Koyama, Y., Nagai, T., Marumo, H. and Ōmura, S. (1975b). *J. Antibiot.* **28**, 868–875.

Tanaka, H., Marumo, H., Nagai, T., Okada, M., Taniguchi, K. and Ōmura, S. (1975c). *J. Antibiot.* **28**, 925–930.

Tanaka, H., Ōiwa, R., Matsukura, S. and Ōmura, S. (1979a). *Biochem. Biophys. Res. Commun.* **86**, 902–908.

Tanaka, H., Shimizu, S., Ōiwa, R., Iwai, Y. and Ōmura, S. (1979b). *J. Biochem.* **86**, 155–159.

Umezawa, S., Umino, K., Shibahara, S., Hamada, M. and Omoto, S. (1967). *J. Antibiot.* **20**, 355–360.

Discussion

Professor Braun: Are antibiotics which inhibit cell wall synthesis at the level of the lipid cycle active against mycoplasma?

Professor Ōmura: We have examined their mode of action against *Bacillus megaterium* but not against mycoplasma.

Professor Braun: The reason for my question is because the lipid cycle is also involved in other kinds of syntheses, such as glycoprotein and glycolipid synthesis. It is possible that what is known to occur with methanobacteria (that is that antibiotics active at the level of the lipid cycle are also active against methanobacteria, despite the absence of a peptidoglycan) may also occur with mycoplasma.

Professor Ōmura: You are probably referring to amphomycin? Amphomycin also inhibits some lipid-linked saccharides which appear in some animal cells or other organisms. I think Professor Braun is right.

Dr. Bost: I was very interested in Professor Ōmura's presentation. With regard to the test on mycoplasma and *Bacillus subtilis*, what type of response is obtained with compounds of the moenomycin family, for instance? Are they active, for instance, on *Acholeplasma laidlawii?*

Professor Ōmura: The moenomycin group of antibiotics is not active against any of the mycoplasma tested, but it is active against *Bacillus subtilis.*

Dr. van Heijenoort: Does Professor Ōmura have any idea of the structure of azureomycin?

Professor Ōmura: We are now studying it, but it is a complex molecule. We expect that azureomycin has a phenolic chromophore, perhaps like vancomycin, also a sugar peptide-containing group. The final structure has not yet been determined.

Dr. Bost: What is the real interest in screening for a cell wall inhibitor with a very narrow spectrum of activity towards Gram-positive bacteria?

Professor Ōmura: If we continue with this screening system, there will be some possibilities of obtaining Gram-negative active compounds because we are checking through the mycoplasma and the bacteria, *Bacillus subtilis* and *Escherichia coli.*

Professor Tomasz: Is KB 152 a *Bacillus subtilis* strain or a *B. megaterium* strain?

Professor Ōmura: The strain has not yet been determined. It is known to be a *Bacillus*, but not whether it is *subtilis* or *megaterium.*

Possible Applications of Genetic Recombination in the Discovery of New Antibiotics in Actinomycetes

D.A. HOPWOOD

John Innes Institute, Norwich, England

Introduction

There are at least two ways in which recombination should be useful in the development of actinomycete strains able to make new anti-biotics (Hopwood and Chater, 1980). The fact that well authenticated examples of such new products of recombination are not yet available does not detract from the potential of a recombinational approach. The necessary techniques of genetic manipulation are so new that there has not been time for them to be applied, let alone seriously evaluated, in an industrial context. However, rapid progress has been made in the development of these techniques, in a few organisms, over the last few years (Hopwood, 1979a); therefore a systematic use of recombination as one of the tools available for the discovery of new antibiotics need not be long delayed. The success of this approach will depend on the effort devoted to the transfer of the new technology from the largely "academic" organisms in which it is being developed to some of the strains most likely to be industrially relevant, but recombination alone will of course not lead to a successful new product. As in all antibiotic discovery, imaginative screening of strains for relevant antimicrobial, pharmacological or other activities is of prime importance. Fortunately, the screening procedures required to investigate a population of recombinants need be no different from those needed to evaluate a group of new wild isolates, and are therefore to a large extent already available.

"Silent" and "Hybrid" Antibiotics

The two possible recombinational routes to a new product both require hybridisation between strains, which may be two different natural isolates of the same species or of different species or even genera. More rarely they will be divergent derivatives of a single wild isolate which has been subjected to such extensive mutation and selection, usually as part of a yield improvement programme for an existing antibiotic, that sufficient genetic diversity may exist between different branches of the pedigree of derivatives of the original isolate to make hybridisation between them worth while. The two routes differ in the types of genes recombined, whether one strain contributes all the (hitherto "silent") structural genetic information for the new product, or whether structural genes come from both strains to produce a "hybrid" product.

"Silent" Antibiotic Genes

Many, perhaps most, actinomycetes produce several chemically different antibiotics. In general, the more intensively a strain is investigated the more antibiotics are discovered. For example, the first antibiotic characterised in the genetically well known A3(2) strain of *Streptomyces coelicolor* was identified only four years ago (Wright and Hopwood, 1976), but now at least five (Rudd, 1978) and probably more (Troost *et al.*, 1979) distinct antibiotics have been recognised in this strain and there is no reason to suppose that the list is complete. Streptomycetes have two to three times more apparently unique DNA than *Escherichia coli* has and probably only a small part of the extra DNA is needed to code for the complex morphogenetic cycle which distinguishes streptomycetes from enterobacteria (Chater and Merrick, 1979), so a considerable amount of genetic information could be available for antibiotic synthesis (Hopwood and Chater, 1980).

Probably much of this information is not expressed, except under particular environmental conditions which may be hard to predict and therefore to reproduce in artificial culture, because of the existence of regulatory circuits operated by the products of control genes. Thus mutation in such regulatory genes should lead to the expression of normally repressed biosynthetic pathways and so to the appearance of new antibiotics. However, even after the most efficient mutagenesis, many thousands of individuals would need to be screened for putative new antibiotic activities arising as a result of the mutational inactivation of negatively acting control circuits.

A more efficient approach could involve random recombination between pairs of strains likely to differ in both structural and regulatory antibiotic genes, so as to free the structural genes from their regulators. Such an approach will probably require generalised chromosomal recombination which (in contrast to the introduction of specific "foreign" genes on vectors: see below) will diminish rapidly in frequency as the evolutionary distance between two strains increases. In practice, we may be forced to work with groups of strains within the same species or "species group". However, there is considerable evidence that members of the same species often produce different antibiotics (for example different strains of *Streptomyces griseus* make aminoglycosides, polyenes, β–lactams, and several other classes of antibiotics) and so a series of crosses between different isolates of the same species, or fairly closely related species, should be the best strategy to discover new antibiotics by separating the structural from the regulatory genes of a particular strain through recombination with a strain that does not possess them. Provided that the two classes of genes are not too closely linked, the appropriate recombinants should occur amongst comparatively small numbers of progeny.

What is needed, then, is the means to bring about, easily and efficiently, generalised chromosomal recombination between pairs of related strains. (Here is an important role for taxonomic studies since, in this strategy, we need to be able to predict which strains are likely to possess chromosomes sufficiently homologous to recombine rather freely, irrespective of what antibiotics they are known to produce.) While the great majority, perhaps all, of the actinomycetes that have been investigated have a natural system of gene exchange (Hopwood and Merrick, 1977), the frequencies of recombination are low (10^{-5} to 10^{-7}). Such frequencies are capable of enormous improvement – in *S. coelicolor* A3(2) the states of the two sex plasmids which control genetic recombination have been manipulated to give nearly 100% recombination in certain combinations (Hopwood *et al.*, 1973) – but this is a long and unpredictable task.

It is therefore fortunate that protoplast fusion in actinomycetes (in various *Streptomyces* and *Streptosporangium* spp. so far: Hopwood *et al.*, 1977; Baltz, 1980) offers the possibility of achieving very high levels of chromosomal recombination with a minimum of development work. The characteristics of protoplast fusion – high frequency crossing-over between the (almost) complete chromosomes of two (or more) parents (Hopwood and Wright, 1978) – are those required in a strategy of empirical recombination. Moreover, not only the frequency of recombinants, but also that of crossing-over amongst recombinants, can be increased even further by ultraviolet irradiation of the protoplasts of both parent strains immediately before fusion (Hopwood and Wright, 1979). A further development is the irradiation of the protoplasts of one parent, only, before fusion with the unirradiated protoplasts of a second strain (D.A. Hopwood and H.M. Wright, unpub. results). In this way, genetic material from any of a series of unmarked wild types, counter-selected by UV–irradiation, could be introduced into a common strain in which genetic markers for counter-selection were available.

An interesting additional possibility to chromosomal recombination as a component of a strategy of antibiotic discovery by the expression of "silent" genes may be the transfer of naturally occurring plasmids between different strains. While in at least one example (methylenomycin A in *S. coelicolor* A3(2)) structural genes for antibiotic biosynthesis are plasmid-borne, a more general role for plasmids appears to be as regulators of the expression of chromosomally carried structural genes (Hopwood, 1978; Okanishi, 1979). None of the mechanisms of such controls have yet been elucidated, so that the specificity of the interaction between a plasmid and the particular set of chromosomal biosynthetic genes in its host cell is unknown. However, it has been reasoned that it is unlikely to be very specific (Hopwood, 1979b), so that transfer of a "regulatory" plasmid to a new host might well lead to the expression of hitherto "silent" chromosomal genes.

It may be argued that, since in the "silent gene" strategy the structural genes for the biosynthesis of the new antibiotic are derived from a single strain, and the original isolate was potentially capable of making the antibiotic in question, it is not really "new"; with the benefit of hindsight the compound might even be detected in the parent strain. No matter; the objective is to detect antibiotics which would otherwise have been missed, and hindsight, when available, is an excellent way of predicting a suitable course of action!

"Hybrid" Antibiotics

The second recombinational strategy to discover new antibiotics is to transfer genes coding for antibiotic biosynthetic enzymes from one organism to another so as to produce a hybrid genotype capable of making a new antibiotic. An obvious starting point for such an approach would be to choose as parents two strains already known to make different members of the same chemical class of antibiotics – aminoglycosides, macrolides, polyenes, β–lactams, polyethers, etc. – since this would maximise the chance that an enzyme introduced into a new host would find a substrate chemically different from, but related to, its normal substrate, and capable of conversion to an analogue of a natural antibiotic. Extensive studies of "mutasynthesis" or "mutational biosynthesis" (Rinehart, 1977; Daum and Lemke, 1979) have indicated that this expectation is likely to be fulfilled; very many artificial analogues of natural antibiotic moieties can be converted to new antibiotics when added exogenously to mutants blocked in antibiotic synthesis. In the proposed recombinational approach, such addition of chemically synthesised precursors would of course be unnecessary.

Success in this approach would indicate that more speculative attempts to produce "hybrid" products could usefully be the next step. For example an enzyme – a hydroxylase, methylase, decarboxylase, etc. – playing a role in some area of metabolism unrelated to antibiotic production in a donor organism might be capable of intervening in antibiotic biosynthesis if introduced into an antibiotic-producing strain. Eventually one could envisage a battery of cloned genes, coding for enzymes of a variety of different biochemical classes, which could be introduced into a series of antibiotic-producing strains in the expectation that, in certain felicitous combinations, the "foreign" enzymes would interact with the set of enzymes already present in the recipient organism to produce an interesting new product. With sufficient knowledge of structure–activity relationships of the functional groups of an antibiotic, this could perhaps be done rationally.

What of the technology required for "hybrid" antibiotic production? Since the objective is to range widely amongst antibiotic producing, or even non-antibiotic producing, organisms as donors of interesting genes, natural mating and protoplast fusion are unlikely to be very useful; genetic homology needed to recombine a foreign gene into the genome of the recipient organism is not expected between distantly related organisms, unless transposable genetic elements are involved (Kleckner, 1977). Recombinant DNA techniques are therefore called for. The development of DNA cloning technology in actinomycetes is now well under way. Streptomycete protoplasts are readily transformed by plasmid DNA (Bibb *et al.*, 1978) or transfected by phage DNA (Chater, 1979; Krügel *et al.*, 1980; Suarez and Chater, 1980a). Potential plasmid vectors are available for some strains (Bibb *et al.*, 1977; Schrempf and Goebel, 1977; Hopwood *et al.*, 1979; Bibb *et al.*, 1980b). The first cloning experiments using these plasmids have already been carried out (Bibb *et al.*, 1980a; Thompson *et al.*, 1980) and it is only a matter of time before the cloning vectors are refined to facilitate the next step: the cloning of antibiotic biosynthetic genes, rather than the antibiotic resistance and prototrophic genes which were used as test subjects in the first successful cloning experiments. Moreover, even if most actinomycete plasmids have restricted host ranges, so that universal vectors for the genus *Streptomyces* (or other genera) may not be readily developed, the discovery of a suitable plasmid for cloning in any streptomycete of interest, if it does not already possess one, may not be difficult. We (D.A. Hopwood and H.M. Wright, unpub. results) detected plasmid DNA by a rapid physical analysis in 40% of strains closely related to *Streptomyces coelicolor* A3(2) and *Streptomyces lividans* 66; some, at least, of these plasmids were transferrable, by mating and/or by transformation, to these two strains. Moreover, it should be possible readily to attach selectable antibiotic resistances to initially cryptic plasmids by shot-gun cloning of resistances from any one of the many streptomycetes that carry them so as to construct a selectable vector (Thompson *et al.*, 1980).

As an alternative to plasmid vectors, and with advantages for some purposes (Chater, 1980), phage vectors will be available. Viable deletion mutants of at least one actinophage capable of accepting and packaging foreign DNA have been isolated and used to construct a hybrid replicon capable of propagation as a plasmid in *E. coli* and as a phage in *Streptomyces* spp. (Suarez and Chater, 1980b).

Conclusion

I hope that these remarks will convey some of the excitement currently being felt by those of us interested in developing the technology needed for a genetic approach to antibiotic discovery. I have talked specifically about actinomycetes, since the wealth of genetic information for antibiotic production in this group makes them by far the best prospect for such an approach. Similar technology might be used in the other important genus of Gram-positive antibiotic-producing bacteria, *Bacillus*, since protoplast fusion (Fodor and Alföldi, 1976; Schaeffer *et al.*, 1976) and gene cloning (Young and Wilson, 1978) are available. The same is true, to a lesser extent, of filamentous fungi. Protoplast fusion, leading to the frequent production of haploid recombinants, has been reported in *Cephalosporium acremonium* (Hamlyn and Ball, 1979), but gene cloning, although well advanced in yeast (Beggs, 1978; Hinnen *et al.*, 1978), is not yet reported for moulds. However, in principle, the necessary methodology could undoubtedly be developed in such organisms as *Penicillium* and *Cephalosporium* (Hopwood and Chater, 1980).

Acknowledgements

I am grateful to Mervyn Bibb and Keith Chater for letting me have details of results prior to publication and to Keith Chater for fruitful discussion of the ideas in this paper.

References

Baltz, R.H. (1980). *Dev. Ind. Microbiol.* **21**, 43–54

Beggs, J.D. (1978). *Nature* (London) **275**, 104–109.

Bibb, M.J., Freeman, R.F. and Hopwood, D.A. (1977). *Mol. Gen. Genet.* **154**, 155–166.

Bibb, M.J., Schottel, J. and Cohen, S.N. (1980a). *Nature* (London) **284**, 526–531.

Bibb, M.J., Ward, J.M. and Hopwood, D.A. (1978). *Nature* (London) **274**, 398–400.

Bibb, M.J., Ward, J.M. and Hopwood, D.A. (1980b). *Dev. Ind. Microbiol.* **21**, 55–64.

Chater, K.F. (1979). *In* "Genetics of Industrial Microorganisms". (O.K. Sebek and A.I. Laskin, eds), pp. 123–133. American Society for Microbiology, Washington, D.C.

Chater, K.F. (1980). *Dev. Ind. Microbiol.* **21**, 65–74.

Chater, K.F. and Merrick, M.J. (1979). *In* "Developmental Biology of Prokaryotes". (J.H. Parish, ed.), pp. 93–114. Blackwell Scientific Publications, Oxford.

Daum, S.J. and Lemke, J.R. (1979). *Annu. Rev. Microbiol.* **33**, 241–265.

Fodor, K. and Alföldi, L. (1976). *Proc. Nat. Acad. Sci. U.S.A.* **73**, 2147–2150.

Hamlyn, P.F. and Ball, C. (1979). *In* "Genetics of Industrial Microorganisms". (O.K. Sebek and A.I. Laskin, eds), pp. 185–191. American Society for Microbiology, Washington, D.C.

Hinnen, A., Hicks, J.B. and Fink, G.R. (1978). *Proc. Nat. Acad. Sci. U.S.A.* **75**, 1929–1933.

Hopwood, D.A. (1978). *Annu. Rev. Microbiol.* **32**, 373–392.

Hopwood, D.A. (1979a). *In* "Genetics of Industrial Microorganisms". (O.K. Sebek and A.I. Laskin, eds), pp. 1–9. American Society for Microbiology, Washington, D.C.

Hopwood, D.A. (1979b). *J. Nat. Prod.* **42**, 597–602.

Hopwood, D.A. and Chater, K.F. (1980). *Philos. Trans. R. Soc. London, Ser. B.* **290**, 313–328.

Hopwood, D.A. and Merrick, M.J. (1977). *Bacteriol. Rev.* **41**, 595–635.

Hopwood, D.A. and Wright, H.M. (1978). *Mol. Gen. Genet.* **162**, 307–317.

Hopwood, D.A. and Wright, H.M. (1979). *J. Gen. Microbiol.* **111**, 137–143.

Hopwood, D.A., Bibb, M.J., Ward, J.M. and Westpheling, J. (1979). *In* "Plasmids of Medical, Environmental and Commercial Importance". (K.N. Timmis and A. Pühler, eds), pp. 245–258. Elsevier–North Holland, Amsterdam.

Hopwood, D.A., Chater, K.F., Dowding, J.E. and Vivian, A. (1973). *Bacteriol. Rev.* **37**, 371–405.

Hopwood, D.A., Wright, H.M., Bibb, M.J. and Cohen, S.N. (1977). *Nature* (London) **268**, 171–174.

Kleckner, N. (1977). *Cell* **11**, 11–23.

Krügel, H., Fiedler, G. and Noack, D. (1980). *Mol. Gen. Genet.* **177**, 297–300.

Okanishi, M. (1979). *In* "Genetics of Industrial Microorganisms". (O.K. Sebek and A.I. Laskin, eds), pp. 134–140. American Society for Microbiology, Washington, D.C.

Rinehart, K.L. (1977). *Pure Appl. Chem.* **49**, 1361–1384.

Rudd, B.A.M. (1978). Genetics of pigmented secondary metabolites in *Streptomyces coelicolor*. Ph.D. Thesis, University of East Anglia, Norwich.

Schaeffer, P., Cami, B. and Hotchkiss, R.D. (1976). *Proc. Nat. Acad. Sci. U.S.A.* **73**, 2151–2155.

Schrempf, H. and Goebel, W. (1977). *J. Bacteriol.* **131**, 251–258.

Suarez, J.E. and Chater, K.F. (1980a). *J. Bacteriol.* **142**, 8–14.

Suarez, J.E. and Chater, K.F. (1980b). *Nature* (London) **286**, 527–529.

Thompson, C.J., Ward, J.M. and Hopwood, D.A. (1980). *Nature* (London) **286**, 525–527.

Troost, T.R., Danilenko, V.N. and Lomovskaya, N.D. (1979). *J. Bacteriol.* **140**, 359–368.

Wright, L.F. and Hopwood, D.A. (1976). *J. Gen. Microbiol.* **95**, 96–106.

Young, F.E. and Wilson, G.A. (1978). *In* "Genetic Engineering". (A.L. Chakrabarty, ed.), pp. 145–157. C.R.C. Press, West Palm Beach.

Discussion

Professor Tomasz: First, what is the frequency of cell regeneration in the fusion experiments? Secondly, if I may be forgiven my ignorance about lethal zygosis, is that caused even by a totally heterologous plasmid?

Professor Hopwood: The frequency of cell regeneration is between one and 10% – perhaps even 50% under the best conditions.

Secondly, lethal zygosis requires mating – that is, it requires plasmid transfer between cells on the Petri dish. It is a mating reaction, analogous to what happens in *Escherichia coli.* Plasmid-carrying spores on a plate of another species might not mate into the background sufficiently frequently to give these zones. But if the plasmid had been transformed or mated into that same species, and then individuals of that transformation or mating were put on to a background of the same species, lethal zygosis would be seen. It is very medium-dependent. When I said that it is probably universally available, it requires some adjustment of media in order to balance the growth rate of the two components, and so on.

Professor Rinehart: When new antibiotics start to be obtained from these protoplast fusions will they be predictable, or unpredictable, as far as structure is concerned?

Professor Hopwood: They will be unpredictable for me, but predictable for Professor Rinehart! In fact, it depends on how completely the precursors available are known in the various strains. It depends also on the various enzymes that might be present but which are not normally expressed. I expect that the real answer is both predictable and unpredictable; they will be semi-predictable. At least, that will be the first situation where we will want to use this technique and work within one antibiotic family, within aminoglycosides for instance. If that turned out to be profitable, we would then become more wildly optimistic and start to fuse things more at random.

Professor Demain: Could Professor Hopwood comment on any problems that arise because, except in a few cases and perhaps in only one case in his own laboratory, structural genes for antibiotic synthesis are generally not located on plasmids?

Professor Hopwood: If they were on plasmids, and if they were known to be on plasmids, that would put us a step ahead because it would eliminate the need to do a "shot-gun" cloning. We could hope to isolate the plasmid from the donor strain and use that. If they were not on plasmids, but were on the chromosome or in some unknown location, the approach is a shot-gun, or blind cloning, just as was done with the neomycin and thiostrepton-resistance genes in Dr. Thompson's cloning experiments which I described.

Professor Demain: There have been some claims of new antibiotics produced, perhaps not with protoplast fusion or recombinant DNA techniques, but by more traditional recombination. Could Professor Hopwood comment on any examples that have already been claimed? Unfortunately, these are not completely described in the literature but, in view of his interest, he may have some information on some of them.

Professor Hopwood: I know of only one that has been published. That is from the group in Jena, East Germany, which was described at the G.I.M. 1978 Meeting. Professor Demain is probably referring to that. The claim was that a new antibiotic was made by mating between two strains making rather unrelated structures. I think that this may be a case of the expression of a "silent gene"; that by some sort of recombination an antibiotic has been obtained which is perhaps within the genetic capability of one of the parents but was not expressed. The technique is good. It is an example of hybridisation giving a new structure, but I do not think that it is necessarily a hybrid structure — although it might conceivably be one.

I know of one example from a company in which a new antibiotic was produced, that is new as far as those two strains were concerned, although it was not new to science.

Professor Tomasz: In antibiotic-producing actinomycetes is it known whether resistance against the resident antibiotic is carried on plasmids?

Professor Hopwood: We are really talking about very few examples with firm evidence so far. In the case to which Professor Demain referred, methylenomycin, the same plasmid that carries the structural genes for synthesis carries a specific determinant for resistance, although the mechanism is not known. There are other reports; for instance, Professor Davies has some information on plasmid determination of one of the aminoglycoside-modifying enzymes. These are about the only examples so far from actinomycetes.

Professor Richmond: From my experience, which is fairly limited, from the products of a very large number of fusions which I have now done, it appears to me, but it may not turn out to be right, that when fusions are done there are very often spectacular changes in the quantities of antibiotics produced. On occasion, antibiotics are found which are thought to be novel, but on thorough investigation, and with the benefit of hindsight, it can nearly always be shown that one or other of the parents actually made small amounts of that antibiotic. Great care must be exercised about concluding that a new antibiotic is being obtained from a given species, or a given strain that has been constructed by fusion.

Professor Hopwood: I absolutely agree. That is the comment I would make about the example to which I have just referred. However hindsight is very useful. If we had tomorrow's newspaper there would be no need to continue working because we would know the stock prices for tomorrow!

Of course, when we talk about fusion, we are not making very wide crosses because, in order to obtain a recombinant by fusion, by definition, there must be considerable homology between the DNAs of the two interacting parents. It will be interesting to see the results of extensive recombinant DNA experiments, to see whether newer structures will appear.

Professor Richmond: At one stage, I amused myself by fusing streptomycetes with *Bacillus megaterium*, by which it is possible to obtain "cripples" which will not survive in anything other than one form or the other for any length of time. At least, I was unable to get them to survive. It is just a matter of squeezing the situation sufficiently hard; the further apart, the harder the squeezing required. I am not at all convinced that we will not get something which will survive, but it may predominantly be one host or the other.

Professor Hopwood: Or it may be entirely one host. It is possible to get cripples from growing up a single culture and examining it thoroughly. I would not expect to get any recombinants between a bacillus and a streptomycete, but we will have to try it and find out.

Production of New Antibiotics by Directed Biosynthesis and by the Use of Mutants

A. L. DEMAIN

*Massachusetts Institute of Technology, Cambridge,
Massachusetts, U.S.A.*

Introduction

Since enzymes of secondary metabolism are not as specific as those of primary metabolism, broths of antibiotic producing microorganisms usually contain a family of antibiotics rather than a single component. For this same reason, one can often direct the biosynthesis towards one particular member of that family by addition to the medium of precursors or inhibitors. New antibiotics can also be formed by such manipulations. This type of manipulation is called "directed biosynthesis". Another means of producing new antibiotics involves the genetic blockage of the pathway leading to one moiety of the antibiotic and the feeding of analogues of the missing moiety to the mutant in the hope that the modified moiety will be incorporated into a new antibiotic. This is called "mutational biosynthesis". These techniques as well as additional means of using mutants will be described in this paper.

Directed Biosynthesis by Precursor Addition

Penicillins

Directed biosynthesis was first observed during the development of the penicillin fermentation. Without supplementation, it became apparent that several different penicillins were being produced in the same broth and that different penicillins were produced in different media. After elucidation of the basic structure of penicillin as 6–aminopenicillanic acid (6–APA) (Fig. 1), it was realised that each

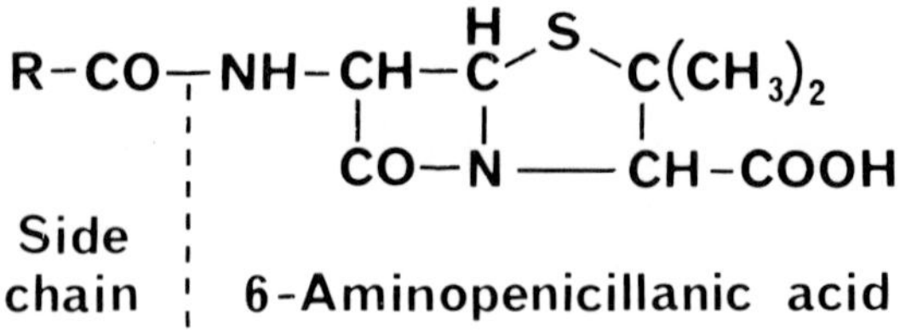

$$R-CO-NH-CH-\underset{|}{\overset{H\quad S}{C}}\diagdown \underset{|}{C}(CH_3)_2$$

$$CO-N \longrightarrow CH-COOH$$

Side
chain   6-Aminopenicillanic acid

FIG. 1   General structure of penicillins.

penicillin contained a unique acyl side chain (R–CO–) attached by amide linkage to the amino group of 6–APA. The particular *Penicillium* strain employed in these early studies used the various acyl compounds which it produced and those present in the complex media as side-chain precursors since side-chain attachment was rather non-specific.

The penicillins produced without any intentional addition of side-chain precursors to the medium are arbitrarily called "natural" penicillins. These include penicillin F (R = Δ^2–pentenyl), G (R = benzyl), X (R = p–hydroxybenzyl) and K (R = heptyl).

After it was discovered that penicillin G was formed "naturally" because the corn steep liquor in the fermentation medium contained precursors of phenylacetic acid, the side chain acid, the intentional addition of phenylacetic acid became standard practice in the industry since supplementation not only directed the biosynthesis to a single member of the penicillin family but markedly increased the total titre of penicillins produced. Soon hundreds of new acids were added to *Penicillium chrysogenum* fermentations by the Eli Lilly group under the leadership of O.K. Behrens (1949) resulting in the formation of over 100 new penicillins. Such penicillins are called "biosynthetic", i.e. those penicillins formed by addition of precursors, but not formed in "normal" media. One biosynthetic penicillin which became commercially important was penicillin V (phenoxymethylpenicillin), formed in response to added phenoxyacetic acid. It reached the marketplace due to its acid-stability which allowed it to be administered orally. Table 1 lists examples of natural and biosynthetic penicillins produced by fermentation. It is not necessary to add the side-chain acid itself, i.e. often a derivative is added which the microorganism converts to the precursor. For example, phenylalanine directs biosynthesis to penicillin G since it is converted via β–phenylethylamine to phenylacetic acid. Toxic precursors are often added as non-toxic derivatives such as esters, amides and triglycerides.

Not all acids are acceptable as side-chain precursors of penicillin. This fact limited the power of the directed biosynthesis technique

TABLE 1

Natural and Biosynthetic Penicillins

Types of precursor	Precursor example	Penicillin obtained (isolation or chromatographic data)
Saturated and unsaturated aliphatic acids	Caproic acid $\beta-\gamma$-hexenoic acid tributyrin tri-n-valerin	penicillin dihydro F penicillin F propylpenicillin butylpenicillin
Dicarboxylic acids	adipic acid	4-carboxy-n-butyl-penicillin
Substituted or unsubstituted phenylacetic acids	N-(2-hydroxyethyl)-p-methoxyphenyl-acetamide N-(2-hydroxyethyl)-o-, m- or p-fluoro-phenylacetamide N-(p-nitrophenyl-acetyl)-Dl-valine Many phenylacetic acid derivatives	p-methoxybenzyl-penicillin o-, m- or p-fluoro-benzylpenicillin p-nitrobenzyl-penicillin benzylpenicillin
Substituted or unsubstituted cyclic, polycyclic or heterocyclic acetic acids	N-(2-hydroxyethyl)-cyclopentylacetamide N-(2-hydroxyethyl)-2-thiopheneacetamide N-(2-hydroxyethyl)-2-naphthylacetamide 5-chloro-2-thiophene acetic acid	Cyclopentylmethyl-penicillin 2-thiophenemethyl penicillin 2-naphthylmethyl penicillin 5-chloro-2-thiophene methylpenicillin
Substituted or unsubstituted mercaptoacetic and oxyacetic acids	N-(2-hydroxyethyl)-phenoxyacetamide N-(2-hydroxyethyl)-p-methoxyphenoxy-acetamide ethylmercaptoacetic acid isopropylmercapto-acetic acid N-(2-hydroxyethyl)-β-naphthylmercapto-acetamide 3-thiophenemercapto-acetic acid phenylmercaptoacetic acid	phenoxymethyl-penicillin p-methoxyphenoxy-methylpenicillin ethylmercapto-methylpenicillin isopropylmercapto-methylpenicillin β-naphthylmercapto-methylpenicillin 3-thiophenemercapto-methylpenicillin phenylmercapto-methylpenicillin

(modified from Cole, 1966; reprinted with permission of the author and of Wheatland Journals Ltd)

but led the way to the development of semi-synthetic penicillins. In this technique, 6-APA produced by enzymatic or chemical deacylation of penicillin G or V is converted chemically into semisynthetic penicillins. All of the new penicillins introduced into clinical practice during the past 15 years belong to this class.

Peptide Antibiotics

Amino acids that are structurally similar to those found in peptide antibiotics as well as analogues of such amino acids have been found to replace certain of the amino acid residues of peptide antibiotics due to the broad specificity of antibiotic synthetases (Katz and Demain, 1977). Often the natural members of a peptide antibiotic family differ only in an aromatic or branched chain amino acid. Supplementation with one of these amino acids can direct biosynthesis so that the mixture will be enriched in the antibiotic containing the supplemented precursor. As an example, tyrocidines A, B and C are normally produced in a ratio of 1 : 3 : 7 by *Bacillus brevis*. These three forms differ solely in the aromatic amino acids present in the peptide. With the addition of tryptophan to the medium, A and B are not produced; tyrocidine C and a new tyrocidine (D) appear instead, these latter two antibiotics being rich in tryptophan. If phenylalanine is added to the medium, only tyrocidines A and B (rich in phenylalanine) are made. Supplementation with tryptophan and phenylalanine leads to the production of all four tyrocidines. Additional examples in *Bacillus* are shown in Table 2. This approach has also been very useful in preparing new

TABLE 2

Directed Biosynthesis in Strains of *Bacillus brevis*

Antibiotic	Additive	Result
Gramicidin S	DL–Thienylalanine	Replaces D–phenylalanine
	DL–Norleucine	Replaces L–leucine to a small extent
	DL–fluorophenylalanine	Replaces D–phenylalanine to a small extent
Tyrocidine	No addition	Tyrocidines A, B, and C formed in ratio of 1:3:7
	L–Phenylalanine (D–phenylalanine)	Tyrocidine A synthesised almost exclusively at expense of B and C; tryptophan replaced
	L–Tryptophan (D–tryptophan)	Tyrocidine C and D produced; little or no A or B formed; phenylalanine and tyrosine replaced
	L–Phenylalanine plus L–tryptophan	Tyrocidines A, B, C and D synthesised
	DL–Thienylalanine	Substitutes for D–phenylalanine
	L–Alloisoleucine, L–isoleucine	Substitutes for L–leucine and L–valine
	L–Pipecolic acid	Replaces proline to a slight extent

(modified from Katz and Demain, 1977; reprinted with permission of American Society for Microbiology) actinomycins with *Streptomyces antibioticus* (Katz, 1974). Ratios of natural actinomycins can be altered by adding hydroxyproline and sarcosine; these are incorporated to some degree at the proline site in the peptide and increase the proportions of actinomycin I, II and III at the expense of actinomycin IV which has two proline residues. Addition of valine to the medium increases the proportion of actinomycin IV (2 valine residues) from 10% to 80% of the actinomycin mixture. L–isoleucine, D–isoleucine or L–alloisoleucine supplementation yields a new biosynthetic actinomycin in which N–methylvaline is replaced by N–methyl–L–alloisoleucine. New actinomycins are also produced by addition of proline analogues such as pipecolic acid, azetidine–2–carboxylic acid, 3–, 4– or 5–methyl proline, 4–fluoro-, bromo-, chloro- or thioproline. Some of these biosynthetic actinomycins have altered therapeutic indices and are showing promise in cancer chemotherapy.

Quinomycin (echinomycin) is a peptide antibiotic family containing two residues of quinoxaline carboxylic acid in addition to amino acid residues. Directed biosynthesis of natural and biosynthetic quinomycins has been achieved by supplementation with amino acids or analogues of quinoxaline carboxylic acid (Yoshida *et al.*, 1968).

Bleomycin constitutes a family of important peptide antibiotics of significant use in cancer chemotherapy. Bleomycin members all possess a common nucleus containing two tripeptides and a disaccharide; they differ in their amine moiety and in their therapeutic indices. There are 12 natural bleomycins produced by *Streptomyces verticillus* with 11 known amine groups (R) as shown in Table 3. Supplementation with amine analogues have resulted in the production of over 42 biosynthetic bleomycins; some of these R groups are shown in Table 3 (Umezawa, 1977).

Novobiocin

Novobiocin analogues can also be produced by directed biosynthesis using *Streptomyces spheroides* (Walton *et al.*, 1962). The structure of novobiocin contains a sugar, a substituted coumarin and a substituted benzoic acid (Fig. 2). Addition of various benzoic acid derivatives to the culture leads to production of biosynthetic novobiocins with altered antibacterial spectra; the precursors are shown in Table 4.

Other Antibiotics

New celestosaminide antibiotics are produced when *Streptomyces caelestis* is fed aromatic acids (Argoudelis *et al.*, 1974). For example,

TABLE 3

Amine Moieties of Natural and Biosynthetic Bleomycins

Natural	Biosynthetic	Biosynthetic
$-NH-(CH_2)_3-SO-CH_3$	$-NH-CH_2-CH_2-CH_2-NH_2$	$-NH-(CH_2)_3-N\bigcirc$ (piperidine)
$-NH-(CH_2)_3-S-CH_3$	$-NH-(CH_2)_3-N\!<^{CH_3}_{CH_3}$	$-NH-(CH_2)_3-N\bigcirc O$ (morpholine)
$-NH-(CH_2)_3-S^+\!<^{CH_3}_{CH_3}$	$-NH-(CH_2)_3-\overset{+}{N}(CH_3)_3$	$-NH-(CH_2)_2-N\bigcirc N$ (piperazine)
$-NH-(CH_2)_4-NH_2$	$-NH-(CH_2)_3-NH-(CH_2)_3-N(CH_3)_2$	$-NH-(CH_2)_3-NH-CH_2-\bigcirc$
$-NH-(CH_2)_3-NH_2$	$-NH-(CH_2)_3-\underset{CH_3}{\overset{|}{N}}-(CH_2)_3-NH_2$	$-NH-(CH_2)_3-NH-\underset{CH_3}{\overset{|}{CH}}-\bigcirc$
$-NH-(CH_2)_2-\text{(imidazole, N–N–H)}$	$-NH-(CH_2)_3-NH-(CH_2)_3-OH$	$-NH-CH_2-\bigcirc-CH_2-NH_2$
$-NH-(CH_2)_3-NH-(CH_2)_4-NH_2$ $\quad\quad -NH_2$, $NH=$	$-NH-(CH_2)_3-NH-(CH_2)_3-OCH_3$	$-NH-(CH_2)_3-NH-\bigcirc$ (cyclohexyl)
$-NH-(CH_2)_4-NH-\overset{\overset{NH}{\|}}{C}-NH_2$	$-NH-(CH_2)_3-N\bigcirc$ (pyrrolidine)	
$-NH-(CH_2)_4-NH-\overset{\overset{NH}{\|}}{C}-NH-(CH_2)_4-NH-\overset{\overset{NH}{\|}}{C}-NH_2$		
$-NH-(CH_2)_3-NH-(CH_2)_4-NH-(CH_2)_3-NH_2$		

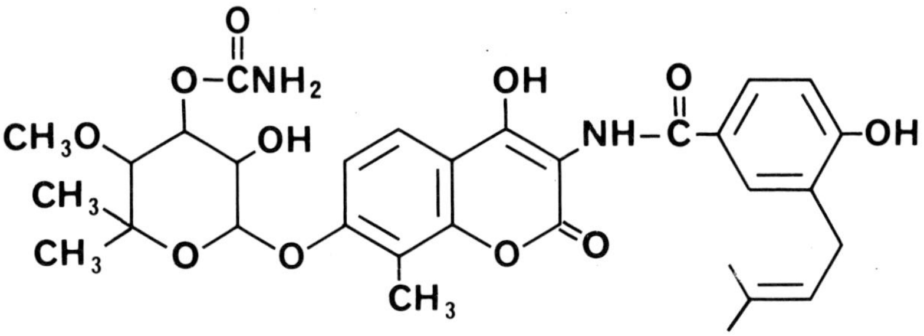

FIG. 2   Structure of novobiocin.

TABLE 4

Precursors of Biosynthetic Novobiocins

3−hexyl−4−hydroxybenzoic acid
4−ethoxy−3(3−methyl−2−butenyl)benzoic acid
4−hydroxy−3(3−phenylpropyl)benzoic acid
3−isopentyl−4−methoxybenzoic acid
4−hydroxy−3−pentylbenzoic acid
4−hydroxy−3−isopentylbenzoic acid
4−acetoxy−3−isopentylbenzoic acid
4−methoxy−3(3−methyl−2−butenyl)benzoic acid
4−hydroxy−3−isobutylbenzoic acid
3−(2, 3−dichloropropyl)4−methoxybenzoic acid
4−hydroxy−3−propylbenzoic acid
4−hydroxy−3−γ−methylallyl) benzoic acid
4−hydroxy−3−(2−methylallyl)benzoic acid
4−hydroxy−3−(α−methylallyl)benzoic acid
3−allyl−4−hydroxybenzoic acid
4−hydroxy−3−methylbenzoic acid
3−ethyl−4−hydroxybenzoic acid
4−amino−3−methylbenzoic acid
3−allyl−4−methoxybenzoic acid

when 4−aminosalicylic acid is the supplement, desalicetin 2′−(4−aminosalicylate) is produced instead of celesticetin (Fig. 3).

Other acids which lead to production of biosynthetic celestosaminides are anthranilic acid, *m*−aminobenzoic acid, N−methylanthranilic acid, *p*−dimethylaminobenzoic acid, *p*−methylaminobenzoic acid and *p*−acetaminobenzoic acid.

Lincomycin, an antibacterial product of *Streptomyces lincolnensis*, contains C−methyl, N−methyl and S−methyl groups (Fig. 4). When ethionine is added to a complex fermentation medium, a

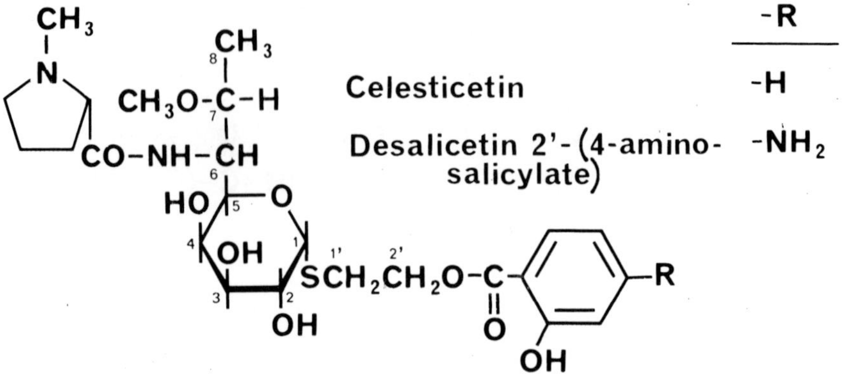

FIG. 3 Structures of celesticetin and desalicetin 2′–(4–aminosalicylate).

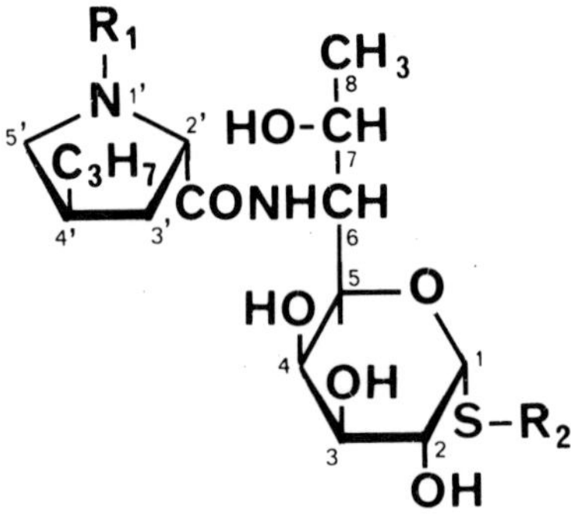

	$-R_1$	$-R_2$
Lincomycin	$-CH_3$	$-CH_3$
N-Demethyllincomycin	-H	$-CH_3$
S-Demethyl-S-ethyllincomycin	$-CH_3$	$-C_2H_5$

FIG. 4 Structures of lincomycin, N–demethyllincomycin and S–demethyl–S–ethyllincomycin.

biosynthetic lincomycin is produced which contains an S–ethyl group (Argoudelis *et al.*, 1970). When ethionine is added to defined medium, both the S–methyl and N–methyl groups are replaced by the ethyl group (Argoudelis *et al.*, 1970).

This effect of ethionine was noted a number of years earlier with the oxytetracycline producer, *Streptomyces rimosus*. Dulaney *et al.* (1962) found that upon ethionine addition, the organism produced the N–ethyl homologue of oxytetracycline along with the parent antibiotic. Another modification in the tetracycline family is the directed biosynthesis of 7–bromotetracycline by adding Br⁻ to the medium of the 7–chlorotetracycline producer (Doershuk *et al.*, 1956).

Pyrrolnitrins are phenylpyrrole antifungal antibiotics produced by species of *Pseudomonas*. The normal precursor is D–tryptophan. Addition of tryptophan analogues substituted with fluorine or methyl results in new biosynthetic pyrrolnitrins (Fig. 5) (Hamill *et al.*, 1970).

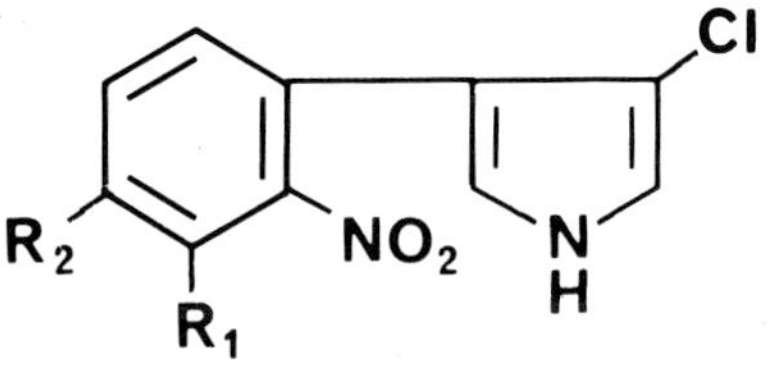

	$-R_1$	$-R_2$
Pyrrolnitrin	$-Cl$	$-H$
4'-fluoropyrrolnitrin	$-Cl$	$-F$
3'-methyl-3'-dechloropyrrolnitrin	$-CH_3$	$-H$

Fig. 5   Structures of pyrrolnitrin, 4'–fluoropyrrolnitrin and 3'–methyl–3'–dechloro-pyrrolnitrin.

Production of polyoxins by *Streptomyces cacaoi* is susceptible to directed biosynthesis. These pyrimidine nucleoside antifungal agents are used as agricultural fungicides in Japan. The pyrimidine bases in natural polyoxins are uracil, thymine, hydroxymethyluracil and uracil–5–carboxylic acid. New biosynthetic polyoxins are formed by 5–fluoro-, 5–bromo- and 6–azauracil supplementation (Fig. 6) (Isono and Suhadolnik, 1976).

Directed Biosynthesis by Inhibitor Addition

There are a number of cases in which inhibitors have been used to block normal methylation steps of secondary metabolism to produce modified antibiotics. When sulfonamides were added to *Streptomyces aureofaciens*, a producer of tetracycline and chlorotetracycline, 6–demethylchlorotetracycline was formed instead (Goodman and Matrishin, 1961; Perlman *et al.*, 1961; Goodman and Miller, 1962). The same result has been achieved with ethionine, aminopterin, D–methionine and analogues such as methoxinine and homocysteine

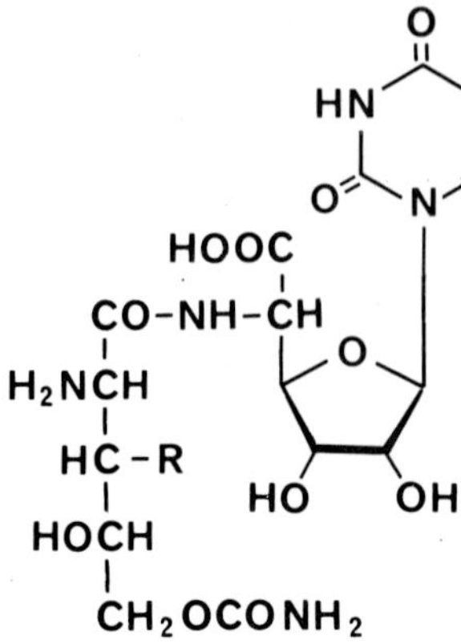

	-X	-R
Polyoxin L	-H	-OH
5-fluoropolyoxin L	-F	-OH
Polyoxin M	-H	-H
5-fluoropolyoxin M	-F	-H

FIG. 6 Structures of polyoxins L and M and of their 5–fluoro derivatives.

derivatives (Goodman and Miller, 1962; Hendlin *et al.*, 1962; Neidleman *et al.*, 1963a and b). Addition of methylation inhibitors to *Streptomyces griseus* leads to the production of the biosynthetic N–demethylstreptomycin along with the natural streptomycin (Heding, 1968). Sulfonamide addition to *Streptomyces lincolnensis* yields N–demethyllincomycin (Fig. 4) (Argoudelis *et al.*, 1973b).

Mutational Biosynthesis Using Idiotrophs

In 1963, Birch suggested that the investigator should be able to produce new antibiotics by the use of mutants which no longer produce a particular moiety of that antibiotic. The work of Shier *et al.* (1969) confirmed the soundness of that suggestion and established the practice of "mutational biosynthesis" (Nagaoka and Demain, 1975). In this process, one first screens for blocked mutants after mutagenesis of a producing culture. The nonproducers are then exposed to the different moieties of the antibiotic and those conditional mutants that can now produce the antibiotic are termed "idiotrophs" (Nagaoka and Demain, 1975), i.e. mutants that can grow without special supplementation but need the supplementation to produce their secondary metabolite. The next step is to feed the idiotrophic mutants analogues of the essential moiety. If the analogue can get into the cell, if it can be accepted by the biosynthetic enzymes to produce the modified antibiotic, and if the modified antibiotic indeed has detectable antibiotic activity, then and only then is the process successful.

Shier *et al.* (1969) announced the production of a new group of aminocyclitol antibiotics which they called "hybrimycins" using

2—deoxystreptamine idiotrophs of the neomycin producer, *Streptomyces fradiae*. By substituting streptamine for deoxystreptamine in the medium, they produced hybrimycins A1 and A2; by substituting with *epi*—streptamine, they obtained hybrimycins B1 and B2. New antibiotics were also produced with the paromomycin producer, *Streptomyces rimosus* forma *paromomycinus* and with the producer of kanamycins, *Streptomyces kanamyceticus* (Shier *et al.*, 1973). In the case of the former organism, substitution of streptamine for 2— deoxystreptamine led to the formation of the hybrimycin C group instead of the paromomycins. With *Streptomyces kanamyceticus*, *epi*—streptamine was used to produce a modified kanamycin. Soon. a similar response was shown by others with deoxystreptamine idiotrophs of the ribostamycin producer, *Streptomyces ribosidificus* (Kojima and Satoh, 1973), the butirosin producer, *Bacillus circulans* (Claridge *et al.*, 1974) and the sisomicin producer, *Micromonospora inyoensis* (Testa *et al.*, 1974). Since 1974, the production of new aminocyclitol antibiotics by the use of deoxystreptamine idiotrophs has continued so that analogues of virtually all deoxystreptamine containing antibiotics have been produced. These developments are described in Table 5.

In the case of aminocyclitol antibiotics containing streptidine, Nagaoka and Demain (1975) obtained a streptidine idiotroph of the streptomycin-producing *Streptomyces griseus*. Of a number of streptidine analogues tested, only 2—deoxystreptidine led to formation of a new antibiotic (Lemke and Demain, 1976). Walker (1978) has found the idiotroph to lack 1D—1—guanidino—1—deoxy—3— keto(*scyllo*)—inositol oxidoreductase, the second dehydrogenase of the streptidine biosynthetic path.

It should be noted that it has occasionally been possible to use a pseudodisaccharide (sugar—aminocyclitol) moiety instead of the aminocyclitol moiety alone. This has been done with certain neamine analogues in *Streptomyces ribosidificus* (Kojima and Satoh, 1973) and *Bacillus circulans* (Takeda *et al.*, 1978a, b, c, d) (Table 5). This ability gives the investigator much more latitude in the options concerning analogue preparation. It is of particular interest that Takeda *et al.* (1978b, c, d) isolated 2 types of idiotroph from the butirosin-producing *Bacillus circulans*. One type responded to deoxystreptamine and the pseudodisaccharides neamine and paromamine. The second type only responded to the pseudodisaccharides.

Although the hybrimycins (Shier *et al.*, 1969, 1973, 1974) were not improved over the original neomycins and paromomycins, there have been compounds prepared by mutational biosynthesis which appear superior. For example, 6—deoxyneomycins, prepared by

TABLE 5

New Aminoglycosides Obtained by Mutational Biosynthesis

Microorganism	Usual antibiotic	Deoxystreptamine analogues yielding new antibiotic	References
Streptomyces fradiae	Neomycin	streptamine 2–*epi*–streptamine 2,6–dideoxystreptamine 3–N–methyldeoxystreptamine streptidine 2,5–dideoxystreptamine 2–bromodeoxystreptamine 6–bromodeoxystreptamine	Shier *et al.*, 1973. Cleophax *et al.*, 1976. Rinehart, 1976.
Streptomyces rimosus var. *paromomycinus*	Paromomycin	streptamine 2,6–dideoxystreptamine	Shier *et al.*, 1974.
Streptomyces kanamyceticus	Kanamycin	1–N–methyldeoxystreptamine 2–*epi*–streptamine	Kojima and Satoh, 1973.
Streptomyces ribosidificus	Ribostamycin	streptamine 2–*epi*–streptamine 1–N–methyldeoxystreptamine 3′,4′–dideoxyneamine	Kojima and Satoh, 1973.
Micromonospora inyoensis	Sisomicin	streptamine 2,5–dideoxystreptamine 5–*epi*–deoxystreptamine 2–*epi*–streptamine 1–N–methyldeoxystreptamine N–methyl–2,5–dideoxystreptamine 1,3,5–triaminocyclohexane–4,6–diol	Testa *et al.*, 1974. Waitz *et al.*, 1978.
Micromonospora purpurea	Gentamicin	streptamine 2,5–dideoxystreptamine	Daum *et al.*, 1977.
Bacillus circulans	Butirosin	streptamine streptidine 2,5–dideoxystreptamine 6′–N–methylneamine 3′,4′–dideoxyneamine 3′,4′–dideoxy–6′–N–methylneamine 3′,4′–dideoxy–6′–C–methylneamine 6′–N–methylgentamine C_{1a} gentamine C_2 gentamine C_{1a}	DeFuria and Claridge, 1976. Takeda *et al.*, 1978a, b, c, d.

feeding 2,6–dideoxystreptamine to *Streptomyces fradiae*, are more active than neomycin C against *Escherichia coli*, *Proteus mirabilis*, *Staphylococcus aureus* and *Salmonella typhimurium* (Cleophax *et al.*, 1976). Also new sisomicin derivatives Mu–1 and Mu–2, produced by *Micromonospora inyoensis* idiotrophs upon feeding streptamine and 2,5–dideoxystreptamine respectively (Testa *et al.*, 1974), are more active than sisomicin against sisomicin and gentamicin-resistant strains. 5–*epi*–sisomicin, prepared using 5–*epi*–deoxystreptamine, shows greater activity against *Pseudomonas aeruginosa* and resistant *Escherichia coli* than does ribostamycin. Many of the butirosin analogues made by feeding pseudodisaccharides to *Bacillus circulans* are more active than butirosin against clinical isolates resistant to butirosin, dibekacin or gentamicin (Takeda *et al.*, 1978b,d). Probably the most promising aminocyclitol antibiotic produced by mutational biosynthesis is Win 42122–2 or 2–deoxygentamicin (Rosi *et al.*, 1977). Win 42122–2 is produced by the feeding of streptamine to idiotrophs of *Micromonospora purpurea*. The new antibiotic has been tested in animals and although somewhat less active than gentamicin, it is considerably less toxic and thus appears to have an improved therapeutic index (Came *et al.*, 1979). The compound is soon to enter clinical tests in man to determine whether it is indeed a safer gentamicin.

Novobiocin production by *Streptomyces niveus* is also susceptible to mutational biosynthesis. Sebek (1974) described the use of a ring B (3–amino–4,7–dihydroxy–8–methylcoumarin) idiotroph to prepare new novobiocins; the compounds added were various analogues of aminocoumarin.

Idiotrophs of the macrolide antibiotic-producing microorganisms have also been obtained. All respond to the addition of the large macrolide lactone rings. *Streptomyces erythreus* idiotrophs form erythromycins when fed erythronolide but when given 8,8a–deoxyoleanolide, produce a new antibiotic (Martin *et al.*, 1974). The platenomycin producer, *Streptomyces platensis*, has been mutated to idiotrophy. The addition of platenolides I and II yields the normal platenomycins A_1, B_1 and C_2 (Furumai *et al.*, 1975). However when narbonolide, the aglycone of narbomycin, is fed, the idiotroph produces 5–0–mycaminosylnarbonolide (Maezawa *et al.*, 1976). Feeding the double moiety, 5–0–desosaminylplatenolide I, results in production of the new antibiotic, 3–0–propionyl–5–0–desosaminyl–9–dihydro–18–oxoplatenolide I (Maezawa *et al.*, 1978).

Use of Auxotrophs to Prepare New Antibiotics

If a group or a moiety of an antibiotic is derived rather directly from a primary metabolite such as an amino acid, an auxotroph can be used to form new antibiotics. For example, griseofulvin biosynthesis by *Penicillium griseofulvum* involves endogenous methionine as a source of a methyl group. A methionine auxotroph fed ethionine plus methionine produced the 2′–ethoxy analogue of griseofulvin which is more active than the parent antibiotic (Jackson *et al.*, 1962).

Production of penicillin N and cephalosporin C by *Cephalosporium acremonium* involves L–α–aminoadipic acid as side-chain precursor.

Since the aminoadipate is an intermediate in the biosynthesis of L—lysine, lysine auxotrophs blocked early (before aminoadipate) can grow with lysine or aminoadipate. When grown with lysine, no antibiotics are produced due to lack of aminoadipate. When fed aminoadipate, the antibiotics are produced. A new penicillin is produced when the aminoadipate analogue, L—S—carboxymethyl-cysteine, is fed to the auxotroph. The new product 6(D)—{[(2—amino—2—carboxy)—erythro]—acetamido}—penicillanic acid (also called RIT 2214), is considerably more active and more stable than penicillin N (Troonen et al., 1976).

Auxotrophs can also be used to produce new antibiotics without the feeding of analogues. In certain cases, the mechanism is well understood. For example, methionine auxotrophs of Streptomyces viridifaciens produce 6—demethylchlorotetracycline under methionine limitation (Neidleman et al., 1963a). Similar auxotrophs of Streptomyces caelestis, the producer of celesticetin and desalicetin, produce the new 7—0—demethylcelesticetin, N—demethyl—7—0—demethyl-celesticetin and N—demethylcelesticetin (Argoudelis et al., 1972, 1973a). Less well understood is the formation of a new antibiotic from the penicillin N producer, Emericellopsis salmosynnemata by an asparagine auxotroph (Fantini, 1962) or production of two new antibiotics by purine auxotrophs of the rubradirin producer, Streptomyces achromogenes (Coats, 1978).

Use of Non-Idiotrophic and Non-Auxotrophic Mutants Blocked in Secondary Metabolism to Produce New Antibiotics

A mutant which is neither an auxotroph nor an idiotroph (i.e. it does not need special factors for either growth or antibiotic production) can still be useful if it has been mutated in a gene coding for an enzyme of secondary metabolism. The simplest case is a blocked mutant which accumulates intermediates which have antibiotic activity. Examples include the production of deacetoxycephalosporin C by mutants of the cephalosporin C-producing Cephalosporium acremonium (Liersch et al., 1976), of demycarosylplatenomycin and 9—dehydromycarosylplatenomycin by a mutant of Streptomyces platensis (Furamai and Suzuki, 1975), of 1—deoxychloramphenicol by a mutant of the chloramphenicol-producer, Streptomyces vene-zuelae (Okagawa et al., 1979), and of demethylrifamycin SV and rifamycin SV by mutants of the rifamycin B producer, Nocardia mediterranei (Lancini and Hengeller, 1969, 1970). In the latter case, the final product (rifamycin B) is devoid of antibiotic activity where-as the intermediates are active. An interesting case was reported by Baud et al. (1977). These workers noted that a mutant of the neomycin producer, *Streptomyces fradiae*, produced ribostamycin which up to that time was known only as a product of *Streptomyces ribosidificus*. However, this discovery revealed that ribostamycin is an intermediate of neomycin biosynthesis. A similar situation was revealed by studies on the butirosin producer, *Bacillus circulans* (Fujiwara *et al.*, 1978). Mutants produce ribostamycin and xylostasin which are butirosins B and A less the α–hydroxy–γ–aminobutyric acid side chain respectively. Up until this investigation, ribostamycin and xylostasin were known only as products of *Streptomyces*.

Somewhat more involved is the situation in which a step of the biosynthetic path is eliminated by mutation, yet the path can still proceed due to the low substrate specificity of secondary metabolism enzymes. Thus a mutationally imposed deficiency in the methylation step in production of tetracycline and chlortetracycline by *Streptomyces aureofaciens* does not stop antibiotic synthesis but leads to the production of the more stable compounds, 6–demethylchlortetracycline and 6–demethyltetracycline (McCormick *et al.*, 1957).

A large number of new compounds are produced by unknown mechanisms as mutationally induced derivatives of known antibiotics. These are shown in Table 6. The most well known of these is the mutation of the daunorubicin producer, *Streptomyces peucetius*, to production of doxorubicin (Arcamone *et al.*, 1969). An interesting case involves the rifamycin producer in which three new rifamycins are produced by mutants (White *et al.*, 1975; Martinelli *et al.*, 1978). One of these, rifamycin P, is the most active rifamycin ever discovered. In other cases, the mutant does not produce a totally new compound but one that is "new" for that species. For example, a mutant of the maridomycin-producing *Streptomyces hygroscopicus* has been found to produce the "new" macrolides leucomycin A_3, carbomycins A and B and SF–837A1 (Uchida *et al.*, 1979). Also the *Streptomyces clavuligerus* culture which normally produces cephamycin C and clavulanic acid has been mutated to a strain which also produces holomycin (Kenig and Reading, 1979). Another interesting case involves mutation of *Streptomyces saganonensis* in which the normal antibiotics, herbicidins A, B, C and E, exhibit herbicidal activity and the new herbicidins (F and G) produced by the mutants are antifungal (Takiguchi, 1979).

TABLE 6

Active Derivatives of Known Antibiotics Produced by Mutants

Normal Antibiotics	New Antibiotics	Organism	Reference
Tetracycline and Chlorotetracycline	2−acetyl−2−decarbox-amidotetracycline and 2−acetyl−2−carbox-amidochlorotetracycline	*Streptomyces aureofaciens*	Miller and Hochstein, 1962.
Cephalosporin C	D−7−(5−amino−5−carboxyvaleramido)−3−methylthiomethyl−3−cephem−4−carboxylic acid	*Cephalosporium acremonium*	Fujisawa, 1977.
Daunorubicin	14−hydroxydauno-rubicin (doxorubicin)	*Streptomyces peucetius* var. *caesius*	Arcamone *et al.*, 1969.
" "	4−O−methyl−13−dihydrodaunorubicin	*Streptomyces peucetius*	Cassinelli *et al.*, 1978.
Polymyxin	new polymyxins	*Bacillus polymyxa*	Nefelova *et al.*, 1974.
Kanamycin	NK−1001, NK−1012−1, NK−1012−3, mono−N−acetyl-kanamycin B, di−N−acetylkanamycin B	*Streptomyces kanamyceticus*	Murase *et al.*, 1970.
Rifamycin B	Rifamycins P, Q, R	*Nocardia mediterranea*	White *et al.*, 1975.
Herbicidins A, B, C and E	Herbicidins F and G	*Streptomyces saganonensis*	Takiguchi *et al.*, 1979.

References

Arcamone, F., Cassinelli, G., Fantini, G., Grein, A., Orezzi, P., Pol, C. and Spalla, C. (1969). *Biotechnol. Bioeng.* **11**, 1101−1110.

Argoudelis, A.D., Coats, J.H. and Johnson, L.E. (1974). *J. Antibiot.* **27**, 738−743.

Argoudelis, A.D., Coats, J.H., Lemaux, P.G. and Sebek, O.K. (1972). *J. Antibiot.* **25**, 445−455.

Argoudelis, A.D., Coats, J.H., Lemaux, P.G. and Sebek, O.K. (1973a). *J. Antibiot.* **26**, 7−14.

Argoudelis, A.D., Eble, T.E. and Mason, D.J. (1970). *J. Antibiot.* **23**, 1−8.

Argoudelis, A.D., Johnson, L.E. and Pyke, T.R. (1973b). *J. Antibiot.* **26**, 429−436.

Baud, H., Betencourt, A., Peyré, M. and Pénasse, L. (1977). *J. Antibiot.* **30**, 720−723.

Behrens, D.K. (1949). *In* "The Chemistry of Penicillins". (H.T. Clarke, J.R. Johnson and R. Robinson, eds), pp. 657−679. Princeton Univ. Press, Princeton, N.J.

Birch, A.J. (1963). *Pure Appl. Chem.* **7**, 527−537.

Came, P.E., O'Connor, J.R., Dobson, R.A., Wagner, R.B. and Fabian, R.J. (1979). *Antimicrob. Agents Chemother.* **16**, 813–822.

Cassinelli, G., Grein, A., Masi, P., Suarato, A., Bernardi, L., Arcamone, F., Di Marco, A., Casazza, A.M., Pratesi, G. and Soranzo, C. (1978). *J. Antibiot.* **31**, 178–184.

Claridge, C.A., Bush, J.A., DeFuria, M.D. and Price, K.E. (1974). *Dev. Ind. Microbiol.* **15**, 101–113.

Cleophax, J., Gero, S.D., Leboul, J., Akhtar, M., Barnett, J.E.G. and Pearce, C.J. (1976). *J. Am. Chem. Soc.* **98**, 7110–7112.

Coats, J.H. (1978). *In* "Proceedings of the Joint US/USSR Seminar on the Genetics of Actinomycetes and Bacilli", p. 31. National Science Foundation, Washington, D.C.

Cole, M. (1966). *Process Biochem.* **1**, 334–338.

Daum, S.J., Rosi, D. and Goss, W.A. (1977). *J. Antibiot.* **30**, 98–105.

DeFuria, M.D. and Claridge, C.A. (1976). *In* "Microbiology – 1976". (D. Schlessinger, ed.), pp. 427–436. American Society for Microbiology. Washington, D.C.

Doershuk, A.P., McCormick, J.R.D., Goodman, J.J., Szumski, S.A., Growich, J.A., Miller, P.A., Bitter, B.A., Jensen, E.R., Petty, M.A. and Phelps, A.S. (1956). *J. Am. Chem. Soc.* **78**, 1508–1509.

Dulaney, E.L., Putter, I., Drescher, D., Chaiet, L., Miller, W.J., Wolf, F.J. and Hendlin, D. (1962). *Biochim. Biophys. Acta* **60**, 447–449.

Fantini, A.A. (1962). *Genetics* **47**, 161–177.

Fujisawa, Y. (1977). *J. Takeda Res. Lab.* **36**, 295–356.

Fujiwara, T., Tanimoto, T., Matsumoto, K. and Kondo, E. (1978). *J. Antibiot.* **31**, 966–969.

Furumai, T. and Suzuki, M. (1975). *J. Antibiot.* **28**, 775–782.

Furumai, T., Takeda, K. and Suzuki, M. (1975). *J. Antibiot.* **28**, 789–797.

Goodman, J.J. and Matrishin, M. (1961). *J. Bacteriol.* **82**, 615.

Goodman, J.J. and Miller, P.A. (1962). *Biotechnol. Bioeng.* **4**, 391–402.

Hamill, R.L., Elander, R.P., Mabe, J.A. and Gorman, M. (1970). *Appl. Microbiol.* **19**, 721–725.

Heding, H. (1968). *Acta Chem. Scand.* **22**, 1649–1654.

Hendlin, D., Dulaney, E.L., Drescher, D., Cook, T. and Chaiet, L. (1962). *Biochim. Biophys. Acta* **58**, 635–636.

Isono, K. and Suhadolnik, R.J. (1976). *Arch. Biochem. Biophys.* **173**, 141–153.

Jackson, M., Dulaney, E.L., Putter, I., Shafer, H.M., Wolf, F.J. and Woodruff, H.B. (1962). *Biochim. Biophys. Acta* **62**, 616–619.

Katz, E. (1974). *Cancer Chemother. Rep.*, Part 1. **58**, 83–91.

Katz, E. and Demain, A.L. (1977). *Bacteriol. Rev.* **41**, 449–474.

Kenig, M. and Reading, C. (1979). *J. Antibiot.* **32**, 549–554.

Kojima, M. and Satoh, A. (1973). *J. Antibiot.* **26**, 784–786.

Lancini, G.C. and Hengeller, C. (1969). *J. Antibiot.* **22**, 637–638.

Lancini, G.C., Hengeller, C. and Sensi, P. (1970). *Progr. Antimicrob. Anticancer Chemother.* **2**, 1166–1173.

Lemke, J.R. and Demain, A.L. (1976). *Eur. J. Appl. Microbiol.* **2**, 91–94.

Liersch, M., Nuesch, J. and Treichler, H.J. (1976). *In* "Proceedings of the Second International Symposium on Genetics of Industrial Microorganisms", (K.D. MacDonald, ed.), pp. 179–195. Academic Press, New York.

Maezawa, I., Kinumaki, A. and Suzuki, M. (1976). *J. Antibiot.* **29**, 1203–1208.

Maezawa, I., Kinumaki, A. and Suzuki, M. (1978). *J. Antibiot.* **31**, 309–318.

Martin, J.R., Egan, R.S., Goldstein, A.W., Mueller, S.L., Hirner, E.A. and Stanaszek, R.S. (1974). *J. Antibiot.* **27**, 570–572.

Martinelli, E., Antonini, P., Cricchio, R., Lancini, G. and White, R.J. (1978). *J. Antibiot.* **31**, 949–951.

McCormick, J.R.D., Sjolander, N.O., Hirsch, U., Jensen, E.R. and Doerschuk, A.P. (1957). *J. Am. Chem. Soc.* **79**, 4561–4563.

Miller, M. and Hochstein, F.A. (1962). *J. Org. Chem.* **27**, 2525–2528.

Murase, M., Ito, T., Fukatsu, S. and Umezawa, H. (1970). *Prog. Antimicrob. Anticancer Chemother.* **2**, 1098–1110.

Nagaoka, K. and Demain, A.L. (1975). *J. Antibiot.* **28**, 627–635.

Nefalova, M.V., Chigaleichik, A.G. and Silaev, A.B. (1974). *Mikrobiologiya* **43**, 307–309.

Neidleman, S.L., Albu, E. and Bienstock, E. (1963a). *Biotechnol. Bioeng.* **5**, 87–89.

Neidleman, S.L., Bienstock, E. and Bennet, R.C. (1963b). *Biochim. Biophys. Acta* **71**, 199–201.

Okagawa, H., Okanishi, M. and Umezawa, H. (1979). *J. Antibiot.* **32**, 610–620.

Perlman, D., Heuser, L.J., Semar, J.B., Frazier, W.R. and Boska, J.A. (1961). *J. Am. Chem. Soc.* **83**, 4481.

Rinehart, K. (1976). Proc. IUPAC, Dunedin, New Zealand, Pergamon Press.

Rosi, D., Goss, W.A. and Daum, S.J. (1977). *J. Antibiot.* **30**, 88–97.

Sebek, O.K. (1974). *In* "Abstracts of the 2nd International Symposium on the Genetics of Industrial Microorganisms (Sheffield)", p. 14. Academic Press, London, New York, San Francisco.

Shier, W.T., Ogawa, S., Hitchens, M. and Rinehart, K.L., Jr. (1973). *J. Antibiot.* **26**, 551–561.

Shier, W.T., Rinehart, K.L., Jr. and Gottlieb, D. (1969). *Proc. Nat. Acad. Sci. (U.S.A.)* **63**, 198–204.

Shier, W.T., Shaefer, P.C., Gottlieb, D. and Rinehart, K.L., Jr. (1974). *Biochemistry* **13**, 5073–5078.

Takeda, K., Kinumaki, A., Furumai, T., Yamaguchi, T., Oshima, S. and Ito, Y. (1978a). *J. Antibiot.* **31**, 247–249.

Takeda, K., Kinumaki, A., Hayasaka, H., Yamaguchi, T. and Ito, Y. (1978b). *J. Antibiot.* **31**, 1031–1038.

Takeda, K., Kinumaki, A., Okuno, S., Matsushita, T. and Ito, Y. (1978c). *J. Antibiot.* **31**, 1039–1045.

Takeda, K., Okuno, S., Ohashi, Y. and Furumai, T. (1978d). *J. Antibiot.* **31**, 1023–1030.

Takiguchi, Y., Yoshikawa, H., Terahara, A., Torikata, A. and Terao, M. (1979). *J. Antibiot.* **32**, 862–867.

Testa, R.T., Wagman, G.H., Daniels, P.J.L. and Weinstein, M.J. (1974). *J. Antibiot.* **27**, 917–921.

Troonen, H., Roelants, P. and Boon, B. (1976). *J. Antibiot.* **29**, 1258–1267.

Uchida, M., Suzuki, M., Takayama, T. and Sugita, N. (1979). *Agric. Biol. Chem.* **43**, 847–852.

Umezawa, H. (1977). *J. Nat. Prod.* **40**, 67–81.

Yoshida, T., Kumura, Y. and Katagiri, K. (1968). *J. Antibiot.* **21**, 465–467.

Waitz, J.A., Miller, G.H., Moss, Jr., E. and Chiu, P.J.S. (1978). *Antimicrob. Agents Chemother.* **13**, 41–48.

Walker, J.B. (1978). *In* "Cyclitols Phosphoinositides" (W.W. Wells and F. Eisenberg, Jr., eds), pp. 423–438. Academic Press, New York.

Walton, R.B., McDaniel, L.E. and Woodruff, H.B. (1962). *Dev. Ind. Microbiol.* **3**, 370–375.

White, R.J., Lancini, G. and Sensi, P. (1975). *In* "Proceedings of Intersect. Congr. of IAMS", Vol. 3. (T. Hasegawa, ed.), p. 483. Science Council of Japan.

Discussion

Professor Rinehart: The hydroxyneomycins are improved, as compared to the neomycins, with respect to their toxicity. The compound from streptamine is only about half as toxic as the neomycins.

Professor Demain: I appreciate that information of which I was not aware.

Dr. Gero: Can *Streptomyces griseus* also take deoxystreptamine, or only deoxystreptidine?

Professor Demain: There is a problem here, as Professor Rinehart has mentioned on several occasions. In merely doing experiments like this it is not known whether these compounds are accepted, or whether the resultant compounds are inactive. He may have done some additional work using labelled precursors to investigate this problem. *Streptomyces griseus* did not make an active antibiotic from 2–deoxystreptamine. That is all we know.

Professor Rinehart: *Streptomyces griseus* would not really be expected to do that because streptamine, for example, is not on the biosynthetic pathway to streptidine. It would be reasonable that it should not be incorporated.

Structure Elucidation of Antibiotics

K.L. RINEHART, Jr.

*Roger Adams Laboratory, University of
Illinois, Urbana, Illinois, U.S.A.*

Introduction

It is difficult to discuss the plethora of methods available for
assigning structures to antibiotics in a short space, given the number
of antibiotics whose structures are presently known and the array of
structural tools available. Nevertheless, it appears that two separate
problems must be addressed: the identification of known antibiotics
and the elucidation of structures of new antibiotics. While the
techniques involved for dealing with the two problems are not
mutually exclusive, they differ sufficiently for them to be dealt with
separately below.

Identification of Known Antibiotics

In the course of searching for new antibiotics a relatively large
proportion of the antibiotics discovered in any screen will be known
compounds; thus, it behoves the scientist involved in screening to be
able to recognise a substance as a known compound and to identify
it as soon as possible. Our own laboratory has not been involved in
classical screening for microorganism-derived antibiotics, but we have
recently carried out extensive screening for antimicrobial, antiviral,
or cytotoxic compounds in crude extracts of marine invertebrates
and algae and many of the techniques required are similar, as
summarised in Table 1.

Probably the technique available at the earliest stage is non-
chemical, involving determination of the antimicrobial spectrum of
the antibiotic. This technique, while crude, nevertheless can narrow

TABLE 1

Techniques for Identification of Known Antibiotics

Technique	Parameter
Bioassay	Antimicrobial spectrum
Paper chromatography	R_f in several systems
Thin layer chromatography	R_f in several systems
Gas chromatography	Retention time and mass spectrometry
High performance liquid chromatography	Retention volume and mass spectrometry
Field desorption mass spectrometry	Molecular formula
Infrared spectroscopy	Spectrum (fingerprint)
^{13}C NMR	Spectrum (fingerprint)

the field considerably with respect to a known antimicrobial substance. This is true, not only for antibiotics isolated from microorganisms, but also for antimicrobial substances isolated from marine
species, as illustrated by the bioactivity spectra of five sponge samples
(Table 2). The very similar spectra suggested that the active compounds in the sponges might be closely related, a suggestion confirmed by subsequent chemical evidence (Rinehart *et al.*, unpub.
results). Indeed, the similar antimicrobial spectra also led to extensive
revisions of taxonomy of the sponges. Table 2 also shows the value
of tissue culture assay as an auxiliary technique in the identification
of bioactive compounds.

Other tools useful for early identification are ultraviolet spectroscopy, very sensitive but limited to compounds containing an
electronic chromophore (Waksman and Lechevalier, 1962), solvent
extractability, and various forms of chromatography (Wagman and
Weinstein, 1978). Extensive libraries exist of paper chromatographic
behaviour in a variety of solvents, and thin-layer chromatography has
become equally valuable. Both paper chromatography and thin-layer
chromatography can, of course, be combined with bioautography vs.
one or more microbial strains. The more powerful separation
techniques of gas chromatography (GC) and high pressure liquid
chromatography (HPLC) have not yet proved as useful for early
identification. Most antibiotics simply do not pass through a gas
chromatograph, while extensive libraries of reproducible retention
volumes are not yet available for high pressure liquid chromatography. However, in principle, each of these methods has the inherent
advantage that it can be combined with mass spectrometry (MS).
GC/MS is a well accepted technique combining the separation power
of GC with the unique ability of a mass spectrometer to identify
compounds by their molecular weights (Milberg and Cook, 1978).
HPLC has only recently been combined with mass spectrometry and

TABLE 2

Bioactivities of Selected Sponge Extracts

	Sponge number				
	59	163	639	650	747
Antimicrobial[a]					
Staphylococcus aureus	15	14	16	17	16
Bacillus subtilis	19	18	24	25	22
Sarcina lutea	15	tr	17	20	15
Klebsiella pneumoniae	17	16	21	21	19
Escherichia coli	0	0	0	0	0
Proteus vulgaris	0	0	0	0	0
Pseudomonas aeruginosa	0	0	0	0	0
Mycobacterium avium	16	0	19	20	17
Saccharomyces pastorianus	0	0	0	0	0
Penicillium oxalicum	0	0	0	0	0
Candida albicans	0	0	14	14	tr
Bacteroides fragilis	18	15	22	24	19
Clostridium perfringens	0	0	tr	15	tr
L1210 Cytotoxicity[b]					
ID_{50}	0.16	0.17	0.16	0.19	0.18
ID_{90}	0.38	0.37	0.37	0.41	0.35
HSV–1 Inhibition[c]	–	–	–	–	–

[a] Activity estimated by the diameter in mm of inhibition zone.

[b] Doses inhibiting 50 or 90% of the growth of L1210 cells in $\mu g/ml$.

[c] Inhibition of *Herpes simplex* virus HSV–1 multiplication; (–): no inhibition.

the results are not yet fully satisfactory (Dawkins and McLafferty, 1978); however, the obvious advantage of HPLC in not being restricted to volatile compounds bodes well for the future of combined LC/MS. Unfortunately, neither GC nor HPLC can be conveniently combined directly with the most characteristic property of the compounds under study, namely, their antimicrobial activity. However, with both techniques one can isolate fractions and determine their antimicrobial activity, as illustrated by an HPLC example from the marine area involving the identification of the antibacterial substances present in the sponge *Aplysina aurea* (Fig. 1), whose bioactivity was shown to be centered in peaks C, F and K (Table 3) (Rinehart and Goo, 1981).

Another relatively new technique of MS, field desorption mass spectrometry (FDMS), appears to be exceedingly promising for potential early identification. FDMS is a gentle technique, giving mainly molecular ions, and is thus useful for analysing impure compounds or mixtures of related compounds. HPLC separation of *Aplysina aurea* components in Fig. 1 was followed closely by FDMS

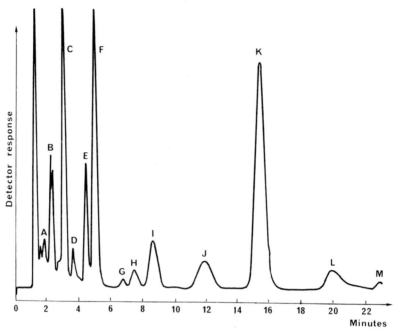

FIG. 1   HPLC separation of components in crude extract of the sponge *Aplysina aurea* (No. 852); refractive index detector.

analysis of the fractions. Although recent attempts to identify antibiotics in fermentation broths proved unsuccessful, extraction of the antibiotic from the broth followed by FDMS gave good results (Rinehart *et al.*, unpub. results). The use of FDMS in identifying a known antibiotic can be illustrated by the recent identification of a pentaene antibiotic. Although it was initially felt to be a new compound, its FD mass spectrum indicated its molecular formula to be $C_{35}H_{58}O_{12}$ and, thus, the compound was suggested to be identical with lagosin (fungichromin). To test this hypothesis, the decahydro derivative of the pentaene antibiotic was treated with periodate, which with lagosin (fungichromin) should give fragments with molecular ions at m/z 410 and 260. These ions were indeed found (M + H at m/z 411 and 261) and, thus, the antibiotic was rather quickly identified as lagosin (fungichromin) (Pandey *et al.*, 1980).

Once an antibiotic is obtained in a higher degree of purity, then a number of spectroscopic techniques can be employed in its identification. Among these, infrared spectroscopy is perhaps the most valuable, both because libraries of infrared spectra are available for identification of antibiotics and because an infrared

TABLE 3

Antimicrobial Activity of Chromatographic Fractions of Ethyl Ether Extracts of
Sponge No 852[a]

| Fraction | Wt, mg | Zone of inhibition[b] | | | | | |
| | | 50 μg | | | 200 μg | | |
		B.s.[c]	*E.c.*[c]	*P.a.*[c]	*B.s.*[c]	*E.c.*[c]	*P.a.*[c]
A	3.3	13	13	- -	22	25	- -
B	3.2	24	23	- -	34	32	- -
C	9.1	36	39	- -	42	48	- -
D	1.7	23	28	- -	31	31	- -
E	2.6	13	13	- -	18	19	- -
F	9.7	31	29	- -	38	37	- -
G	0.5	- -	14	- -	14	20	- -
H	1.0	- -	- -	- -	- -	- -	- -
I	2.3	13	- -	- -	19	14	- -
J	3.2	- -	- -	- -	- -	- -	- -
K	12.9	31	27	- -	39	34	- -
L	1.9	16	- -	- -	25	- -	- -
M	1.0	- -	- -	- -	- -	- -	- -

[a] $C_{18}\mu$–Porasil A; 1/8 in.; MeOH–H_2O : 1–2; 2 ml/min; refractive index detector.
[b] Zone of inhibition in mm.
[c] *B.s.* = *Bacillus subtilis*
E.c. = *Escherichia coli*
P.a. = *Penicillium atrovenetum.*

spectrum has a large number of different bands, providing fingerprint-type identification. The same can be said of the much newer tool of ^{13}C NMR spectroscopy in that the carbon absorptions of a molecule are spread over a wide region and, thus, can also provide a fingerprint with many points of comparison to a known substance. ^{13}C NMR spectroscopy will be discussed in some detail in the next section.

Elucidation of Structures of New Antibiotics

X–Ray Crystallography

Nearly all current structure proofs of antibiotics involve physical tools, especially those in Table 4, and depend on chemical reactions to a lesser extent. The most powerful and most convincing technique is X–ray crystallography, which can provide not only unambiguous proof of the gross structure of the compound but also extensive information regarding relative stereochemistry, bond lengths, and bond angles. If the crystallographic data are sufficiently accurate, then the absolute stereochemistry of the compound can also be ascertained. No technique is, of course, perfect and a caveat also

TABLE 4

Techniques for Elucidation of Structures of New Antibiotics

Technique	Advantages, disadvantages
X–ray crystallography	A: Complete structure, including relative and absolute stereo-chemistry
	D: Crystals required
Mass spectrometry	
PDMS	A: Solid state ionisation of least volatile compounds
	D: Poor resolution
FDMS	A: Solid state ionisation of non-volatile compounds, high resolution
	D: Modest sensitivity
CID	A: Solid state ionisation of non-volatile compounds
	D: High resolution not yet available
CI	A: Gentle ionisation in vapor state, high sensitivity
	D: Volatility required
FI	A: Gentle ionisation in vapor state
	D: Low sensitivity, volatility required
EI	A: High resolution in vapor state
	D: High sensitivity, volatility required
NMR spectroscopy	
^{13}C NMR	A: Wide dispersion of signals
	D: Modest sensitivity by Fourier transform method
^{1}H NMR	A: First order coupling patterns at high field, high sensitivity
	D: Sometimes complex spectra

needs to be applied to X–ray crystallography in that the computer drawn stereochemical formulas are sometimes mistranslated to planar projection formulas. It is also sometimes difficult to distinguish between adjacent atoms in the periodic table, for example, between carbon and boron (Nakamura *et al.*, 1977). The most significant difficulty with respect to use of X–ray crystallography, however, is that the compound must be obtained in satisfactory crystalline form before X–ray crystallography can be successful. Not only must the compound be crystalline *per se*, but it must also be in a satisfactory space group for analysis and the crystals must not be twinned. One must always attempt to obtain suitable crystals, since the information garnered from a successful X–ray crystallographic analysis is so definitive, but it can be frustrating to work many months, or even years, attempting, unsuccessfully, to obtain crystals.

Antibiotics in general seem to be relatively refractory to crystal-lisation. For example, only one polyene antibiotic, amphotericin B (Mechlinski *et al.*, 1970), has thus far been crystallised to a degree satisfactory for X–ray analysis, in spite of extensive attempts on the part of many workers to obtain good crystals. A complicating problem is that antibiotics often occur as mixtures of closely related materials inseparable by chromatography, and single components do not crystallise easily from the mixtures, making an X–ray crystallographic analysis essentially impossible. Although by no means complete or even perhaps statistically significant, a survey of the antibiotics whose structures were assigned in the *Journal of Antibiotics* in 1979 reveals that most were assigned by ordinary spectroscopic and chemical techniques and only about 20% of the assignments involved X–ray crystallography. The failure to make greater use of X–ray crystallography is presumably due to the difficulty in obtaining crystals.

Mass Spectrometry

For those compounds which do not crystallise and whose structures cannot, hence, be established by X–ray crystallography, the first physical method to be employed in assigning their structures must inevitably be mass spectrometry (MS), since the very first parameter one wishes to have at hand is the molecular formula of the compound. Fortunately for the study of antibiotics, there are a number of new techniques available which increase the range of applicability of mass spectrometry towards non-volatile, polar compounds. At the present time, the most useful of these techniques is field desorption mass spectrometry (FDMS), developed at the University of Bonn by Beckey and his co-workers (1977), and shown early to be of value for antibiotics (Rinehart *et al.*, 1974). The FD technique involves applying a solution of the sample to be studied to a specially prepared emitter wire and then applying a high voltage to the emitter wire so that the sample is, conceptually at least, ionised in the solid state. Some control can be exercised over the energy imparted to the sample by varying the current (hence the temperature) flowing through the emitter wire. FD, as noted above, normally gives predominantly molecular ions and, hence, is a valuable technique for analysing mixtures. At higher temperatures, however, fragmentation ions can be made to predominate so that FD can also be employed for studying structures of compounds. The upper mass range obtainable depends mainly on the range of the magnet, but with current magnets it can extend to approximately m/z 3000. FD can also be employed to obtain high resolution data and, hence, molecular formulas for an unknown compound.

An ionisation technique alternative to field desorption is plasma desorption (PD), developed by Mac Farlane and Torgerson (1976), which involves bombarding the sample on a thin film with fission fragments from ^{252}Cf. This source of exceedingly high energy can cause vaporisation of the sample without fragmentation and has been used to obtain molecular ions as high as m/z 12,000.

PDMS has also been shown to be successful in obtaining molecular ions with some compounds difficult to analyse by FD, e.g., bleomycin (MacFarlane, 1980), and polyene antibiotics. On the other hand, PDMS is not amenable to high resolution and, indeed, due to a present resolution limit of approximately 400, a molecular ion at m/z 2000 would be approximately 5 atomic mass units (amu) broad. Where FD works, it is the method of choice; where it does not, PD must be employed. Unfortunately, there are still only a very few operating PD mass spectrometers in the world.

Other mild ionisation techniques are also available. Field ionisation employs the same emitter wires used for FD, but the molecule is first vaporised and ionised in the gaseous state. Electron impact (EI) ionisation, which still provides the best high resolution data, can be employed at reduced ionising voltages. An especially valuable gentle ionisation technique is chemical ionisation (CI). Here instead of bombarding the sample molecules with high energy electrons (EI), a reagent gas present in high concentration is instead ionised by EI and its charge is then transferred (sometimes with a charged particle) to the sample under study. By varying the choice of reagent gas, ionisation can be effected under a variety of conditions. Argon CI, for example, gives spectra much like EI spectra, with much fragmentation, while isobutane CI gives mainly molecular ions or t-butylated molecular ions. A modification of the CI technique which is promising for non-volatile compounds is chemical ionisation desorption (CID), in which the sample in the solid state is treated with ionised reagent gases. In some cases, CID seems to be competitive with FD.

Nuclear Magnetic Resonance

The major innovation in nuclear magnetic resonance (NMR) techniques in recent years has been the introduction of the Fourier transform (FT) method, in which all nuclei of a particular type are excited and allowed to undergo decay simultaneously, with the results being sorted out by computer (Farrar and Becker, 1971). FT increases the sensitivity of an NMR spectrometer enormously, so that either a much smaller sample or a much lower isotopic abundance is required for obtaining a spectrum. Specifically, FT has allowed the development of ^{13}C NMR spectroscopy into its present status as probably the most useful NMR tool for structural investigations (Stothers, 1972). By irradiation of all the protons in the molecule simultaneously, they are decoupled from the ^{13}C nuclei so that ^{13}C signals appear as single lines in an ordinary ^{13}C spectrum. Moreover, through the operation of the nuclear Overhauser effect, such broad band irradiation enhances most of the signals' intensity. Since individual carbon atoms appear over a range of 200 ppm (vs. 10 ppm for protons), it is unusual for two carbons to appear at exactly the same position. It is, in fact, often possible to determine the number of carbon atoms present by counting the signals. ^{13}C NMR spectra, for example, have proved exceedingly useful in studies of aminocyclitol antibiotics (Naito *et al.*, 1980), in which nearly all of the carbon atoms appear in a very narrow range. Off-resonance decoupling, which only partially decouples the protons, allows one to count the number of protons attached to each carbon by the pattern of the carbon (quartet for $-CH_3$, singlet for $-\overset{|}{\underset{|}{C}}-$, etc.). FT spectroscopy has also allowed the study of other nuclei present in low abundance, e.g., ^{15}N, although other nuclei have by no means achieved the prominence of utility of ^{13}C.

With respect to ^1H NMR spectroscopy, the major advance in recent years has involved the development of superconducting magnets operating at exceedingly high fields. Standard high field spectrometers now operate at 360 or 470 MHz (for protons) and spectrometers operating as high as 600 MHz have been constructed. The main virtue of a high field for antibiotics is that it serves to separate individual protons and give easily interpretable first-order spectra, as opposed to the more complex second-order spectra previously observed. Spreading the proton signals out at higher fields has the additional advantage of allowing more selective decoupling of individual protons from each other. Selective decoupling of individual protons, thus enhancing through the nuclear Overhauser effect only the signal of the carbon atom which is coupled to those particular protons, is also rendered easier.

Other Spectroscopic Tools

While the major spectroscopic weapons for investigating structures of new antibiotics are mass spectrometry and nuclear magnetic resonance, as discussed above, some structural parameters are still best investigated with the classical spectroscopic tools of infrared and ultraviolet spectroscopy, which can also be employed to confirm or refute individual structural features assigned; for example, conjugated polyenes through ultraviolet spectroscopy, carbonyl groups through infrared spectroscopy. Moreover, none of the other spectroscopic tools thus far noted can give any information about the absolute configuration of a compound (with the exception of X—ray crystallography). For assigning absolute configurations, the twin tools of circular dichroism and optical rotatory dispersion are invaluable (Crabbé, 1972). Circular dichroism, which depends upon the selective absorption of left or right circularly polarised light, provides more readily interpretable spectra, while optical rotatory dispersion, depending on the relative speeds of left and right circularly polarised light, gives spectra more readily recognisable for their relationship to ordinary optical rotation at a single wavelength. Such rotatory measurements can be used either to assign the absolute configuration of a chiral center in the vicinity of a chromophore or to assign the overall configuration of a molecule whose relative stereochemistry has been determined.

Chemical Methods

Most structures of antibiotics are now assigned almost exclusively by the physical methods described above. However, the intact antibiotic is often simply too large to be assigned from spectroscopic means alone. In those cases, it is necessary to degrade the molecule to one or more smaller or simpler molecules whose structures can then be assigned by spectroscopic means. Although synthetic organic chemistry has made enormous strides in recent decades, with specific emphasis laid on developing regiospecific and stereoselective reagents, little attention has been accorded to the development of similarly selective reagents for chemical degradations, probably because of the development of the spectroscopic tools noted. Thus, the classical methods of cleavage, hydrolysis and oxidation remain the methods of choice.

Prognosis

The techniques described above for determining structures of organic compounds are very powerful. They have reduced the time required for structure elucidation from years to months or from months to days. They have also reduced the sample requirement for structure determination by several orders of magnitude. Indeed, there is little doubt that any compound which can be obtained pure can have its structure determined if there is sufficient interest in the compound. One area for major future improvements can be expected to be in methods of purification, since the purification of a compound is often the rate-limiting step.

References

Beckey, H.D. (1977). "Principles of Field Ionisation and Field Desorption Mass Spectrometry". Pergamon Press, Oxford.

Crabbé, P. (1972). "ORD and CD in Chemistry and Biochemistry. An Introduction". Academic Press, New York.

Dawkins, B.G. and McLafferty, F.W. (1978). *In* "GLC and HPLC Determination of Therapeutic Agents". (K. Tsuji and W. Morozowich, eds). Part 1, pp. 259–275. Dekker, New York.

Farrar, T.C. and Becker, E.D. (1971). "Pulse and Fourier Transform NMR". Academic Press, New York.

MacFarlane, R.D. (1980). *In* "Biochemical Applications of Mass Spectrometry, Supplementary Volume". (G.R. Waller and O.C. Dermer, eds), pp. 1209–1218. Wiley-Interscience.

MacFarlane, R.D. and Torgerson, D.F. (1976). *Science* **191**, 920–925.

Mechlinski, W., Schaffner, C.P., Ganis, P. and Avitabile, G. (1970). *Tetrahedron Lett.*, 3873–3876.

Milberg, R.H. and Cook, J.C., Jr. (1978). *In* "GLC and HPLC Determination of Therapeutic Agents". (K. Tsuji and W. Morozowich, eds). Part 1, pp. 235–258. Dekker, New York.

Naito, T., Toda, S., Nakagawa, S. and Kawaguchi, H. (1980). *In* "Aminocyclitol Antibiotics". (K.L. Rinehart, Jr. and T. Suami, eds). ACS Symposium, Series 125. American Chemical Society, Washington, D.C.

Nakamura, H., Iitaka, H., Kitahara, T., Okazaki, T. and Okami, Y. (1977). *J. Antibiot.* **30**, 714–717.

Pandey, R.C., Kalita, C.C., Aszalos, A.A., Geoghegan, R., Jr., Garretson, A.L., Cook, J.C., Jr. and Rinehart, K.L., Jr. (1980). *Biomed. Mass Spectrom.* **7**, 93–98.

Rinehart, K.L., Jr. and Goo, Y.M. (1980). Manuscript in preparation.

Rinehart, K.L., Jr., Cook, J.C., Jr., Maurer, K.H. and Rapp, U. (1974). *J. Antibiot.* **27**, 1–13.

Stothers, J.B. (1972). "Carbon–13 NMR Spectroscopy". Academic Press, New York, N.Y.

Wagman, G.H. and Weinstein, M.J. (1978). "Chromatography of Antibiotics". J. Chromatogr. Library, Vol. 1. Elsevier, Amsterdam.

Waksman, S.A. and Lechevalier, H.A. (1962). *In* "The Actinomycetes. Vol. III. Antibiotics of Actinomycetes", pp. 141–412. Williams and Wilkins Co., Baltimore, MD.

Discussion

Professor Demain: What are the problems with these newer techniques, in terms of mixtures? As a microbiologist, I think of streptomycetes and fungi making many different compounds at the same time. Is that a real problem or not?

Professor Rinehart: I think it depends on whether we are simply trying to establish the molecular formulae or the structures. From that standpoint, field desorption is a beautiful technique, and the same is true of plasma desorption, in that they both give insight quickly into the fact that we are dealing with mixtures, also some idea about the sort of mixtures and the proportions of compounds that are present. Assigning structures, however, remains a problem. The individual components have to be separated, and worked on separately if they are new compounds.

Professor Demain: Is it possible to give some idea of the amount of compound that must be in the broth to be picked up by these techniques?

Professor Rinehart: Field desorption is successful on neomycin with 10 ng of material: that is a very small sample which is required. On the other hand, an attempt was made to do it directly on the broth, but the problem is that there are salts in the broth which tend to occlude the antibiotic.

Professor Sabath: Would Professor Rinehart comment further about mixtures? He has talked mainly about the identification, but I gather that in the industrial production the three gentamicins are very difficult to separate. I also understand that *Streptomyces aureofaciens* co-produces tetracycline as well as chlortetracycline. Which of these techniques would have picked up these mixtures early — perhaps they all would — and which of the analytical techniques are applicable to production systems?

Professor Rinehart: Field desorption mass spectrometry is an ideal technique for following those. The gentamicins are rather unusual as aminocyclitols. Mass spectra of gentamicins can be obtained by electron impact, and even that method would give the information at an early stage. Field desorption, however, would do it much more easily, and that technique would also give good information with regard to the tetracycline problem. If the broth is simply extracted with butanol — or whatever is used — and the emitter wire dipped into the butanol and put into the mass spectrometer, the answer is obtained within 30 minutes. It is very straightforward.

The Design of Antagonists of Natural Processes

F. LE GOFFIC

CNRS–CERCOA, Thiais, France

Introduction

Most of our useful chemotherapeutic agents are not the product of deliberate and rational design; the majority of them have been discovered by the systematic screening of series of molecules synthesised by organic chemistry or isolated from the growth medium of filamentous fungi and actinomycetes.

The rational design of new drugs able to interfere with fundamental biological processes may, however, represent a valuable approach which has not been sufficiently explored.

Let us consider a metabolite S and its biological receptor E. This molecule is able to recognise specifically its receptor site and gives rise to an $E_{III}S$ complex by a binding process which is usually reversible (see Fig. 1(a)).

If E is a receptor without catalytic activity, the biological response

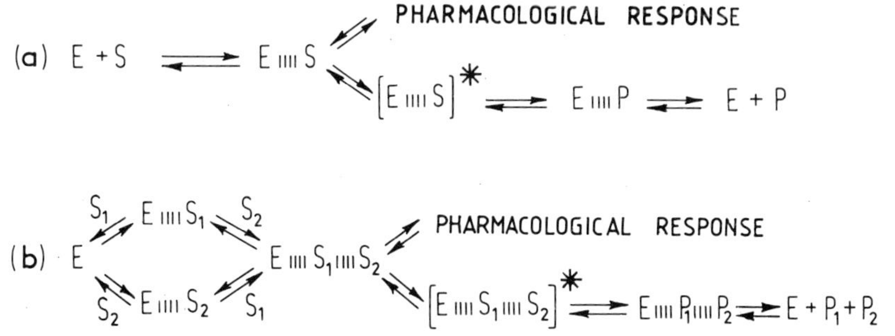

FIG. 1   Scheme of interaction between one receptor (E) and one (S) or two (S_1 and S_2) ligands.

will be elicited during this binding. If E is an enzyme, the EⅢS complex (also called the Michaelis complex) will move to a high energy complex [EⅢS]*, called the "transition state", which has a short half-life. This transition state will transform again into a new and more stable complex EⅢP which will eventually dissociate and release product P.

Another more complicated scheme of interaction may often occur, and is represented in Fig. 1(b). Here two ligands, S_1 and S_2, recognise (either successively or in a random manner) receptor E to give the Michaelis complex EⅢS$_1$ⅢS$_2$ which may elicit a biological response if E possesses no catalytic activity (such a case can be found with molecules acting synergically). But if E is an enzyme, a high energy intermediate [EⅢS$_1$ⅢS$_2$]*, also called a transition state, is obtained. It will also transform into a more stable complex, EⅢP$_1$ⅢP$_2$, to release finally the products P_1 and P_2.

Thus Fig. 1 represents a ligand–receptor interaction or, rather schematically, mono and bi-molecular enzymic reactions. It leads to the definition of three types of substance: K_S reagents, transition state analogues, and K_{cat} inhibitors or suicide substrates, which can interfere with these processes and disturb the overall function of a cell.

K_S Reagents

K_S inhibitors are molecules structurally related to S or P. From an enzymological viewpoint, these molecules are termed reversible inhibitors. They can give rise to reversible complexes close in structure to EⅢS, EⅢS$_1$ⅢS$_2$, EⅢP or EⅢP$_1$ⅢP$_2$.

The most familiar K_S reagents are undoubtedly those which have been designed to disturb tetrahydrofolic acid biosynthesis. Most bacteria are unable to use exogenous sources of folate and must synthesise the vitamin *de novo* from pteridine, p–aminobenzoic acid (p–ABA) and glutamic acid. This synthetic ability is lacking in mammals, including man, which need exogenous folic acid or a precursor of this cofactor derived from plant foods.

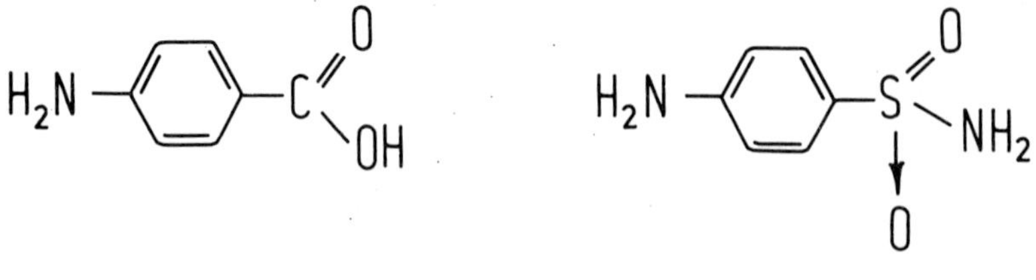

FIG. 2   Structures of (A) p–aminobenzoic acid (p–ABA) and (B) sulphanilamide.

The sulphonamide drugs possess electronic and steric properties very similar to those of p—ABA (see Fig. 2) and competitively inhibit dihydropteroate synthetase. Since dihydropteroate synthetase is absent from mammals, the sulphonamides can interfere with the development of bacteria without concomitant toxicity to the host. Thus sulphonamides are ideal drugs in the sense that they have as their target an enzyme specific to bacteria.

If one now considers the event which occurs after dihydrofolic acid biosynthesis and leads to tetrahydrofolic acid, the importance of dihydrofolic acid reductase is readily appreciated. This enzyme catalyses the reduction of dihydrofolic acid synthesised in bacteria, or supplied by the external medium or even released during thymidylic acid biosynthesis. In contrast to dihydrofolate synthetase, this enzyme is present in both procaryotic and eucaryotic cells. The function of this enzyme is thus extremely important and its inhibition should have dramatic effects on procaryotic as well as eucaryotic cells.

Several K_S inhibitor molecules have been synthesised. Three of them are particularly selective, trimethoprim (T), methotrexate (M) and pyrimethamine (P). (T) is selectively toxic for bacteria, (M) is an effective anticancer agent and (P) has powerful antimalarial properties.

The problem is then to understand this selective toxicity: is it a question of selective permeability, or of metabolism, or a difference of selectivity in enzyme recognition?

These various hypotheses have been tested. (T) recognises specifically bacterial dihydrofolate reductase, whereas (M) recognises dihydrofolate reductases from procaryotic as well as eucaryotic cells, and (P) is specific for *Plasmodium berghei* enzyme. This example shows that it is therefore possible today to design molecules able to recognise specifically a receptor providing that structural and functional data concerning the relevant receptor are available.

A consequence of that is that in the future the biochemical research field should be more and more implicated in the rational design of new drugs.

The majority of K_S inhibitors generally have weak biological activity, often because of their poor affinity for the receptor. However, this biological activity may be easily enhanced in some particular cases. When two metabolites S_1 and S_2 bind to a biological receptor (for example in the case of bimolecular reactions), it is sometimes possible to combine them with a covalent bond or to combine two K_S inhibitors of S_1 and S_2 or one of the inhibitors of this reaction with one of the substrates.

This type of approach appears to be of considerable interest because of a large potential increase in the affinity of these inhibitor molecules for their receptor site. This concept can be illustrated by the following example: the aminoglycoside antibiotics are inactivated by different enzymatic processes in strains resistant to these drugs. The N–acetylation of these molecules is of great importance. This reaction occurs by the transfer of an acetyl residue from acetyl coenzyme A to the aminoglycoside antibiotic. Thus it follows that the design of powerful inhibitors of aminoglycoside acetyltransferases should be a useful means of protecting these antibiotics from inactivation. Northrop bound gentamicin covalently to acetyl coenzyme A and obtained a "bisubstrate complex" with high inhibitory potency ($Ki = 10^{-12} M$). Unfortunately, this substance does not show its inhibitory properties *in vivo* because it cannot penetrate the bacterial cell to a sufficiently high concentration.

Transition State Analogues

During an enzymic reaction a number of intermediates are produced before the substrate(s) is (are) converted into product(s). The complex possessing the highest energy (the most transient one) is called the "transition state complex".

It is obvious that, at the level of the transition state, the enzyme and the substrate have structures quite different from those of the substrate and the native enzyme; furthermore, the transition state theory leads to the conclusion that catalysis can only occur if the enzyme-ligand interaction is much stronger than in the fundamental state (Michaelis complex).

The conclusion to be drawn from this theory is very important, for if it is possible to tailor stable structures similar to those involved in the transition state, these structures will bind tightly to the enzyme and consequently possess powerful inhibitory effects. From this concept arise two important consequences relevant to the design of new drugs. Since there is a correlation between the affinity of a drug for its receptor and its therapeutic effect, it can be expected that at equal concentrations $(K_S)^*$ inhibitors will be much more effective than K_S analogues. $(K_S)^*$ inhibitors will be much more specific than K_S inhibitors. Consider an important metabolite S which can give rise enzymatically to four products P_1, P_2, P_3 and P_4. In these enzymic reactions will appear four transitory states $[E_1 \text{iiii} S_1]^*$, $[E_2 \text{iiii} S_2]^*$, $[E_3 \text{iiii} S_3]^*$, $[E_4 \text{iiii} S_4]^*$ (Fig. 3), in which S will assume transiently four structural states $[S_1]^*$, $[S_2]^*$, $[S_3]^*$, $[S_4]^*$. A structural analogue A of S may not be able to discriminate between the four enzymes E_1, E_2, E_3, E_4; and thus, in addition to

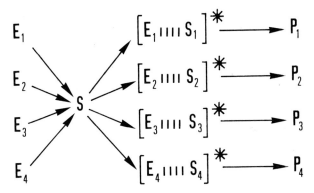

FIG. 3   Scheme of interaction between one metabolite (S) and four enzymes (E_1, E_2, E_3, E_4).

the desired primary effect (due for instance to inhibition of E_1), side effects due to the binding of A to E_2, E_3, E_4 may occur. The situation will be quite different with a molecule T_1 related in structure to $[S_1]^*$. This molecule will be able to recognise only E_1, and thus all side effects will be eliminated.

Such a concept has already been made use of, and has led to the design of interesting molecules like N—(phosphonoacetyl)—L—aspartic acid (PALA) and 9—β—D—ribofuranosyl—6—hydroxy-methyl—1,6—dihydropurine.

Aspartate transcarbamylase (ATCase) catalyses the condensation of aspartic acid with carbamoyl phosphate to give carbamoyl aspartate (Fig. 4, structure 4). The structures of the substrates and of the products strongly suggest that an intermediate of structure 3 can be transiently formed during this process. PALA (Fig. 4, structure 5) was synthesised to imitate this transition state. Its affinity for ATCase was measured and shown to be considerably higher than that of either substrate. It was also shown to have promising antineoplasic potential.

1—β—D—arabinosyl adenine (ARA—A) is a powerful antiherpetic agent. It is, however, inactivated by a specific deaminase, according to the scheme shown in Fig. 5. The rate-determining step in this inactivation is the addition of water to ARA—A. This gives a high energy transient intermediate which then stabilises by elimination of ammonia. By developing a stable molecule closely resembling this intermediate structurally, it should be possible to obtain a good inhibitor of adenosine deaminase. This led to the synthesis of two isomers of 9—β—D—ribofuranosyl—6—hydroxymethyl—1,6—dihydropurine. One of them was a powerful inhibitor of the enzyme, whereas the other isomer had no effect at all.

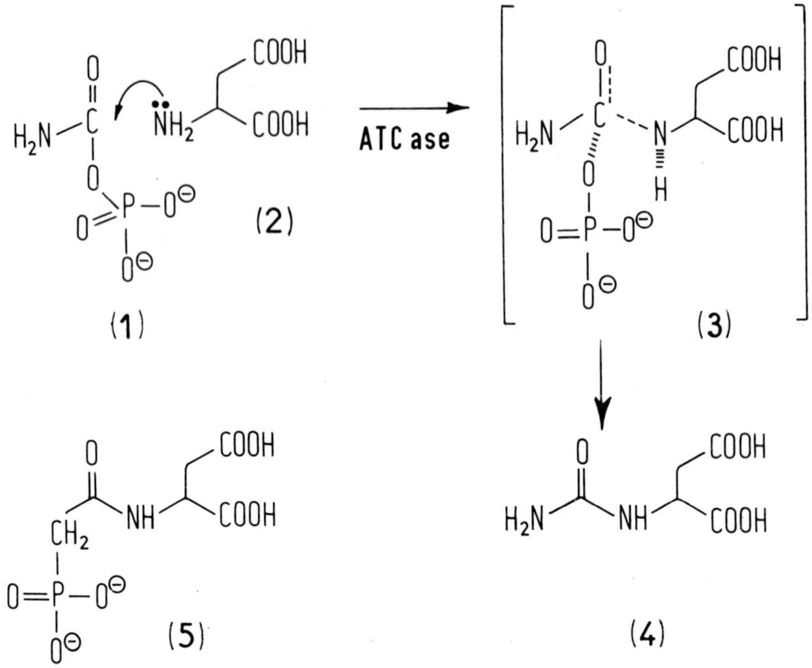

FIG. 4   Biosynthesis of carbamoyl aspartate (4) by condensation of carbamoyl phosphate (1) with aspartic acid (2), in presence of aspartate transcarbamylase (ATCase). PALA (5), an analogue of the transition state (3), is an inhibitor.

It should also be noticed that nature itself has tailored such transition state analogues. Coformycin (Fig. 5) is a powerful inhibitor of adenosine deaminase, for instance.

K_{cat} Inhibitors or Suicide Substrates

The irreversible and specific inactivation of enzymes has been used for a long time (in affinity labelling) to obtain information about their active sites. The molecules used in such experiments cannot be employed as drugs either because of their intrinsic reactivity or because they require prior activation, for instance, by UV light.

There remains a third possibility for the design of effective molecules which can be used as exploratory reagents as well as effective drugs. Figure 6 summarises the way how such molecules can operate: a K_{cat} reagent S' must be an enzyme pseudo-substrate which gives rise to a reactive molecule P'. As a consequence, if the diffusion rate of P' is low as compared to its chemical reactivity, it can react with some nearby amino acid residue on the enzyme and therefore

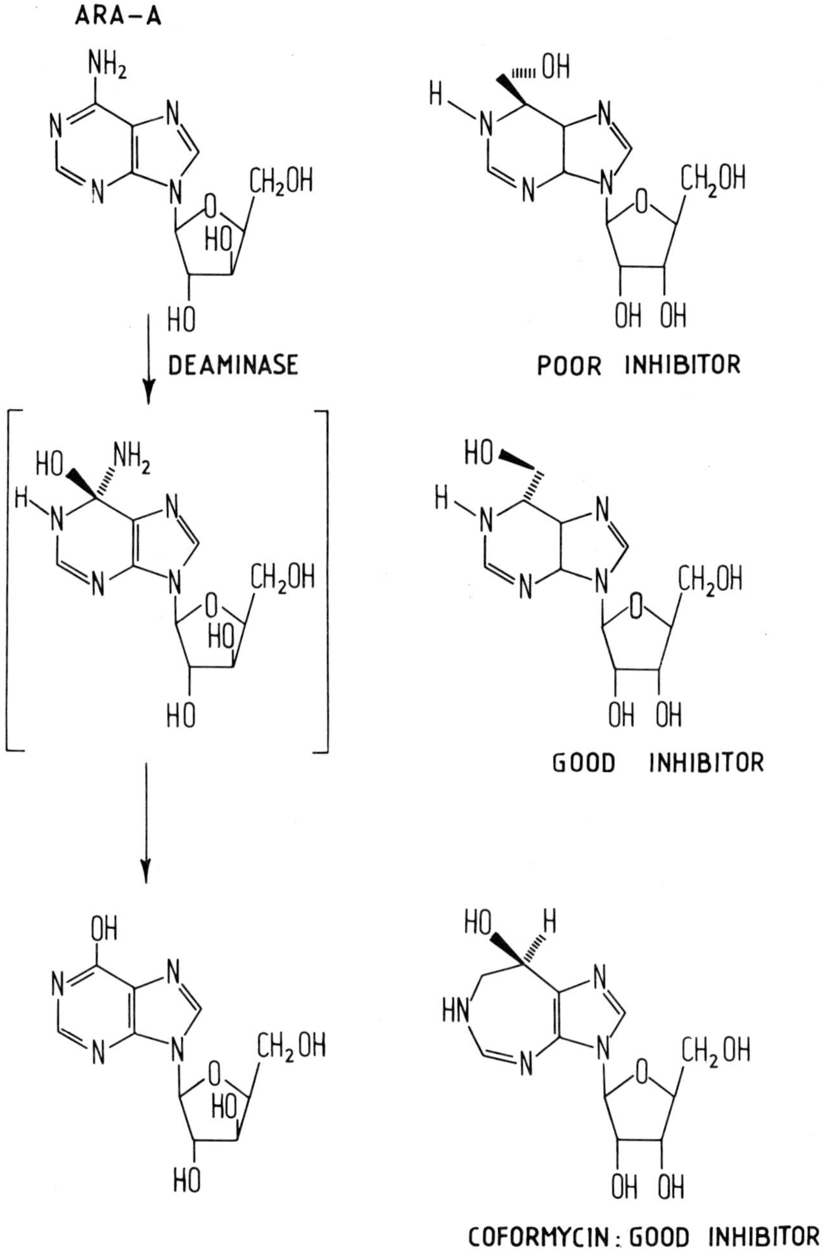

FIG. 5   Enzymic deamination of 1–β–D–arabinosyl adenine (ARA–A). Structures of synthetic and natural inhibitors of adenosine deaminase.

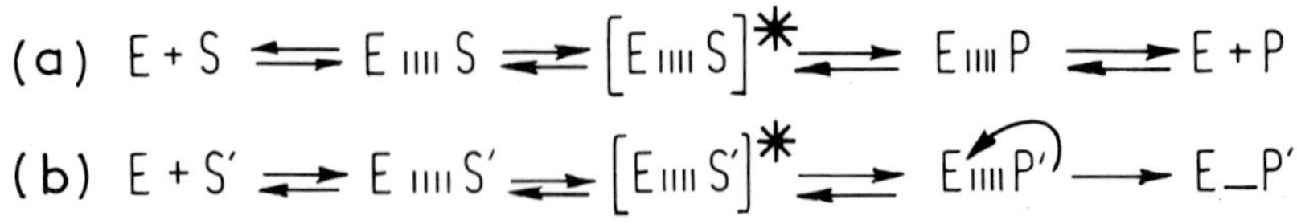

(a) $E + S \rightleftharpoons E_{\text{\tiny III}} S \rightleftharpoons [E_{\text{\tiny III}} S]^{*} \rightleftharpoons E_{\text{\tiny III}} P \rightleftharpoons E + P$

(b) $E + S' \rightleftharpoons E_{\text{\tiny III}} S' \rightleftharpoons [E_{\text{\tiny III}} S']^{*} \rightleftharpoons E_{\text{\tiny III}} \overset{\frown}{P'} \longrightarrow E\_P'$

FIG. 6   Scheme of interaction between an enzyme receptor E and (a) a normal substrate S, or (b) a suicide substrate S'.

inactivate the enzyme irreversibly, giving successively one $E_{\text{\tiny III}}\overset{\frown}{P'}$ and one E–P' complex.

Drugs of this class were already known before they were recognised to be suicide substrates: examples are pargylin and cycloserine. Other molecules of this class have been isolated from nature or have been synthesised. Some of them are under clinical trial now and will probably become valuable drugs.

Clavulanic acid (Fig. 7) belongs to this class. It inactivates irreversibly the β–lactamases which are responsible for the hydrolysis

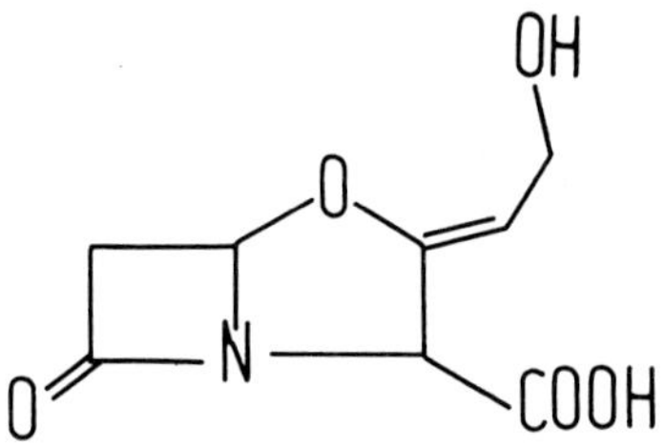

FIG. 7   Structure of a suicide substrate, clavulanic acid.

of penicillins in bacteria. The association of clavulanic acid and penicillin is in fact an efficient combination to treat infections due to bacteria resistant to penicillin.

Conclusion

It is clear today that the new concepts presented here should greatly help the laboratories involved in the development of new therapeutic agents. However, this type of approach requires a better knowledge of the biological receptors to be antagonised.

Discussion

Dr. Courvalin: Concerning transition state analogues, how can you say that $[S_1]^*$ structure is very different from $[S_2]^*$ and $[S_3]^*$ etc.?

Professor Le Goffic: It is obvious, otherwise you would get the same product at the end. In other words, it is the transition state that determines which kind of product you get at the end of the enzymatic reaction.

Dr. Bost: In the case of cycloserine, do we know whether toxicity is associated with a mechanism identical to that responsible for its activity?

Professor Le Goffic: No, we do not know. In fact, I am not even sure that the inactivation mechanisms I have presented have actually been proven experimentally.

Part 4
General Discussions

Part 1

M.H. RICHMOND

It seems from talking to people in the pharmaceutical industry that at the moment one detects, as far as antibacterial agents are concerned, that matters are reaching a crisis point. We know that over the last few years a number of different companies with big stakes in the field of antimicrobial chemotherapy have had agonising reappraisals of whether to remain in this field. Certain very big operators decided some years ago that the prospects from the commercial point of view were so difficult that they would drop out.

It seems to me that crisis is coming from two factors. First, some points which have been touched on at this meeting only briefly. One is the cost of the agents, which is inevitably increasing as they become more sophisticated. Professor Milhaud talked at some length about the impact of legislation, which brings in its train additional costs. Very strong economic forces are also at work — the increased price of oil, which means that the price of products also increases. Of course, there is more and more the insertion of politics into this field, which came to the surface in the course of some of the comments made by Dr. Braude. To take one example, certain antibiotics are not available in some countries, such as India, because of government decisions that, if they are introduced, they can be sold only at a certain price — and that price is below the world price. Therefore people tend not to introduce such compounds into that country. Thus, certain, perhaps rather arbitrary, political decisions come in here, and everything adds up to the fact that profit margins are being squeezed extremely tightly.

The second factor in the crisis, which relates much more to what we heard in the first part of this Round Table, and which was highlighted by Professor Williams and Professor Kunin, as well as others, is the question whether we actually need any more antibacterial antibiotics. This question is often raised these days. To try to summarise the contributions here, the feeling seems to be that, if we use the antibiotics which we have at the moment in the right way, it can be argued that no more agents are needed against bacterial infections. I think it is a real point which we must face up to. As Professor Sabath outlined, there may be some areas of need, in relation to *Pseudomonas*, and some small areas in relation to certain oral antibiotics; there may be possibilities for growth promoters in farm animals, as came out in the contribution from Professor Ruckebusch. However, in general, many people would argue, including Professor Acar, that the doctor at the moment has the necessary antibacterials at his disposal. Where perhaps he does need greater help, and perhaps more time, is to ensure that the right agent is used in the right way.

What about the question of resistance? We had papers from Professor Humbert, Professor Duval and Professor Frottier, which documented for us the fact that there are very many resistant micro-organisms. This fact being generally accepted across the world, two things can also be said.

First, in many cases the incidence of resistance in a particular species has probably not increased enormously over the years. *Staphylococcus aureus*, for example, reached a situation in hospitals within 10 years of the introduction of benzylpenicillin where 70% of the strains were resistant because they made penicillinase, and the situation remains much the same today. The invention of methicillin, cloxacillin, dicloxacillin, oxacillin and other compounds has allowed us to treat those infections with some success.

Secondly, the importance of resistance matters much less to the clinician, bearing in mind the armamentarium of antibiotics that he has at the moment. I would argue that the question of resistance has been greatly highlighted by those who wish to find some new "cachet" to give to their new compound and claim that it is "active against resistant strains". Outside the hospitals, resistance is certainly found, but probably it is not of enormous clinical impact.

The idea that I would put to this meeting is that the time has perhaps come for people in the pharmaceutical industry who are interested in designing anti-infectives to think again, to change their point of attack and not to look for more aminoglycosides or for more derivatives of that kind. If they are to look for anything of the old-fashioned type, I think that the future must lie with the $\beta-$ lactams, if only because of their great effectiveness and, in general, their lack of toxic side effects. Particularly, if the rumours of very effective oral cephalosporin materialise, we may soon have an armamentarium of nitroimidazoles, trimethoprim plus sulphonamides and a good range of β—lactams which will meet the needs of a very great number of cases.

Over the years, since antibiotics were first introduced, there has been an enormous emphasis on trying to sophisticate agents which will kill bacteria. Certainly, people who have tried to sterilise bacterial cultures with penicillin will know that this is impossible. It is too often overlooked that people who are treated with antibiotics basically cure themselves; in other words, the antibiotics give the defences of the host the time and opportunity to respond and to effect the cure.

If we are to think of the future, the area for investigation should be the interaction of the organisms and the host, paying more attention to the host side. To trespass briefly on to Professor Davies' subject, the impact of antibiotics, or other molecules, on immunomodulation is one of the fields in which a great deal has to be learnt, and where many of the techniques and approaches that have been so fruitful in designing and finding new antibacterial agents may be turned to some considerable profit. Similarly, Professor Chabanon's approach to the question of adherence, which is a particular example of the investigation of the interaction of microorganisms and the host, is another area which might well produce compounds with potential therapeutic value. They may not necessarily kill bacteria, but they may have some considerable therapeutic value, even conceivably prophylactic value.

If we are to succeed in this new area and to try to find agents which are active in these new respects (the interaction of microorganisms and the host, or the stimulation of the host), then the old-fashioned methods of screening and of evaluation of antibiotics, have to go out of the window. We have to start assessing compounds in a totally new and different way.

As I said at the beginning, I feel that pharmaceutical companies are in a very crucial phase at the moment. Things are changing fundamentally, in relation to the treatment of infection. At least, as far as innovation is concerned, there are extremely big challenges to microbiologists, doctors, biochemists and to everyone who would be involved in the programme and these challenges have to be taken up.

Discussion

Professor Kunin: I agree with Professor Richmond's remarks, but I want to add that physicians do not always use antibiotics rationally. For that reason, I suspect that there is plenty of marketing room. We should do a better job with the present drugs and we probably do not need very many more. If they were used properly, the resistance problem would not be a major one. However, I doubt that, given the complexity of medical practice, this will be achieved readily. Therefore, there are many opportunities for preparing drugs that will meet some of these needs. They will not solve any major problems, in terms of saving any more lives, but there will certainly be a market for such agents.

Professor Richmond: So Professor Kunin sees that there are some commercial opportunities, even if those opportunities may be rather superficial from the point of view of an objective scientist or doctor.

Professor Kunin: Yes. I can give many examples of this. For example, there is almost no need for cephalexin, an oral cephalosporin and yet, it has made a major impact on the market. New oral cephalosporins, although they are probably not needed, will definitely do well in the market. For example, there will be some new oral cephalosporins that have activity against *Haemophilus influenzae* and the pneumococci and they will certainly capture a large part of the market for treatment of chronic bronchitis which is a very common problem in office practice. The only element which will prevent this will be whether the insurance schemes in various countries will permit its use. Perhaps it will not be permitted in Britain, but it will certainly do extremely well in the United States – even though it is not absolutely needed.

Secondly, if promotion of drugs is studied, companies have been remarkably adaptable to the circumstances. There is an enormous number of cephalosporins, all of which are highly effective. They have decided to develop a strategy, not of stressing sales but rather of stressing costs to the buyer. A good example would be the tactics used by Bristol Laboratories, since there has been almost no advertising of its cephalosporin. Instead, it is simply priced 10% below that of the nearest competitors. In that way a large part of the market has been seized. The truth is that there will be plenty of marketing opportunities for the competitive individual who can see where something can be insinuated in this complex market.

Professor Richmond: There is no doubt that the impact of governments in this business is an important factor – perhaps not in the United States, but certainly in Europe. From Professor Trouet, we hear that the Belgian Government has limited the use of certain antibiotics. Sometimes reasons are laudable, but sometimes, they are simply emotional.

Professor Davies: With respect to the question of oral cephalosporins, they could be both a tremendous benefit and a real danger. Once there is an oral antibiotic that is a broad-spectrum compound and which is very effective, it moves out of the hospital. It is a real danger, at least in prospect, that the oral cephalosporin would then be used by the general physician. I wonder whether that would lead to tremendous problems of resistance. The problems of resistance are not as bad as they have been made out to be in general, but they are certainly very bad in specific instances. Are we likely to kill the goose that is laying the golden eggs, when an antibiotic like a cephalosporin which most physicians might want to use is made generally available?

Professor Kunin: That is already done: the cephalexin sales are enormous. Another example is oral carbenicillin. When this agent was introduced on the market this was thought to be of great advantage for the hospitalised patient with severe *Pseudomonas* sepsis. However, the oral form which is available to all practitioners is widely used for urinary tract infections, although much less expensive and even more effective drugs are available. This is not good with respect to *Pseudomonas* infections in hospital.

Professor Sabath: In my opinion, the future belongs to the β–lactams, because of the lack of toxicity, the low cost of monitoring proper levels and the limited dependence to *in vivo* conditions, principally pH, protein binding and hypoxia.

A totally new concept is needed of antimicrobial agents that by themselves will cure the patient without involving his specific defence, for instance, patient with agranulocytosis, usually secondary to treatment for neoplastic disease, but occasionally due to aplastic anaemia of other sources. It is a fact that, until now for all practical purposes, cultures are not really sterilised but, *a priori*, somebody could today produce a new class of agents able to do that. That is a totally new world for which a need does exist, and very strikingly so in large medical centres.

Professor Kunin: I would not discount the developments of the aminoglycosides. Essentially, the limitations of aminoglycosides are those pointed out by Professor Sabath, but the dominant one is toxicity. There was a structure shown here earlier with three amino groups.

At least from work in our laboratory, there is a reasonable association between toxicity of the drugs and the number of free amino groups that are present on the molecule. That is a generalisation and, even though not exact, it may be helpful. A structure with three amino groups with relatively low toxicity seems very exciting. Also, perhaps some of the binding to mammalian tissue may be influenced by those amino groups. The aminoglycosides remain promising, perhaps with the discovery of an oral aminoglycoside ester-type compound. With respect to the different organisms that may be involved in severe Gram-negative sepsis the aminoglycosides remain the first choice. Research for a less toxic derivative should continue.

Professor Richmond: What seems to be good about the aminoglycosides, from the *in vitro* point of view, is their very hard knockdown effect. The new cephalosporins perhaps tend to be slightly softer in their action. We will have to demonstrate whether this has clinical implications. What is always so impressive, as Professor Sabath said, is the value of the therapeutic index (toxicity over m.i.c.); for β–lactams it could be one million, and for conventional aminoglycosides 12 to 20. Even if this increased to 200, it is still far short of one million. Apart from their immunological side effects, which is perhaps a problem, the β–lactams are so extremely safe.

Professor Sande: In this conference on the future of antimicrobial therapy, it is slightly surprising that there was no presentation on the therapy of infection in the impaired host. Certainly our oncologist colleagues will get better at treating patients with antitumoural and toxic drugs for longer periods of time, and therefore the challenge will be to keep alive the patients with recurrent infections by giving them bactericidal drugs for longer periods of time.

Today polypharmacy is applied to patients who are impaired hosts and who have sepsis, but with dreadful problems of toxicity. All these patients are in renal failure. All of them are given aminoglycosides, and many of them go deaf or become ataxic. That is the single most important area in the future.

It is correct to say that penicillin, or a drug that is bacteriostatic to the pneumococcus, is probably all right to treat 99% of the infections in the non-impaired host. The challenge remains in the impaired host.

Professor Richmond: It is a very clear statement, often underestimated by non clinicians, that for people with very impaired defences, there is a need for drugs with rapid knockdown.

May we turn again to the question of resistance with a comment from Professor Acar?

Professor Acar: Apparently, many of us are interested in products more active, less toxic, given more easily and over a larger period of time to impaired patients much more than by products, as marketed for a while, which are active against classes of resistant bacteria and have a large antimicrobial spectrum. Undoubtedly, products could have a restricted spectrum, like cephalosporins active against *Pseudomonas* and virtually inactive against other species. Today, the appearance of resistant strains is not a serious argument to ground research for new products.

Now, regarding β–lactamases, there are at the present time not so many indications in epidemiology on the time frequency of β–lactamases producing strains and on the role of such enzymes in resistance phenomena. It has been said that in hospital 10% of enterobacteria produce β–lactamases. In these organisms, β–lactamases are not responsible for all the resistance phenomena. So, new leads of research are necessary.

Professor Richmond: Staphylococcus and perhaps gonococcus are species where inactivating enzymes are clearly involved. The cases are perhaps less than might be assumed from the literature.

Professor Demain: One of the points of the discussion is that the future of aminoglycosides, if indeed there is a future for new compounds, would deal with toxicity. Those of us who are not involved in the clinical application of these compounds need advice about simplified or rapid methods of estimating toxicity such as ototoxicity and nephrotoxicity. It is very difficult and very expensive for the people who are trying to produce new drugs to determine the extents of these toxicities. It costs millions of dollars, and many kilograms of material have to be made, before those tests can be performed. Is any work going on in the area of toxicology concerning new and improved methods to determine early how toxic a compound is?

Professor Richmond: Several people suggested that an area that would be sufficiently non-controversial and sufficiently important to be worth a joint approach might be the development of reliable laboratory methods for trying to assess toxicity problems. Unquestionably, the major cost of developing any agent at the moment is the toxicity testing. This has a very real knock-on consequence, as far as the patient is concerned, because it has a major impact on the price that the person has to pay. I am sure that if the toxicity testing could be reduced very significantly, a large number of conditions would become accessible to the design of agents which are ruled out at present because of the cost.

It is an area in which industry might be prepared to get together because it would be very much everyone's advantage to do so. In the United Kingdom there occasionally arises the question of whether there are any research areas in which pharmaceutical companies could cooperate in doing joint research. One that came up some time ago, and which has been pursued, is the question of Ames testing, or broadly speaking, laboratory methods for assessing potential carcinogenicity and mutagenicity.

Professor Kunin: Many people will be familiar with some of techniques now used to measure toxicity of the aminoglycosides. One of the most widely used, unfortunately not helpful at the present time, is enzymuria. The reason why enzymuria, i.e. the appearance of large numbers of various kinds of enzymes from the renal tubules, is not a good toxic screen at the moment is that as soon as a few injections of an aminoglycoside are given to someone, enzymuria will appear. It is so sensitive a test that all its appearance means is that there is some irritation present, not disease. It is not until there are multiple doses of an aminoglycoside over a prolonged period of time that clinically important renal toxicity is actually seen.

On the other hand, if there was a new compound which did not elicit enzymuria, or required a high dose to do so, this would be an exciting opportunity to observe that it was quite different from all the other compounds.

There are many very sophisticated renal function tests that relate to glomerular filtration rate, tubular secretion of organic ions, acidification mechanisms and so on, which are affected long before loss of potassium in the urine, long before there is clinical renal disease that may be observed. The best animal in which to test nephrotoxicity is man because of the heterogeneity of the toxic sensitivity in various experimental animals. A battery of renal function tests which are a prelude to eventual clinical renal dysfunction is highly desirable. That is the way in which these compounds should be screened.

Professor Trouet: The best animal in which to test the toxicity of drugs is the cell. For drugs such as the aminoglycosides it is easier with cells to try to find some correlation between their distribution and their activity, for example, on lysosomal enzymes or other enzymes. All that is required are cultures of cells and some biochemistry.

Professor Richmond: Professor Sebald gave a very interesting paper, on anaerobes, and particularly on β–lactamases and penicillin resistance in anaerobes. Can the people say whether anaerobic infections are important, or whether they are increased out of their proportion by the sort of pressures about which we talked earlier?

Professor Sabath: The importance of anaerobic infections depends from what point of view they are considered. Sometimes they may be over-emphasised, with that well-known problem of the presence of colonisation or isolation versus a role in disease. On the other hand in spite of the attention that they have received, they may be grossly under-emphasised, and many patients have very serious illnesses in which the responsible people are not aware that anaerobes are playing a major role.

Professor Kunin: I think the subject of the reservoir of anaerobes and when they are important deserves further discussion. Anaerobes are not a mystery, nor is Gram-negative sepsis a mystery. Anaerobes will grow in areas where tissue is dead, also only in certain selected parts of the body: the abdomen, the pelvis and occasionally in the upper respiratory tract.

Anaerobic sepsis, in fact, can be devided into abdominal, pelvic, chronic pulmonary and necrotic site infections. In most cases, the pelvic and the abdominal problems are surgical problems, requiring the best treatment against anaerobic infections — which is the knife. We have to remember that oxygen is the best antibiotic of all for anaerobic infections.

An anaerobic infection, however, does not necessarily mean a specific anaerobic drug should be given. For example, in bronchopulmonary infections, despite everything we have learnt about anaerobes, all the evidence indicates that penicillin G is still as effective as any other specific antianaerobic agent that is available. Therefore, a large proportion of anaerobic infections are still curable by our oldest agent. These points need to be stressed.

Professor Richmond: Perhaps, finally, we might address briefly this question of veterinary use of antibiotics. Professor Davies urged the development of specific antibacterials in that field.

Dr. Braude: May I bring back the discussion to the animal. First, from the pharmaceutical companies' point of view, there is an enormous market here for them to exploit. Practically, we are still using antibiotics on "healthy" animals, which means that the population benefiting from the use of these drugs is the total population. Therefore, the field is enormous and there is room for competition. What is important is cost and effectiveness. That is one major difference between the veterinary and human fields.

The second major difference is that we are generalising on the use of antibiotics as feed additives to such an extent because their mode of action is still not known. That opens the door for new products, and provided they are effective in terms of growth performance and feed conversion rather than of activity one does not worry about their effect on specific microorganisms. Until we understand the mode of action, this attitude will remain.

Professor Richmond: It is right, that in the veterinary field there are considerable possibilities, perhaps not only in relation to antibacterials but to a slight wider range of compounds. The cost effectiveness is of absolutely paramount importance, and it is here that we really come up against legislation which makes the cost of introducing the agents so high, whereas users are only prepared to pay a low price for them.

Part 2

J. DAVIES

In trying to think through what was said during the second part of this Round-Table Conference I have come up with a number of questions which I will pose in an effort to be as provocative as Professor Richmond was, and also to make some (probably) naïve statements.

The first question is: who should decide what drugs we want? It seems at the moment that it is the pharmaceutical companies who decide what drugs we want. I wonder whether physicians should not have a great deal more to say what drugs are needed, and also veterinarians. I am rather disturbed by the present rather militaristic approach to chemotherapy. It seems that if a group of drugs are being used, when things start to go slightly wrong with respect to resistance the "big guns" are brought in, and when things start to go wrong again another group of "big guns" is brought in. Therefore, a decision has to be taken about who chooses what kinds of drugs are needed in the first place.

Perhaps it is time for us to be slightly more selective and retrospective about the way in which drugs are used. Today there are drugs for other uses that are not being developed properly, for instance, for all agricultural purposes, not only for animals, but plants too. There is an enormous market in antibiotics involved in all aspects of human life on earth.

Secondly, how do we screen for new compounds and activities? Having once told the pharmaceutical industry the kind of compounds we want, how can they be screened for? I am a "mode of action person" myself but, even though the study of the mode of action of drugs is very exciting, I find it extremely difficult to believe that mode of action studies *per se* will be very helpful in the search for new compounds.

Of course, it is possible to screen for drugs by using mode of action studies. Professor Tomasz showed some interesting approaches to this, and Professor Vazquez talked about some applications to protein synthesis inhibitors. The problem we always have to face, however, is that unless we are working with the whole organism there will always be the problem of permeability. Everybody knows there are antibiotics that are effective against a particular macromolecular process in cell-free extracts, but which are absolutely useless against the whole organism. Neomycin and kanamycin, for example, inhibit protein synthesis in extracts of *Pseudomonas*, but they are not effective against *Pseudomonas* (probably) because they do not penetrate the organism.

There are also problems with regard to the use of more sophisticated methods for looking for drugs. Referring to Professor Ōmura's presentation in particular, what many pharmaceutical companies are doing very well is to try to have their screen provide antibiotics that might affect protein synthesis, cell wall biosynthesis or something similar, and then to select and use the required organism. But we will have to be extremely intelligent and very careful about the mode of action studies; perhaps the pharmaceutical industry has not given sufficient thought to the subject.

But in the meantime are we not becoming too sophisticated in our screening for new compounds? We are trying to use all sorts of fancy methods when, in reality, what is wanted is a compound that will be active in curing disease. Although pharmacokinetics and studies of drug binding in animal cells, animal models and so on may seem to be very sophisticated, they can give us some very important answers with respect to how drugs are really working. Everybody knows that there are marvellous compounds which will inhibit bacteria in a test-tube, but which will do absolutely nothing in a whole animal. More studies are required on why things do not work when they should work. Although these approaches may be difficult, they can provide much basic information required for the development of chemotherapeutic agents.

With regard to the problem of resistance, this is one which will be with us for a long time although it may not be an enormous problem. The problem of resistance is most crucial with respect to the spectrum of antibiotic effectiveness: why are antibiotics effective against some organisms and not against others? We must ask why do some antibiotics fail to get into *Chlamydia, Pseudomonas* and so on?

From this point of view, we must think a great deal more about the kind of experiments discussed by Professor Braun and Professor Gilvarg. Many bacteria are known which seem incapable of taking up our favourite drugs, so why not change those drugs in such a way that they can get into some of these bacteria? We must begin to investigate the specificity of uptake in some of the organisms which are presently the problem organisms; we must be able to find out how to get antibiotics into them.

With respect to the animal models, and the work described by Professor Trouet, one area which has been mentioned already as having been ignored over the years is toxicity. We do not have good means of studying toxicity that can be accepted by everybody. When Schering Co. compares tobramycin and gentamicin, its model shows that gentamicin is less toxic than tobramycin, but when E. Lilly Co. makes the same comparison its model says that tobramycin is less toxic than gentamicin! One chooses the model to suit oneself. Simple models are needed for the testing of toxicity which are not directed towards a self-interest; they must be non subjective. For this reason, perhaps we have to think about having non-interest groups of scientists to develop and do this kind of research.

With respect to the militaristic approach to chemotherapy, the point has been made at this meeting, that much better use should be made of the agents that we have now. Instead of trying to make ever bigger bombs to throw at smaller organisms, why not start looking at the compounds that are available now, using them better, perhaps changing them? If we know that particular antibiotics have deficiencies, and if we are aware of what those deficiencies are, and if something is understood about the basic biochemistry and cell physiology involved, perhaps some of the compounds that we now have could be made better by chemical modification? Let us use our knowledge of cell biology and of biochemistry and try to apply this, asking the organic chemists to give us something that might be what we want.

Do we need so many broad-spectrum antibiotics? If narrow-spectrum antibiotics are used properly, many diseases can be cured. This leads into the question of backing up our medical therapy with much better microbiology. If we are to be faced increasingly with the problem of organisms which have to be hit specifically, we must be able to recognise these organisms. There is a tremendous future for rapid microbiological detection. It is something which is going on now, but it has to be improved substantially.

The pharmaceutical industry has actually done a marvellous job in providing us with very many good compounds, but there are many things that it has not done because it is not interested in doing them. The pharmaceutical industry is interested in producing a compound that could be effective for one purpose or another. The work that the industry does is expensive in both time and money and I wonder whether there needs to be much greater collaboration between universities and industry. There is not a good relationship at the moment, and I think that industry should do much more in the universities. A lot of things could be done inexpensively and quickly: cell biology, and much of the basic biology could be learned through the medium of supporting graduate students.

I can give many examples of this. For instance, mutasynthesis was developed very quickly in a university. Useful or, at least, improved compounds came out of this study after about one year's work. I doubt whether industry would have done that same kind of work in a year. It really worries me that industry is so slow, and seems to take such a long time to get anything done. If industry wants faster results, perhaps it should invest in universities; if it invested in a graduate student at a university, it would often be possible to learn a great deal of useful basic biology very rapidly.

In addition to asking for collaboration between physicians and the pharmaceutical industry, and between biochemists and cell biologists, it is time that we looked back a little on some basic biology. The best way to learn the basic biology of a system is in a university. Suppose we asked someone in a university department to try to work on screening methods for measuring the toxic effects of aminoglycosides, that might provide a way of developing reasonable methods which would not favour one drug over another. There is a lot of merit to this suggestion. If industry suddenly decided that the way to go forward on a particular project was in genetic engineering, and wanted a cloning vector, the fastest way to get it would be to ask a university to make it. A postdoctoral fellow would come up with it in a year; I doubt whether industry would do it so well. The cloning vector could then be available to all in the field.

Of course industry has a self-interest like each of us. Both things could be done slightly differently, and then, everyone can be well served.

I believe that one of the problems with antimicrobial drugs at the moment is that much background biochemical information is lacking. The detailed mode of action of no antibiotic is known in chemical terms. I am not sure whether the knowledge would help, but we would certainly like to know something about the mode of action as it applies to animals, to toxicity, to absorption and similar aspects. It has to be decided who would be the best people to provide this information.

To summarise: a few questions have been raised about who decides what drugs should be made, how to look for them, how to determine whether they are toxic or active and so on, and how to support various aspects of the work that will lead to the development of these new drugs.

Discussion

Professor Kunin: Professor Davies stressed throughout his presentation the importance of permeability, that is, getting the drug into the microorganism. Does he know of any examples of success in that regard, or where there is even a potential for enhancing permeability and, if so, what would be the next step?

Professor Davies: The peptide transport system is one where there has been success in getting otherwise impermeable compounds into an organism, although not to the extent of finding a chemotherapeutic agent. But the fact remains that the biological basis is now established, and we should perhaps try to develop that possibility now.

Another example is ampicillin. Penicillin was not active against Gram-negative organisms unless huge amounts of it were used. However, ampicillin was a true development in which a chemical modification of an antibiotic led to another compound which would now be taken into a different organism and would be effective against that organism. That was a highly successful example and there is no reason to believe this is unique. If peptide transport, ion transport, and other transport systems are used, which may exist in a variety of organisms such as *Pseudomonas*, it might be possible to get other compounds into cells.

Professor Gilvarg: As usual, nature is always ahead of us. A few years ago, Höltje, in Tübingen, showed that the aminoglycosides are in fact representative of what is an illicit form of transport because they are entering cells by a transport portal that is intended for polyamines. There probably are many opportunities if only we could be as clever as evolution in mimicking transport portals to serve our own interests.

Professor Davies: I think that this research applied fairly closely to strepto-mycin more than to the aminoglycosides in general — but the example is well taken.

Professor Tomasz: I would like to re-emphasise a point I was trying to make in my presentation; it concerns the potential usefulness of mode of action type studies for drug development and drug improvement. Clearly, complex exper-imental designs — some of which I described in my talk — are too time consum-ing and expensive to be used as assays for new beta-lactams. On the other hand, these types of assays might be helpful in another sense. There exist a very large number of beta-lactams and very little is known about why specific structural differences among these compounds can cause the very considerable variation in antibacterial spectrum and in specific biochemical effects (such as in the capacity to induce bacterial lysis, cause sensitisation of bacteria to immune factors, selectively bind to certain penicillin-binding proteins, inhibit trans-peptidation, diffuse through the surface in some bacteria, but not in others, etc., etc.). A systematic application of mode of action type studies to various "branches" of the beta-lactam tree may provide useful clues for some of those questions and such information may eventually be fed back into improved drug design and even into screening.

Actually, Dr. Ōmura's presentation illustrated how mode of action type assays may even be used for the early screening of antibiotics. The use of envelope mutants, intrinsically resistant mutants or some of the tolerant bacteria, or the monitoring of morphological effects could provide still further resolution to the efforts to identify an inhibitor detected in a fermentation broth.

Professor Davies: I do not want to give the impression that I am opposed to mode of action studies; they are very important. As Professor Tomasz said, they can then be used as a basis for the screening method by picking the right organisms. This is clearly a way of finding new drugs.

Professor Braun: I would like to emphasise that perhaps we should look more for support from the natural defence mechanisms. There are hints on how this could be done, one of which is to limit iron, as I stressed in my presentation. Another point worth making is that cell wall material apparently induces the immune system, certainly in a non-specific way, but it triggers the immune defence mechanism. This is probably a mechanism which has evolved over millions of years. I am very sorry that there has not been a discussion on immune mechanisms, and on attempts by industry in this direction.

Professor Richmond: In answer to Professor Davies' question about who should decide what drugs we want, one of the problems about leaving it to the medical profession is the following. The whole economic pressure means that if we are to try to produce a new agent, it has to be sold on a worldwide scale. As I understand it, the practices of medical people across the world vary enormously. Italy is classically a market in which everything is injected; in the United Kingdom everything possible is put into people's mouths; in France, there are apparently other routes which are used: this does not lead to a very uniform view about what is a worldwide commodity.

Professor Sabath: Professor Davies has been rather hard on the pharmaceutical industry. The productivity of this meeting shows that good can come out of getting together people from different backgrounds and areas of expertise. I have spent all my career in academia and there I have met people with vested interests which are as difficult to deal with as in industry. Further, adding a third corner to the triangle, as suggested by Harry Dowling, in a book called "Medicines for Man", that there should not only be a flow of information between academia, industry and government, but also a flow of personnel. People should work in one area for one part of their career and in another for another part. I suggest that none of the triangle has the monopoly of wisdom or of the solutions to the problems, and that it is improper to suggest that major decisions be made by only one corner of the triangle.

Dr. Videau: Since we discussed antibiotics of the future, I wonder what the future of antibiotherapy is going to be and I wonder if an improved knowledge of pharmacokinetics of antibiotics in patients would not improve our knowledge because we usually study drugs in healthy people. We have also discussed associations of antibiotics, but the pharmacokinetics of associations is very poorly understood. I recall studying combinations of aspirin and antibiotics: the results were very surprising and the opposite to what would have been observed if we had simply assumed the release of the antibiotic bound, for instance, on serum proteins.

Professor Chabbert: I wish to support Professor Davies in his courageous attempt to get more money for his university, because there is no doubt that in countries like France, official agencies that provide grants to research organisations assume that all studies of antibiotics should be supported by the industry. We are rarely funded by the government to study new antibiotics, to develop an experimental model, or to make an adequate clinical study. And hitherto, we turn to fundamental studies, because antibiotics have enabled us to understand protein synthesis or cell wall structures and functions. It is surprising to note that we have understood certain modes of action of beta-lactams or aminosides, but we still do not know how bacteria die. Three years ago, I heard Luigi Gorini saying that he did not know how aminosides kill, and right now Dr. Tomasz is asking again how penicillin kills microbes. So, obviously, we are entering a new era in which progress for antibiotics must be based on more accurate study of all cell wall mutants. This is impossible nowadays because the government will not help us unless industry does. So, if industry works on a short time basis and only with traditional methods of screening, it will not find anything extraordinary. To take a new step forward, industry will have to finance fundamental research.

Professor Davies: I think Professor Chabbert is absolutely right. Professor Demain just received his first NIH grant in eight years, to work on β–lactam biosynthesis. I have to agree with Professor Sabath that there must be agreement and collaboration all around. In the United States there was no point in writing a grant application to the NIH for chemical or biochemical work on an antibiotic, since such work should have been supported by industry.

In this respect there is another example that I did not mention. Dr. Labia spoke about using combinations. Although many people are opposed to combinations, some like the sulphonamide/trimethoprim combination work very well. But perhaps other combinations could be devised that would be more active against organisms that are resistant to trimethoprim and to sulphonamide.

Professor Trouet: We are just coming from a period where antibiotics were discovered by chance with classical screening techniques, we are not yet in an era in which we can develop antibiotics on the basis of accurate knowledge of enzymatic action and of structure activity studies. We are now in an intermediate stage where we work on the basis of substances that are available, by investigating their fundamental action, their penetration, their interaction with cells. Then, by using all these data we must try in a more rational manner to modify the available antibiotics.

Part 3

A. L. DEMAIN

Before starting to discuss the last part of the programme I would like to mention the importance of permeability in improving the antibiotics that we already have. Any of the mechanisms that have been discussed is to be encouraged in terms of bringing these antibiotic molecules into the cell via transport systems. However, unfortunately, there is a lack of industrial interest in studies of permeability of compounds through the Gram-negative outer-membrane. There are excellent non-toxic antibiotics which work in the test-tube on targets in Gram-negative cells, but which cannot get into such cells. More research is needed to find inhibitors of outer-membrane synthesis, such compounds to be used either in combination with narrow-spectrum drugs, or by themselves if they have activity in aiding host defences to attack infectious bacteria.

Like the people in the pharmaceutical industry, I feel rather confused concerning the importance of resistance. Although I do not work on it myself, I read articles which state that resistance is so bad that all of our current antibiotics will soon be extinct. Yet, at this meeting, the general feeling is that perhaps now resistance is not the major problem that it was once thought to be. This is rather difficult to understand. I feel that it is important to encourage the continuance of the search for new antibiotics since it would be rather dangerous and irresponsible to stop doing so.

When joining the Merck Sharp and Dohm Laboratories upon leaving graduate school in 1954, I was assigned a problem of penicillin biosynthesis. I discussed this project with some of my professors before leaving graduate school, since I knew the project on which I would be working. The question they asked was why study β–lactam biosynthesis? The penicillins had been available for about 10 years, and what more was there to learn about them? Of course, very soon afterwards, came the discovery of 6–aminopenicillanic acid, leading to the semisynthetic penicillins. There was also the discovery of the cephalosporins at Oxford. Certainly no one had anticipated their appearance.

Some years later (in the early 1960s), I was put back on a project involving β–lactam biosynthesis by the same organisation, i.e. to study cephalosporin biosynthesis. The question raised then by some colleagues was: why study cephalosporin biosynthesis since certainly all of the semisynthetic penicillins coming on the market would solve the current problems and make cephalosporins unnecessary. However, the continual study of β–lactams has led to a tremendous number of surprises. After the demonstration that semisynthetic cephalosporins would be of clinical use, there came the completely surprising discovery of the ability of streptomycetes to make cephalosporins and penicillins. In recent years, this has led to the development of the cephamycins, for example cefoxitin, about which we have heard much; also the discovery of thienamycin, about which we hope to hear more in the future because it is an exciting extremely potent molecule, structurally between the penicillins and the cephalosporins; and also the discovery of β–lactamase inhibitors such as clavulanic acid, another aspect in our battle against infectious bacteria.

Professor Lechevalier, who has spent much of his career in the area of actinomycetes and antibiotic discovery, supports the approach being used in many pharmaceutical companies of isolating rare actinomycetes as a means of increasing the chance of finding new antibiotics. He pointed out that the most prolific producers of anti-biotics are the actinomycetes and the bacilli. In thinking about screening, I wonder why we have not applied the same concept into looking at bacilli as sources of new antibiotics. They were studied early on, for instance, the tyrothricin discovery by Dubos many years ago. Some companies have spent short periods of time looking at *Bacillus* and other unicellular bacteria, but I do not think that they have committed a great deal of either money or time to studying these bacteria. This is in spite of the interesting discovery made a few years ago that the aminoglycoside butirosin was made by a *Bacillus*. This was the first and the only aminoglycoside to be made by *Bacillus*; and it was a novel aminoglycoside. Thus, we suddenly saw in *Bacillus* the ability to make what is normally considered to be an actinomycete-type molecule. This makes me slightly uneasy about our screening, in that we are not looking broadly enough perhaps.

Professor Lechevalier noted the production of compounds with novel structures by *Actinoplanes*. This is quite encouraging.

Another interesting concept that he raised was that of antibiotics being produced under unusual conditions. Companies have been wrestling for many years with the problem of the production of an antibiotic activity on agar but not in submerged culture, an experience that is certainly not uncommon. It is interesting that at least in one case this was solved in terms of the morphological differentiation. The Japanese workers, whose paper he described, were eventually able to make the antibiotic in liquid culture by the use of conditions which allowed for the same morphological form to develop.

This raises the question concerning the following possibility: is it better to screen many thousands of cultures, and concentrate on the major compound in each particular culture broth? Or might it be better to exhaustively study one or a few particular cultures to discover every possible compound made by these few cultures? For instance, the discovery of cephalosporins did not come from a mass screening programme. Most people will probably remember that the cephalosporins were discovered by Abraham and Newton in Oxford as a contaminant peak in a column effluent in which the purification of penicillin N was being carried out. It certainly was a very minor part of the population of antibiotic compounds in that *Cephalosporium acremonium* broth.

Certain other findings of interest have been mentioned during the meeting. For instance, the finding by Pogell, at St-Louis University, with the puromycin producer, *Streptomyces alboniger*, of additional interesting compounds which at first were called "germination activators" or "stimulators of aerial mycelium formation" and which were later found to have antibiotic activity. Ensign, at Wisconsin, has found that the germination inhibitor of *Streptomyces viridochromogenes* has antibiotic activity.

I remember discussing *Streptomyces coelicolor* with David Hopwood perhaps 10 years ago, when we all thought that it made no antibiotic. I asked him why he was working on the genetics of a streptomycete that makes no antibiotic, and why not on one that has more commercial appeal? Professor Hopwood told me today that at least five antibiotics are made by this same strain that at one time was thought to make no antibiotics at all. They include actinorhodin, methylenomycin A (which is interesting because it is coded by a plasmid), and three others.

Also, let us consider the interesting culture, *Streptomyces clavuligerus*, which the Eli Lilly Company described a number of years ago as making cephalosporins and penicillins. At first, it was revealed that this culture made penicillin N, cephamycin C, and another cephalosporin. Some years later, it was found to make clavulanic acid, and perhaps about two years later to make holomycin. Recently, workers have described additional β–lactam molecules found in *Streptomyces clavuligerus* broth which, amazingly, do not have antibacterial activity but have antifungal activity.

Thus, we have to consider that many of the cultures that have been studied and discarded over many years might have some trace components which are very interesting molecules.

Professor Ōmura told us about his very interesting methods of looking for new antibiotics by way of mode of action studies. We have had a discussion about that. When Professor Davies said that perhaps these might not be utilisable, I think what he meant was not so much mode of action *per se* but perhaps mode of action tests in the test-tube as opposed to mode of action tests using the intact organism. This has been a controversial point in many different screening groups around the world, especially in regard to the use of a mode of action test as a primary screen instead of as a secondary or tertiary part of a programme to establish priorities.

Those people who are against using mode of action as a primary screen for new compounds feel that a compound which has a certain mode of action might not be useful if it does not inhibit the growth of the whole cell; if it does inhibit growth then why not use growth inhibition as the primary means of demonstrating activity? I think that Professor Ōmura's presentation brought out much light on this point. Perhaps a mode of action test can be valuable if used with an intact organism. This approach has become valuable. I would guess that some of these mode of action screens have been involved in the interesting discoveries of the cephamycins, olivanic acids, clavulanic acid, and thienamycin, as well as other compounds. We might wonder why it took 20 years to discover these compounds when it is now known that many of these β–lactams are produced by a large number of streptomycetes. The methodology must have changed in some way and possibly screening tests have become more sensitive; for instance, thienamycin may have been present on many occasions but, because of its low concentration and its instability, it was not picked up in the more conventional type of assay.

Professor Hopwood described some new possibilities in which genetics might be used to give us some new structures. His discussion is rather useful, because it is rather difficult to think of how new concepts and techniques, such as recombinant DNA, could be applied to the antibiotic field. It is fairly easy to see how genetic engineering could be used to make interferon, but to make streptomycin, which is the product of perhaps 20 or 30 enzymes (and thus 20 or 30 genes), one wonders how these concepts and techniques can be used. There is the possibility, however, that the genes coding for enzymes of these biosynthetic pathways are arranged in clusters, and that some of this technology could be used. The expression of silent genes sounds very interesting. Undoubtedly some organisms have parts of pathways, or almost complete pathways that are not being expressed and need some genetic material or signal to turn on these pathways. Certainly, protoplast fusion will become very important. It is already being used, and has been published, as a means of antibiotic producing strain improvement. It will be interesting to see whether some new compounds are generated along the way.

In my own talk, I dealt with the directed biosynthesis. It is an old technique, but one that is still useful. There is also the mutational biosynthesis and the technique of bioconversion. These options give the microbiologist a chance to contribute, along with the synthetic chemist, to the generation of new and perhaps less toxic modifications of known antibiotics.

Concerning Professor Rinehart's paper, it is encouraging to hear that the chemists are making such marked progress in the area of antibiotic identification. I say this with great sincerity because the major problem of all antibiotic screening groups is what is known in the industry as the "old friends" problem, i.e. the problem of eliminating the possibility that a "new" antibiotic that is found is one which has been discovered previously. With some 3000 known antibiotics, and the fact that most of them are not available, i.e. there is no way of obtaining these compounds for reference, this is a tremendous problem. I certainly welcome the new chemical methods because they will free a lot of time for more productive work, if it is possible to make a very early identification of a compound by techniques such as field desorption mass spectrometry.

Of course, microbiologists alone should not have to carry the entire burden of development of new drugs. Professor Le Goffic's presentation was encouraging, in that he described how biochemists and enzymologists are also progressing in the area of the discovery of new compounds by more rational means. However, these groups of researchers have the same problem as microbiologists who have shown that very potent natural inhibitors for any enzyme can be found in the broth of microorganisms. Umezawa's group has certainly demonstrated that, and part of Professor Ōmura's work deals with natural enzyme inhibitors. The general problem here is the lack of information concerning the relevance of a particular enzyme in a disease condition. This is why there must be a great deal of communication between the medical people, the biochemists and the microbiologists, so that we will know what is worth going after in terms of the enzyme inhibition concept.

Discussion

Professor Lechevalier: First, I would like to make the general comment that this meeting was entitled "Antibiotics of the Future", but as Professor Richmond pointed out earlier, it has been limited, in fact, to antibacterial antibiotics. When we are trying to think about the future of antibiotics, we must remember that bacteria are not the only microorganisms which cause disease and that at any time one-quarter of the world's population is suffering from some kind of protozoal disease. If we are looking for new antibiotics, we should not be looking only for antibacterial antibiotics, and specifically not for antibiotics which are especially well suited for the bacteria that are found in Paris, London, New York and Minnesota. This is something to be kept in mind. There are many opportunities in the search for useful drugs, and the important basic question is what are the important targets? In my view, this question has not been answered at all at this meeting, except that I have been vastly reassured by hearing that resistance is no problem.

   Although my former boss was very proud of the fact that he coined the word "antibiotic", I prefer to think of "natural products". It is very important to know as much as possible about natural products. We eventually find then that certain of them have this or that property which is useful for this or that application. There is a multitude of applications. The only problem about knowing more about natural products is that there are so many natural products. That is why we have screening programmes. Although our chemists now have marvellous instruments — as long as they have sufficient money to buy them — instruments permitting them to determine structures using amazingly small amounts of compounds, we still must have targets in our screening programme to be able to determine what should be looked for first.

Professor Demain: I might add that certainly we have heard nothing about viral diseases and antiviral agents at this meeting. It is certainly an area for which it has not been easy for industry to develop compounds. In fact, most of the industry gave up the attempt some years ago. Perhaps much more basic investigation is needed in that area in order to discover some targets that might encourage the pharmaceutical industry to start working in it again.

Professor Tomasz: With regard to bacterial resistance — I have not heard anything at this meeting that would make me less concerned about the emergence of antibiotic resistant bacteria. Just to the contrary. We have heard various clinical reports that entire bacterial flora have been taken over by bacteria which are now resistant to some of the most useful antibacterial agents. We also learned that an antibiotic resistant population once established will not necessarily disappear from a natural environment upon the removal of the antibiotic from the milieu. Bacterial species capable of inactivating or not taking up antibiotics, are wide-spread. I briefly described the penicillin resistance of the South African strains of pneumococci that show still another kind of resistance mechanism involving the decreased affinity of penicillin binding proteins for the beta-lactam molecules. Studies in our laboratory indicate that the intrinsic beta-lactam resistance of gonococcal and staphylococcal isolates involves a similar mechanism. All these should be arguments for continued drug development. In view of the wide-spread occurrence of beta-lactamases, it would seem important to extend the search for antibiotics that may inhibit other selective procaryotic targets such as early steps in the synthesis of cell walls or other bacterial surface components. Still other novel strategies were outlined in the talks of Professors Gilvarg and Braun.

Professor Richmond: On the question of the disappearance of resistance, I would personally think the use of all antibiotics would have to be stopped in order to have a major impact. Of course, I have in mind particularly that to stop the use of antibiotics as feed additives, while maintaining their use for prophylaxis or therapy, is not something which will produce a major change.

As far as the importance of resistant organisms is concerned, I would be very interested if the clinicians would affirm or deny my feeling that if a problem of resistance is found, there is usually an acceptable alternative. Fairly sophisticated laboratory facilities may be required, for instance in meningitis or analogous situations, to decide which alternative should be used. However I have the impression that although the alternative may be slightly more expensive, and produce a few more side effects, I do not often hear of doctors that they are totally without defences in the presence of a resistant organism.

Professor Sande: About four or five years ago we developed a tremendous out-break of aminoglycoside-resistant *Klebsiella* in our medical intensive care unit. At that time, we happened to be studying amikacin, so we used it immediately. But, if we had not had amikacin, there was no other antimicrobial agent or combination available which we could have used. Although I tend to agree that, in the past, resistance has been overstated, it can still be a severe problem. We are now also faced with methicillin-resistant staphylococci. The only two drugs — as mentioned earlier by Professor Duval — available for use against those organisms are rifampicin and vancomycin. These problems keep arising, and they should continue to be a stimulus to search for new drugs.

Professor Kunin: I agree with Professor Sande. Like all questions, it must be considered in some detail. For instance, with the cephalosporins, a new cephalosporin is added to the market because it has a slightly different spectrum, or it is slightly more active against one or two strains. The question to ask is whether those new cephalosporins are a major advance as compared, for instance, to amikacin or a drug like thienamycin, that is a drug with a novel activity spectrum or resistance to inactivation. I am not very excited about the cephalosporins, but I am excited about novel compounds, and I hope that what has been said here will not inhibit people from looking for novel compounds with new properties and modes of action, rather than looking for old compounds with slightly different advantages.

Professor Demain: For those people who are not familiar with the history of amikacin, I might point out that it would not be available today without the strange finding of a *Bacillus* making an aminoglycoside which had an unusual side chain not previously observed in any streptomycete or actinomycete aminoglycoside. It was the Bristol—Banyu chemists who decided to put that side chain on all the known aminoglycosides, changing kanamycin B which is scarcely used any longer into a compound which is very active against resistant organisms. This is another stimulus for continuing to try to find some new natural modifications of known drugs.

Professor Sabath: May I add to Professor Sande's comment that resistance remains a big problem. I would not be so extreme as to say that we are rapidly running out of antimicrobial agents. However it is a rare day in a large hospital, probably anywhere in the Western world, when the choices do not appear to be close to exhaustion. People with long experience can often work out a way of coping, but ordinary practitioners may have difficulty in so doing.

Secondly, with regard to Professor Lechevalier's comment about the needs for which to search, may I enumerate the following:

1) Forty % of coagulase-negative staphylococci in American hospitals are resistant to methicillin. The choices of antibiotics are relatively limited. In American hospitals, those organisms are the major cause of endocarditis from prosthetic valves.
2) The effective drugs for use against anaerobes are relatively limited, so this would be another interesting area in which to look for new compounds.
3) Reference has already been made to *Pseudomonas*.
4) Antifungal compounds are greatly needed.
5) There is no time to discuss the antivirals, but there is a great need for them.

Professor Lechevalier: Turning to a slightly different field and Professor Demain's comments, I would not like to give the impression that I believe rare actinomycetes are the only kind of organisms to look at as a source of natural products and antibiotics. I simply mentioned them because we happen to know more about them than other groups of bacteria or other groups of microorganisms.

There is a vexing problem with the rare actinomycetes which plagues us. It might be helpful if more was known about the basic properties of the actinomycetes. Many of the rare actinomycetes grow very slowly. If it was known what are the basic differences between slow-growing and fast-growing organisms, and if we knew how to handle the former to speed up their rate of growth, it might be possible to find a whole new collection of natural products which could be examined. Some of them would probably be found to eventually have interesting properties. That would be a field of study for geneticists, physiologists and would probably require a large amount of different sorts of talent which I do not have. It might give us some idea about these organisms which are very interesting, but which grow so slowly.

Professor Demain: I might add that the cost of gentamicin today is closely associated with that slow growth rate. It is extremely frustrating working with organisms such as *Micromonospora*, at least with *Micromonospora purpurea*, because experiments take weeks rather than days, which, of course, costs money. Strain improvement programmes take decades rather than only a few years of intensive effort.

Professor Rinehart: With regard to slow-growing organisms, probably a number of people are aware that Okami in Tokyo is studying many microorganisms that are growing on the sea bottom. Some of these come from rather deep waters and are slow-growing because they are used to rather low temperatures. That is a promising new area for investigation. Secondly, with regard to the antivirals, the sponge and tunicate extracts seem a fairly promising area for antiviral agents.

Conclusion

L. NINET

Because he succeeded in putting Death
temporarily in chains, Sisyphus was
condemned by the gods perpetually to
roll his rock uphill.

(from Greek mythology)

At the end of the present book it is tempting to evoke the legend of
Sisyphus, one of the best known myths of the ancient Greeks, such
fine experts of the human condition, in order to depict our own
situation. Unfortunately, despite the subtle analysis of the psychology
of the hero by Albert Camus in 1942, we do not know from the
legend whether Sisyphus passively executed his punishment or
secretely hoped that, when rolling down again, his rock would once
run over Death. However if we intend to compare Sisyphus' position
with ours, we must adopt the second hypothesis unreservedly, since
in every field, but probably more in Medicine than anywhere else,
Man continuously rolls the rock upward, with the steady but possibly
foolish hope of success.

The recent introduction of antibiotics into medicine has afforded
a new and excellent proof that the myth is perennial, and our daily
experience has shown that in the treatment of bacterial diseases
nothing is ever final, even though many spectacular and real
successes have been achieved.

This book deals only with a relatively small number of topics, but
these are sufficiently varied to reveal the complexity of the theoretical and practical situations and the small chance of finding the
perfect solution by a single approach.

As a matter of fact, the situations offered by each patient, by each
bacterium and by the environment are so different that it seems
impossible at present to foresee from which field the solutions will

come and how extensive and ultimate they could be. Moreover, as far as the biochemistry and physiology of bacteria, the pharmacology and toxicology of drugs, and the pathological and immunological state of patients are concerned, the relevant basic knowledge is too often rudimentary and dispersed or cannot be directly and quickly applied to daily practical situations.

Therefore, it would be risky and even dangerous to believe that in the future a single natural antibiotic, semisynthetic compound or synthetic antagonist of a natural process will become the definitive "deterrent" of infectious diseases. We shall probably witness the appearance of more and more active and sophisticated drugs, almost conforming to the definition of the ideal antimicrobial agent. But experience gained in laboratories and in medical practice gives too many warnings on the great variety of conditions and on the extraordinary adaptability of bacteria to adverse conditions to support fully the possibility of a total victory.

Two conclusions should meet general acceptance: first, new antimicrobial agents are needed and we must learn to make more judicious use of existing and future ones; second, if we slacken the intensification of our efforts to acquire the basic knowledge and to study different approaches, we shall miss the convenient solutions to the present and future problems, and we might even find ourselves facing a worsening situation.

It becomes trite to say that a close cooperation between all the people engaged in the battle is necessary, since apparently everybody heartily agrees with this proposal. However, in spite of generous intentions the situation in practice is far from satisfactory and a serious effort has to be made by all the different partners in this direction. To this end, we hope that the attempt made on the occasion of the Second Rhône–Poulenc Round Table Conference will be echoed and will modestly contribute to the exciting discovery of the antibiotics of the future.

Having probably heard of Taylor, Sisyphus has today changed his methodology. He has burst his heavy rock into an infinite number of small fragments which, one after the other, must be brought to the top of the hill. Moveover he has gathered his fellow men as anxious as himself to defeat Death, in order to share and relieve his effort, with the firm belief of a common success. But meanwhile, the gods laughed up their sleeves, since they alone are able to master Infinity...

Meaning of abbreviations following genus and species names:

AP : antibiotic producer
PB : pathogenic bacterium
SS : screening strain